Health Psychology in Practice:

Exploring Behavior, Meaning, and Resilience

Agathi Argyriadi
American University, UAE

Alexandros Argyriadis
https://orcid.org/0000-0001-5754-4787
Hellenic Mediterranean University, Greece

IGI Global
Scientific Publishing
Publishing Tomorrow's Research Today

Vice President of Editorial	Melissa Wagner
Director of Acquisitions	Mikaela Felty
Director of Book Development	Jocelynn Hessler
Production Manager	Mike Brehm
Cover Design	Jose Rosado

Published in the United States of America by
IGI Global Scientific Publishing
701 East Chocolate Avenue
Hershey, PA, 17033, USA
Tel: 717-533-8845 | Fax: 717-533-7115
Website: https://www.igi-global.com E-mail: cust@igi-global.com

Library of Congress Cataloging-in-Publication Data

LCCN: 2025046667 (CIP Data Pending)
ISBN13: 979-8-3373-6294-6
Isbn13Softcover: 979-8-3373-6295-3
EISBN13: 979-8-3373-6296-0
British Cataloguing in Publication Data
A Cataloguing in Publication record for this book is available from the British Library.

Table of Contents

Detailed Table of Contents

Trauma-Informed Care (TIC) represents a gradual but important reorientation in how mental-health professionals understand distress and healing. Rather than asking "What is wrong with you?", TIC invites a different kind of question: "What happened to you?" and "What would help you feel safe again?" This approach brings together psychological knowledge about trauma with ethical commitments such as autonomy, dignity, and non-maleficence. It emphasizes collaboration, trust, and empowerment as central conditions for recovery. This chapter discusses the theoretical background, practical applications, and ethical-cultural dimensions of trauma-informed work. It draws on recent global literature (2020-2025) to identify the conditions under which TIC reduces re-traumatization, strengthens therapeutic relationships, and supports the well-being of both clients and practitioners. Attention is given to the importance of reflective supervision, organizational culture, and social justice as part of trauma-informed systems of care.

Psychological health of the people is highly essential to achieve their desired tasks. While the practice of forgiveness enables individuals to focus on inner peace, mindfulness, quality of life, and satisfaction with life. This chapter, therefore, assesses how negatively reinforced feelings can affect physiological wellbeing and health of youth? It is based on previous studies which explored the association of

provides a list of indicators that are leading to mental disorders. This chapter makes a significant contribution in the theoretical literature in medical psychology.

Ethics plays a foundational and indispensable role in health psychology practice, shaping how professionals interact with clients, conduct research, design interventions, and contribute to public health. Health psychology, as an interdisciplinary field concerned with the relationships among biological, psychological, and social factors in health and illness, deals with sensitive aspects of human life such as physical well-being, mental health, cultural values, coping with illness, adherence to treatment, and end-of-life care. In this context, ethical principles act as guiding frameworks to ensure that practices are fair, respectful, and beneficial to clients, while minimizing harm and protecting vulnerable populations. Without strong ethical grounding, For example, pushing a patient toward behavior change without respecting their readiness or cultural context could lead to resistance, guilt, or distress. Ethical practice therefore involves striking a delicate balance between supporting growth and avoiding unnecessary harm.

This chapter integrates Positive Psychology Interventions (PPIs) into health psychology shifts the focus from pathogenesis to salutogenesis. Rooted in frameworks like SOC, Broaden-and-Build, and PERMA, PPIs build resilience and well-being. Evidence shows they reduce anxiety and depression, supported by neurobiology (e.g., vagal tone). The chapter discusses their application across settings, addresses methodological issues, the "tyranny of the positive," and the need for rigorous,

Preface

INTRODUCTION

Health psychology has undergone a remarkable transformation over the past few decades. Once primarily concerned with the psychological factors associated with illness and treatment adherence, it has developed into a broad and interdisciplinary field that seeks to understand how thoughts, emotions, relationships, culture, and lived experience influence health across the lifespan. This shift reflects an equally important change in healthcare itself. Increasingly, health is viewed not merely as the absence of disease but as a process of adaptation in which people strive to maintain wellbeing while facing illness, adversity, and uncertainty.

The chapters brought together in this volume were selected with this broader perspective in mind. Although they approach health psychology from different theoretical traditions and professional settings, they share a common interest in understanding how people respond to challenging life circumstances and how psychological science can contribute to more compassionate and effective care. Rather than presenting resilience, coping, or meaning-making as abstract concepts, the contributors examine how these processes unfold in real clinical, family, and community contexts.

CHAPTER OVERVIEW

Several chapters focus on the experience of trauma and the implications it has for healthcare practice. Others explore the psychological significance of forgiveness, emotion regulation, and adaptive coping, demonstrating how these factors influence wellbeing across different age groups and cultural environments. Together, they remind us that psychological adjustment is rarely explained by a single variable.

Instead, it emerges from the ongoing interaction between individual characteristics, interpersonal relationships, social environments, and the wider cultural context in which people live.

Resilience occupies a central place throughout the book, yet it is presented in many different forms. Readers will encounter discussions of families raising children with intellectual disabilities, individuals coping with prenatal diagnoses, people living with chronic illness, therapists supporting survivors of child sexual abuse, and communities facing migration and social change. Although these experiences differ substantially, they reveal a common reality: resilience is not simply a personal quality that some individuals possess and others lack. It develops through relationships, supportive environments, opportunities for growth, and the capacity to construct meaning from difficult experiences.

Another important contribution of this volume lies in its international perspective. Health psychology cannot be fully understood without considering the cultural, social, and economic conditions that shape people's experiences of health and illness. The inclusion of chapters addressing South Asian populations, migrant communities, and cross-cultural perspectives reflects the growing recognition that psychological theories and interventions should be interpreted within diverse cultural frameworks. Such diversity strengthens the field by encouraging dialogue across disciplines, healthcare systems, and societies.

The volume also addresses areas that have become increasingly significant in contemporary practice, including pain psychology, ethical issues in research and professional practice, and the application of positive psychology to health promotion. These topics illustrate the breadth of modern health psychology and highlight its contribution not only to clinical treatment but also to prevention, rehabilitation, and the promotion of long-term wellbeing.

While each chapter stands on its own, the collection has been organized to encourage readers to appreciate the connections between them. Questions concerning trauma, adaptation, resilience, ethics, meaning, and psychological growth appear repeatedly from different perspectives, gradually forming a broader understanding of the challenges faced by individuals, families, healthcare professionals, and societies. It is this dialogue between diverse viewpoints that gives the volume its coherence.

This book is intended for psychologists, physicians, nurses, psychotherapists, allied health professionals, researchers, educators, and students who wish to deepen their understanding of the psychological dimensions of health and healthcare. We also hope that policymakers and professionals involved in designing health services will find ideas that support more person-centered and culturally responsive approaches to care.

Finally, this volume is the product of collaboration among scholars whose expertise spans multiple disciplines and geographical regions. Their contributions reflect both scientific rigor and a genuine commitment to improving people's lives through research, education, and clinical practice. We are deeply grateful for their willingness to share their knowledge and perspectives.

It is our hope that the chapters collected here will encourage thoughtful reflection, stimulate new research questions, and support clinical practice that recognizes the complexity of human experience. Health psychology continues to evolve alongside the changing needs of society, and its future will depend on the ability to integrate sound scientific evidence with empathy, cultural awareness, and respect for the unique stories that every individual brings to the healthcare encounter.

Agathi Argyriadi
American University, UAE

Alexandros Argyriadis
Hellenic Mediterranean University, Greece

Chapter 1
Trauma-Informed Care in Clinical Practice:
Effectiveness, Implementation Barriers, and Future Directions

Agathi Argyriadi
American University in Dubai, UAE

Prince Kouamelan Kouassi
http://orcid.org/0009-0001-3663-6460
American University in Dubai, UAE

Alexandros Argyriadis
http://orcid.org/0000-0001-5754-4787
Hellenic Mediterranean University, Greece

ABSTRACT

Trauma-Informed Care (TIC) represents a gradual but important reorientation in how mental-health professionals understand distress and healing. Rather than asking "What is wrong with you?", TIC invites a different kind of question: "What happened to you?" and "What would help you feel safe again?" This approach brings together psychological knowledge about trauma with ethical commitments such as autonomy, dignity, and non-maleficence. It emphasizes collaboration, trust, and empowerment as central conditions for recovery. This chapter discusses the theoretical background, practical applications, and ethical-cultural dimensions of trauma-informed work. It draws on recent global literature (2020-2025) to identify the conditions under which TIC reduces re-traumatization, strengthens therapeutic

DOI: 10.4018/979-8-3373-6294-6.ch001

relationships, and supports the well-being of both clients and practitioners. Attention is given to the importance of reflective supervision, organizational culture, and social justice as part of trauma-informed systems of care.

1. INTRODUCTION

Over the past few decades, the concept of trauma has expanded far beyond its original clinical definition. What was once seen mainly as an individual pathology is now recognized as a pervasive influence on emotions, thoughts, and relationships throughout life. Trauma-informed care emerged as a comprehensive and humane framework designed to acknowledge these long-term effects and to ensure that care environments promote safety, trust, and empowerment rather than fear or control (Substance Abuse and Mental Health Services Administration [SAMHSA], 2014).

Evidence from psychology, psychiatry, education, and public health consistently links early and repeated trauma to difficulties in emotional regulation, attachment, cognitive performance, and physical health (Felitti et al., 1998; Hughes et al., 2021). The global experience of the COVID-19 pandemic intensified public and professional awareness of trauma, highlighting how collective uncertainty and isolation can trigger or deepen pre-existing vulnerabilities (Horesh & Brown, 2020). Against this background, the call for trauma-informed systems has become increasingly urgent across disciplines.

Trauma-informed care shifts the focus of mental-health services from asking "What's wrong with you?" to "What happened to you?" and "What do you need to feel safe again?" This reframing represents more than a change in language; it marks a transformation in professional ethics and power dynamics. Instead of viewing distress as pathology, trauma-informed care interprets behavior as an adaptation to adversity and aims to create conditions that support recovery through choice, collaboration, and compassion. It combines scientific knowledge with moral principles such as autonomy, non-maleficence, and justice, situating care within a context of respect for human dignity.

In practice, implementing trauma-informed care has been associated with positive outcomes for both clients and professionals. Studies show that when practitioners integrate its core principles—safety, trust, collaboration, empowerment, and cultural awareness—clients report stronger engagement in therapy, improved emotional regulation, and lower dropout rates (Isobel & Edwards, 2017; Johnson et al., 2021; Champine et al., 2023). A meta-analysis by Lotzin et al. (2022), reviewing twenty-six studies with more than ten thousand participants, found moderate but meaningful improvements in post-traumatic symptoms, daily functioning, and satisfaction with care. At the same time, therapists trained in this approach demonstrate greater empathy, stronger boundaries, and reduced burnout (Menschner & Maul, 2023).

Despite this encouraging evidence, trauma-informed care is still unevenly applied. Differences in professional training, institutional readiness, and policy support create wide variation in implementation quality (Bunting et al., 2021). In many clinical contexts, risk-management and diagnostic models continue to dominate, sometimes replicating the same hierarchies of control and disempowerment that retraumatize clients (Bloom & Farragher, 2018). Sustained change requires more than good intentions; it depends on systemic alignment, reflective supervision, and organizational cultures that value safety for both clients and staff.

Current scholarship tends to move in three main directions. The first focuses on effectiveness, exploring measurable outcomes of trauma-informed care in therapy, psychiatry, and community services. The second examines training and implementation, emphasizing practical tools and readiness frameworks to support adoption (Bendall et al., 2020). The third investigates organizational transformation, seeking to embed trauma-informed values in leadership, policy, and everyday practice (Leitch, 2022). Collectively, these strands reflect a growing recognition that trauma-informed care is not a technique but a culture shift.

However, several questions remain open. Comparative data are still lacking on which forms of implementation—top-down institutional programs or bottom-up practitioner learning—achieve more sustainable results (Dimitros et al., 2025). There is also limited research on how trauma-informed principles operate within the therapeutic relationship itself, particularly in complex or culturally diverse settings. Moreover, much of the existing evidence comes from high-income Western contexts, leaving uncertainty about how the approach can be adapted to low-resource or non-Western systems (Yehuda et al., 2023).

This chapter addresses these gaps by reviewing recent international literature published between 2020 and 2025. It examines theoretical foundations, empirical evidence, and ethical-cultural dimensions of implementation, while also identifying barriers and enablers for success. Above all, trauma-informed care is presented as a profoundly human approach to healing—one that reconnects science with empathy and calls for a shared responsibility to create environments where recovery becomes possible.

2. THEORETICAL FRAMEWORK AND CORE PRINCIPLES OF TRAUMA-INFORMED CARE

Trauma-informed care is a broad and holistic framework developed to support individuals who have experienced trauma. Rooted in humanistic and psychodynamic traditions, it understands trauma as an ongoing process that continues to shape the body, emotions, and relationships in the present (van der Kolk, 2014). Its foundation draws from psychotherapy, neurobiology, systems theory, and social psychology, bringing together scientific understanding with compassion and ethical awareness.

Originally created in response to domestic violence and abuse, trauma-informed care has evolved into a flexible model that can be applied across many care environments. At its core lies the idea that behaviors often labeled as resistant or dysfunctional are survival strategies that developed in response to threat. Rather than asking "What is wrong with this person?", the trauma-informed perspective asks "What happened to them, and how have they learned to survive?" (SAMHSA, 2014). This shift in questioning recognizes the adaptive function of coping mechanisms that emerge after trauma and reframes them as signs of resilience rather than pathology.

The theoretical background of trauma-informed care is supported by research in attachment theory, emotional regulation, and the neurobiology of stress. Repeated or early trauma disrupts the body's ability to regulate stress through its influence on the hypothalamic–pituitary–adrenal axis and on brain regions such as the amygdala, hippocampus, and prefrontal cortex (Argyriadi et al., 2025; McEwen, 2021). These physiological changes affect emotional stability, concentration, and behavior, explaining why trauma can profoundly alter how a person perceives and responds to the world (Porges, 2022). This understanding grounds trauma-informed care in the recognition that healing is both psychological and biological.

SAMHSA's Six Core Principles of Trauma-Informed Care

The Substance Abuse and Mental Health Services Administration identified six key principles that define trauma-informed practice and guide its application across settings. These principles are safety, trustworthiness, choice, collaboration, empowerment, and cultural sensitivity. Together they form the ethical and practical foundation of trauma-informed care.

Safety is the first and most essential condition for healing. Both physical and emotional safety must be intentionally cultivated in therapy and care environments. Practitioners promote safety through consistency, clear boundaries, and a pace that allows the client to remain regulated and present. Research has shown that when clients feel secure, therapy outcomes improve significantly (Bloom, 2019; Isobel et al., 2021).

Trustworthiness and transparency are equally important. Because trauma often involves betrayal or violation of trust, restoring predictability becomes a therapeutic goal in itself. Clinicians can build trust by explaining procedures clearly, communicating openly about therapeutic intentions, and encouraging clients to anticipate emotional reactions (Leitch, 2022).

The principle of **choice** reinforces agency. Clients who are given meaningful options regarding the pacing of sessions, the use of specific interventions, or the level of disclosure experience a greater sense of control, which directly counteracts trauma-related helplessness (Sweeney et al., 2018).

Collaboration replaces hierarchical dynamics with shared responsibility. Instead of the therapist acting as an expert who corrects or directs, the process becomes co-created through dialogue and shared decision-making (Knight, 2021). This balance of power fosters trust, transparency, and authentic engagement.

Empowerment is central to all trauma-informed work. It means focusing on strengths and capacities rather than deficits. By recognizing behaviors as adaptive responses to adversity, practitioners can validate survival skills and support the client's natural ability to recover (Champine et al., 2023). Empowerment restores confidence and encourages self-efficacy, which are critical to long-term resilience.

Finally, trauma-informed care demands cultural, historical, and gender sensitivity. Trauma never occurs in isolation; it is shaped by the social and cultural environment. Practitioners must remain aware of how factors such as racism, discrimination, poverty, and gender inequality affect the experience of trauma and healing (Yehuda et al., 2023). This sensitivity requires humility and a rejection of uniform interventions, ensuring that care is responsive to the lived realities of each client.

From Theory to Practice: The Therapeutic Relationship

Translating trauma-informed theory into everyday practice requires more than theoretical knowledge. It calls for a transformation of professional culture. Traditional therapy models often focus on analyzing behavior or correcting dysfunction, while trauma-informed care places the relationship itself at the center of healing. Therapists must structure sessions carefully, avoid overwhelming clients with traumatic material, and offer grounding or self-regulation tools when distress arises (Courtois & Ford, 2020).

Empirically supported therapies such as Trauma-Focused Cognitive Behavioral Therapy, Eye Movement Desensitization and Reprocessing, and Somatic Experiencing all integrate trauma-informed principles by emphasizing safety, gradual exposure, and empowerment (Schwarz et al., 2021). Yet research consistently shows that the therapist's attitude, including empathy, flexibility, and non-judgment, matters as much as the specific technique (Isobel et al., 2021). This evidence underscores that trauma-informed care is not confined to one therapeutic approach but can be woven into any modality, from cognitive-behavioral to existential.

At the organizational level, trauma-informed care extends beyond individual sessions. Institutions that adopt its principles commit to shared values of safety, transparency, and staff well-being. Administrators, clinicians, and support personnel all play a role in creating an environment that reflects these values. Organizations that embrace reflective supervision and prioritize staff mental health report lower burnout and higher job satisfaction (Bloom & Farragher, 2018; Menschner & Maul, 2023). This demonstrates that trauma-informed systems protect both clients and caregivers.

In essence, trauma-informed care redefines healing as a collaborative and relational process. Recovery becomes possible when professionals help clients rediscover their capacity for safety, meaning, and connection. This vision aligns with philosophical and ethical traditions such as Martin Buber's dialogical ethics, which view human encounter as the foundation of transformation, and with mindfulness-based practices that emphasize presence and non-judgment. By placing human connection at the center of the therapeutic process, trauma-informed care restores the possibility of healing through understanding rather than control.

Although trauma-informed care is often presented as a set of principles or guidelines, in practice it constitutes a distinct way of thinking that shapes how professionals approach every dimension of the therapeutic relationship. Beyond technical skills, it involves a deeper shift in stance. Therapists are asked to move away from the traditional assumption that behavioral difficulties, fluctuations in emotional regulation, or sudden changes in cooperation are signs of indifference or unwillingness. Instead, they are encouraged to view such reactions as traces of a past that continues to echo in the present. This perspective is not simply more compassionate; it is more accurate, aligning with contemporary understandings of psychological functioning and the ways in which individuals integrate or wall off painful memories.

Fundamentally, a trauma-informed perspective urges professionals to remain attuned to what is not explicitly spoken. The body, gestures, silences, and subtle behavioral patterns often reveal far more than words alone. Thus, the therapist becomes not merely an interpreter but a witness to the person's internal experience. This shift from "analysis" to "witnessing" carries significant implications for how the therapeutic space is constructed. The therapist's presence is not intended to correct but to acknowledge, and through this acknowledgment, the possibility of relief and processing slowly emerges.

A central aspect of this shift is the gradual cultivation of trust. Trust does not arise immediately, nor can it be imposed. It develops slowly through consistency, transparency of intention, and repeated encounters with safety. Many individuals who have experienced trauma are accustomed to environments where unpredictability was the norm. Even small changes in pace, tone, or interpersonal rhythm may evoke a sense of threat. Practitioners must be sensitive to these subtleties and work with deliberate steadiness, setting a tempo that allows the person to settle psychologically at each step of the process.

The application of trauma-informed thinking is not confined to individual therapy. Systems such as schools, hospitals, mental health services, and social welfare agencies are deeply influenced by how they conceptualize trauma's role in human behavior. When a system remains anchored in disciplinary or punitive logics, it inevitably fails to recognize the forces that shape the reactions of the people it serves. Conversely, when a more reflective institutional culture develops—one that allows space for individuals' lived experiences—relationships of cooperation, tolerance, and shared purpose become more likely.

Equally important is the idea of self-regulation. Self-regulation is often misunderstood as a purely individual skill, as if it can be acquired through the right instruction alone. Trauma-informed perspectives recognize that regulation is profoundly interpersonal. Human nervous systems are shaped by signals of safety or danger from the environment and from others. The presence of a calm, steady, emotionally available professional can function as an external regulator. Over time, repeated experiences of such regulation support the internal development of the capacity to self-regulate.

Within this context, the significance of embodied experience becomes evident. People do not live trauma solely as narrative; they experience it in the body—through tightened muscles, interrupted breath, or reflexive reactions that arise without conscious intent. The therapeutic process aims to create a space where these embodied memories can be acknowledged and transformed. Verbal processing alone is often insufficient. Bodily awareness, relaxation techniques, and gradual activation or deactivation strategies contribute to a deeper reorganization of experience. These are not peripheral methods but essential dimensions of healing.

At the same time, trauma-informed practice requires continuous self-reflection from the professional. Confronting human suffering is not easy, and it can stir personal memories or lead to fatigue and emotional strain. A therapist's ability to recognize personal limits, seek support when necessary, and care for their own physical and psychological health is essential to the sustainability of the work. A depleted system cannot provide genuinely therapeutic conditions for the individuals who depend on it.

Moreover, trauma-informed care extends into an ethical domain related to social justice. Trauma is not distributed evenly across society. It often accumulates in communities burdened by poverty, marginalization, or limited access to essential services. Through this lens, the therapist is not restricted to the individual role of supporter; they are often encouraged to see themselves as potential agents of social change—whether through education, organizational reform, or advocacy for policies grounded in dignity and respect.

Finally, trauma-informed care reminds us that healing is not linear. Progress and regression coexist, and some of the most meaningful changes occur not within the session itself but in daily life—in a quiet moment of connection, in a renewed sense of safety, in a night of restful sleep. These seemingly small shifts often signal profound internal reorganizations. When a person begins to feel worthy of care, capable of trust, and welcomed into a space where their experience is not dismissed but honored, the therapeutic process has already achieved something significant.

3. EMPIRICAL EVIDENCE ON THE EFFECTIVENESS OF TRAUMA-INFORMED CARE

Recent research on trauma-informed care has moved from theoretical exploration to measurable outcomes in clinical and community settings. Evidence now supports the idea that trauma-informed approaches across psychotherapy, psychiatry, education, and public health contribute to improvements in both client and practitioner well-being (Bendall et al., 2020; Champine et al., 2023). The level of effectiveness depends largely on how carefully the model is applied, the quality of training, and the broader institutional climate.

A meta-analysis by Lotzin and colleagues (2022) reviewed twenty-six studies with more than ten thousand participants. The findings indicated consistent reductions in post-traumatic symptoms, improvements in daily functioning, and stronger therapeutic relationships. The most effective programs combined professional training with organizational support and ongoing supervision.

In psychotherapy, trauma-informed principles have produced measurable progress. A study involving survivors of abuse found that adaptations of cognitive-behavioral therapy grounded in trauma awareness reduced anxiety and avoidance more than standard treatment after twelve sessions (Johnson et al., 2021). Work with clients who have experienced complex trauma shows that approaches based on safety, trust, and collaboration increase engagement and lower dropout rates (D'Andrea et al., 2020).

Similar patterns appear in psychiatric contexts. Implementing trauma-informed practices has been linked to fewer aggressive incidents and a decline in the use of physical restraints. In a multicenter study in Sweden, Khalifeh and colleagues (2022) reported that after staff completed trauma-informed training, the use of restraints dropped by thirty-five percent while patient satisfaction rose by twenty percent. The best results were found in organizations that maintained supervision and peer consultation after training.

Research by Isobel and collaborators (2021) in acute psychiatric wards showed that introducing trauma-informed practices shortened hospital stays by seventeen percent and improved nurse–patient relationships. These improvements were accompanied by higher staff resilience and reduced occupational stress. Taken together, these results show that trauma-informed care strengthens both therapeutic outcomes and workplace well-being.

Studies in educational and youth contexts show comparable benefits. Kim and colleagues (2023) reviewed fifteen school-based mental health programs and found that trauma-informed approaches reduced behavioral problems and enhanced social and emotional learning. Programs that involved teachers and parents achieved the strongest results. For children exposed to violence, cognitive behavioral therapy informed by trauma-sensitive principles improved emotional control and reduced aggression (De Candia et al., 2022). The therapist's consistency, warmth, and respect for boundaries were crucial in sustaining these outcomes.

Professionals themselves benefit from working in trauma-informed environments. Exposure to trauma survivors can lead to compassion fatigue and emotional strain (Figley, 2021). Organizations that adopt reflective supervision and emphasize staff well-being reduce these risks. In a survey of four hundred and eighteen psychotherapists, those employed in trauma-informed organizations reported lower burnout and higher job satisfaction (Menschner & Maul, 2023). A similar study of six hundred mental health nurses across Europe found a thirty percent decrease in emotional exhaustion and increased confidence in managing trauma-related cases after specialized training (Bunting et al., 2021).

Qualitative studies enrich these findings. Clients describe trauma-informed therapy as respectful, collaborative, and empowering (Knight, 2021). They often emphasize the importance of stability, clear communication, and emotional validation, explaining that these elements help them feel safe and committed to treatment (Leitch, 2022; Isobel et al., 2021). Practitioners report that mindfulness and reflective practice protect them from compassion fatigue and help them maintain empathy in complex clinical situations (Isobel & Edwards, 2017).

Levels of Intervention

Champine et al. (2023) categorize TIC interventions into three levels:

- Micro: Staff education and clinical training
- Meso: Adjusting daily clinical practices and protocols
- Macro: System-wide organizational transformation

The micro level involves staff education and clinical training. The meso level focuses on daily practices and routines within organizations. The macro level addresses leadership, policy, and cultural transformation. Research shows that meaningful and lasting change occurs when all three levels are addressed together. Programs limited to isolated training events tend to produce short-term results (Bendall et al., 2020).

As evidence accumulates, studies highlight that the greatest impact occurs when trauma-informed care is seen as an organizational culture rather than an isolated clinical method. Findings from Isobel et al. (2021), Lotzin et al. (2022), and Menschner and Maul (2023) converge on the same point: alignment of values across all levels of a system sustains improvement over time. When trauma-informed principles are integrated into supervision, leadership, and governance, the benefits extend from individual sessions to the wider organization.

Researchers are also refining the criteria used to define success. Earlier evaluations focused mainly on symptom reduction, but newer studies include relational indicators such as trust, emotional safety, and empowerment. These dimensions are now recognized as key markers of progress because they influence participation and long-term recovery. Improvements in perceived safety and mutual trust often appear before measurable changes in symptoms, suggesting that emotional connection is the foundation of healing (Johnson et al., 2021; D'Andrea et al., 2020).

At the institutional level, trauma-informed systems display higher staff morale, better collaboration, and lower turnover. Organizations that prioritize open communication and emotional safety report greater stability and improved performance (Menschner & Maul, 2023). These outcomes show that trauma-informed care promotes both ethical integrity and organizational health.

Evidence from community and public health programs further supports this perspective. Studies show that trauma-informed community initiatives increase engagement and trust among populations affected by systemic discrimination and marginalization (Bloom, 2019; Knight, 2021). Successful programs address social and economic factors such as poverty and inequality alongside psychological recovery (Berring et al., 2024).

Recent work also explores how trauma-informed models adapt to cultural contexts. While early studies were based mainly in Western countries, newer research confirms that the values of safety, trust, empowerment, and cultural humility are relevant across societies when adapted sensitively to local norms (Kim et al., 2023; Bunting et al., 2021). Respect for cultural beliefs and community definitions of safety strengthens both engagement and effectiveness (Yehuda et al., 2023).

Longitudinal studies indicate that benefits become stronger with time. Initial program evaluations often show moderate effects, but consistent application over several years produces deeper change. Ongoing supervision, feedback, and professional reflection help maintain empathy and prevent desensitization among practitioners (Isobel & Edwards, 2017).

Researchers have begun linking these findings with neurobiological evidence. McEwen (2021) and Porges (2022) describe how safe and predictable environments help regulate the parasympathetic nervous system, improving emotional balance and cognitive flexibility. This bridge between neuroscience and psychology confirms that trauma-informed care supports healing through both relational and biological pathways.

The ethical dimension of trauma-informed practice has also received attention. Studies by Figley (2021) and Bloom and Farragher (2018) emphasize that workplaces ignoring the emotional impact of trauma risk repeating harmful dynamics within their systems. In contrast, organizations that value fairness, compassion, and transparency create conditions that foster collective well-being and moral integrity (Bloom, 2019). These insights affirm trauma-informed care as not just a therapeutic framework but also an ethical stance in human services.

Recent studies extend these ideas into digital spaces. With the rise of telehealth and online therapy, new challenges emerge around privacy, presence, and emotional connection. Research by Isobel et al. (2021) and Leitch (2022) suggests that while online services expand access, they also require new strategies to preserve safety and empathy. Future work needs to explore how technology can sustain genuine connection in remote care.

Overall, the research consistently shows that trauma-informed care improves outcomes when adopted as an integrated and sustained practice. It enhances recovery, protects professionals, and builds organizational strength. The growing body of evidence portrays trauma-informed care as both a practical and ethical model for creating environments where people can heal with safety and respect.

4. BARRIERS TO IMPLEMENTATION AND SUCCESS FACTORS IN TRAUMA-INFORMED CARE

Although trauma-informed care has gained wide recognition as an effective and ethical framework, its implementation across settings often encounters obstacles. The challenges stem from structural, cultural, and professional factors that limit consistency and sustainability. Understanding these barriers is essential for developing strategies that ensure trauma-informed approaches become integrated and enduring practices.

Many institutions face difficulties in translating theory into practice. Limited funding, rigid administrative systems, and high staff turnover often undermine consistent application (Menschner & Maul, 2023). Organizations may endorse trauma-informed values in policy documents but lack the resources or time to provide adequate training and supervision. In such environments, trauma-informed initiatives risk becoming symbolic rather than transformative (Bloom & Farragher, 2018).

A recurring challenge lies in organizational culture. Environments dominated by hierarchy, control, or risk management can unintentionally reproduce the very dynamics that contribute to trauma (Knight, 2021). Staff who feel unsupported or pressured by performance demands may struggle to apply relational and compassionate approaches. Without reflective supervision and emotional safety for professionals, the principles of trauma-informed care remain theoretical rather than lived practice.

Another structural issue concerns staff workload and burnout. Implementing trauma-informed systems requires time for reflection, collaboration, and training, yet many institutions operate under constant time pressure (Figley, 2021). When staff are emotionally exhausted or lack stability in their roles, maintaining empathy becomes difficult. Studies show that without attention to staff well-being, trauma-informed care loses much of its effectiveness (Bunting et al., 2021).

Many practitioners value the philosophy of trauma-informed care but feel unprepared to implement it. Training programs are often short or fragmented, offering limited opportunities to develop deep understanding and skill. Research by Isobel and Edwards (2017) shows that a single workshop rarely leads to meaningful change unless followed by supervision and practice-based reflection. Professionals who do not feel confident in their ability to manage trauma-related reactions may revert to traditional, symptom-focused methods.

A related issue is the lack of integration between trauma-informed knowledge and existing professional models. In some clinical and educational contexts, practitioners still operate under diagnostic or behaviorist frameworks that view distress primarily as dysfunction. This disconnect can create internal tension between institutional expectations and trauma-informed values (De Candia et al., 2022). Overcoming it requires not only knowledge but also permission from leadership to practice differently.

Cultural adaptation remains another major challenge. Trauma is shaped by social and historical contexts, yet many trauma-informed frameworks were originally developed in Western societies (Yehuda et al., 2023). When applied in non-Western or low-resource settings, some concepts may not align with local understandings of safety, authority, or community. For example, collectivist cultures may interpret empowerment or self-expression differently from individualist models (Kim et al., 2023).

Language can also be a barrier. Translating terms such as "trauma," "recovery," or "empowerment" into local languages sometimes alters their meaning or emotional tone. Practitioners who are not sensitive to these nuances may unintentionally alienate clients. This highlights the need for cultural humility and for co-designing interventions with local communities (Berring et al., 2024).

Trauma-informed principles can lose strength when introduced into systems that prioritize compliance, efficiency, or crisis management over human connection. Hospitals, schools, and social service agencies are often bound by bureaucratic procedures that limit flexibility. In such contexts, trauma-informed care may be seen as an "add-on" rather than a guiding philosophy (Bloom, 2019).

A policy gap also exists between endorsement and implementation. Many national health strategies reference trauma-informed care, but few include detailed frameworks for evaluation or accountability. Without measurable indicators, organizations may claim to be trauma-informed without truly changing their practices (Bendall et al., 2020). Long-term success depends on embedding these values in policy, budgeting, and leadership structures.

Despite these barriers, numerous studies identify conditions that enhance the sustainability of trauma-informed care. Leadership commitment is consistently cited as the strongest predictor of success (Leitch, 2022). When senior administrators actively model trauma-informed values such as respect, transparency, and empathy, staff are more likely to internalize and sustain the approach.

Comprehensive and ongoing training is equally important. Programs that combine theoretical learning with experiential components, case discussions, and reflective supervision produce deeper and more lasting change (Isobel et al., 2021). In contrast, isolated workshops tend to raise awareness but not competence.

Creating emotionally safe work environments is another crucial factor. Staff who feel supported and valued are more able to offer empathy to clients. Organizations that establish peer support groups and regular debriefing sessions report higher morale and lower turnover (Menschner & Maul, 2023).

Collaboration across disciplines strengthens implementation. Integrating trauma-informed practices across health, education, and social care allows professionals to share language and understanding (Champine et al., 2023). This alignment reduces fragmentation and ensures that clients experience consistency across services.

Evaluation and feedback mechanisms also contribute to long-term success. Data collection on client experiences, staff well-being, and service outcomes helps organizations identify gaps and celebrate progress. Regular reflection promotes accountability and continuous improvement (Lotzin et al., 2022).

Finally, cultural humility and inclusivity are fundamental success factors. Effective trauma-informed systems honor diversity and remain sensitive to the intersections of trauma with race, gender, and social class (Yehuda et al., 2023). When professionals approach clients and colleagues with openness and respect, trauma-informed care becomes more than a framework—it becomes an ethos of humanity.

Implementing trauma-informed care is a gradual process that unfolds through learning, reflection, and shared commitment. Sustainable change depends on consistent leadership, supportive supervision, and alignment between individual practice and organizational culture. Studies show that when institutions embrace these elements collectively, trauma-informed principles become part of daily life rather than temporary initiatives (Bloom & Farragher, 2018; Menschner & Maul, 2023).

At its heart, trauma-informed care requires a shift in how systems view both clients and staff. It invites organizations to replace control with compassion, judgment with understanding, and rigidity with flexibility. Success is not defined by perfection but by the continuous effort to create environments where healing, trust, and dignity are possible for everyone involved.

5. ETHICAL AND CULTURAL DIMENSIONS OF TRAUMA-INFORMED PRACTICE

Trauma-informed care extends beyond a clinical model and into an ethical and cultural framework for human interaction. It invites professionals and organizations to recognize the moral responsibility inherent in caring for people who have experienced harm. The approach emphasizes empathy, respect, and human dignity as guiding values in every stage of assessment, treatment, and organizational practice.

The ethical dimension of trauma-informed care aligns closely with the fundamental principles of autonomy, beneficence, non-maleficence, and justice (Beauchamp & Childress, 2019). Respecting autonomy means allowing individuals to make choices about their care and recognizing their capacity for self-determination. Beneficence calls for actions that promote healing and growth, while non-maleficence reminds practitioners to avoid interventions that might re-traumatize. Justice emphasizes fairness and the equal right of every person to safety and support.

Trauma-informed practice also builds on relational ethics, which focus on trust, presence, and authentic human connection (Buber, 1958). Healing occurs in relationships where power is shared and vulnerability is met with empathy. This perspective reframes professional boundaries not as distance but as containment that ensures emotional safety for both parties. The ethical goal is to create conditions where people can rediscover agency without fear of judgment.

Transparency and accountability are further ethical imperatives. Clients have the right to understand how decisions about their care are made. Professionals are responsible for explaining interventions, obtaining informed consent, and inviting collaboration throughout the process (Knight, 2021). These practices reinforce trust and reduce the sense of powerlessness that often follows traumatic experiences.

An ethic of care also demands reflection on professional well-being. Working with trauma affects the emotional lives of practitioners. Burnout, vicarious trauma, and compassion fatigue can compromise ethical judgment and empathy (Figley, 2021). Trauma-informed systems therefore include safeguards such as supervision, peer consultation, and space for emotional processing. Attending to the well-being of professionals is not self-indulgent but a moral requirement that ensures the safety of clients.

Culture shapes how trauma is experienced, expressed, and healed. Effective trauma-informed practice must therefore reflect cultural humility, which involves awareness of one's own biases and respect for the perspectives of others (Yehuda et al., 2023). Instead of assuming a single model of recovery, practitioners need to approach each client's story as embedded in a cultural and social world.

Research has shown that trauma intersects with race, ethnicity, gender, and social class in complex ways (Berring et al., 2024). For example, individuals from marginalized communities often experience trauma not as a single event but as a repeated exposure to systemic discrimination or economic hardship (Kim et al., 2023). In such contexts, healing must include advocacy for justice and equity. Cultural competence alone is not enough; cultural humility calls for ongoing self-reflection and dialogue.

Language and meaning are central to this process. Words like "trauma," "resilience," or "empowerment" may not exist in every language, and when they do, their emotional resonance varies. Practitioners must pay attention to metaphors, rituals, and community practices that express suffering and recovery in culturally specific ways. Integrating these perspectives fosters inclusion and belonging, which are themselves healing.

Gender and sexuality also influence how trauma is understood and addressed. Women and LGBTQ+ individuals often face unique forms of violence that require sensitive and inclusive responses (De Candia et al., 2022). Trauma-informed systems must ensure that spaces are physically and psychologically safe for all identities. Policies that acknowledge diversity in gender and sexual orientation strengthen both ethical integrity and effectiveness.

Beyond individual experiences, trauma can be collective, transmitted across generations, or embedded in historical injustices. Examples include colonization, slavery, war, and forced displacement. Trauma-informed care that ignores these legacies risks treating symptoms without addressing causes (Bloom, 2019). Recognizing collective trauma involves listening to stories of communities and validating their experiences as part of the healing process.

Community-based trauma-informed programs have demonstrated how collective recognition of pain can lead to empowerment and social change (Leitch, 2022). Rituals, storytelling, and shared memory help transform private suffering into communal resilience. Practitioners who engage with these narratives must do so with humility and respect, acknowledging that healing can take cultural forms different from clinical interventions.

Ethical principles apply not only to individual interactions but also to the structures that govern organizations. Institutions that aspire to trauma-informed care must ensure fairness, transparency, and shared responsibility at every level. Leadership plays a decisive role in setting the moral tone. When leaders model empathy and openness, ethical behavior spreads throughout the organization (Menschner & Maul, 2023).

Policies should be developed collaboratively, with attention to the voices of both clients and staff. Open communication about goals, risks, and decision-making fosters a sense of shared ownership. Organizations that practice self-reflection and seek feedback from service users are more likely to identify blind spots and make ethical corrections (Bloom & Farragher, 2018).

Accountability mechanisms are essential. Evaluation tools that include ethical indicators such as safety, inclusion, and respect can help ensure that trauma-informed principles are not reduced to rhetoric. These indicators align moral responsibility with measurable standards of care (Lotzin et al., 2022).

As trauma-informed care expands internationally, ethical considerations become even more complex. Practitioners must navigate differences in culture, religion, and value systems while maintaining the universality of human dignity. In some societies, discussing trauma openly may be seen as inappropriate or disrespectful. Professionals must balance cultural sensitivity with the commitment to safety and justice (Yehuda et al., 2023).

International collaboration can enrich trauma-informed practice by allowing mutual learning among cultures. Western models emphasize individual healing, while many non-Western traditions view recovery as a collective process involving family and community. Integrating these perspectives broadens the ethical scope of trauma-informed care, making it more responsive to the diversity of human experience (Kim et al., 2023).

6. CONCLUSIONS AND FUTURE DIRECTIONS

The ethical and cultural dimensions of trauma-informed practice remind professionals that healing is not only a psychological or physiological process but also a moral and social one. Ethics without empathy can become rigid, and culture without reflection can perpetuate harm. True trauma-informed care seeks balance: it honors individual choice, acknowledges collective history, and promotes justice within and beyond the therapeutic setting.

Ultimately, the ethical goal of trauma-informed care is to restore dignity. It challenges systems to move from reaction to reflection, from procedure to presence, and from control to compassion. By grounding professional action in empathy and cultural understanding, trauma-informed care affirms the shared humanity that makes recovery possible.

Trauma-informed care has evolved from a clinical initiative into a comprehensive philosophy that redefines how individuals and systems approach human suffering. Its foundations in safety, trust, collaboration, empowerment, and cultural humility have reshaped professional ethics and organizational practice. The evidence reviewed across previous chapters demonstrates that trauma-informed approaches benefit clients, practitioners, and institutions alike, offering measurable improvements in mental health, engagement, and workplace well-being (Lotzin et al., 2022; Menschner & Maul, 2023).

The growing body of research confirms that the effectiveness of trauma-informed care depends on the consistency of its application. Programs that embed trauma-informed values across all levels of an organization achieve more sustainable results than those that limit the approach to individual training sessions (Isobel et al., 2021; Bendall et al., 2020). The integration of these principles into supervision, leadership, and policy allows care systems to move from isolated interventions to a culture of compassion and accountability.

The theoretical and empirical evidence presented in this work highlights several key insights. First, trauma-informed care changes the focus of professional practice. It reframes distress as an understandable human response to adversity and emphasizes recovery through safety and connection. This shift challenges traditional models that treat trauma as a disorder located within the individual. Instead, it views healing as a social and relational process supported by trust and choice (Bloom, 2019; Knight, 2021).

Second, the success of trauma-informed systems depends on leadership and staff well-being. Professionals who feel safe, supported, and valued are more capable of creating environments that foster recovery (Figley, 2021; Menschner & Maul, 2023). Reflective supervision and peer collaboration remain central to sustaining empathy and preventing burnout.

Third, trauma-informed care operates not only within therapy rooms but across communities and institutions. When applied to education, health care, and social policy, it contributes to a broader culture of respect and inclusion (Champine et al., 2023). The approach thus bridges psychology with social justice, reminding professionals that care and equity are inseparable.

Despite strong evidence, trauma-informed care faces challenges related to implementation and evaluation. Many organizations adopt the language of trauma-informed care without transforming underlying structures (Bloom & Farragher, 2018). Short-term training without systemic support often fails to produce lasting change. The absence of clear evaluation tools also limits accountability and consistency (Bendall et al., 2020).

Another challenge concerns cultural adaptation. The global expansion of trauma-informed practice demands sensitivity to diverse cultural meanings of safety, healing, and autonomy (Yehuda et al., 2023). Practitioners must balance universal principles with local traditions, ensuring that interventions are respectful and relevant to each community.

Digitalization presents new ethical and relational questions. Online therapy and telehealth expand access but also create distance that can weaken the sense of presence essential to trauma recovery (Leitch, 2022). Future work should explore how technology can support genuine connection and emotional safety in virtual environments.

Directions for Future Research

Research on trauma-informed care continues to evolve. Future studies should focus on longitudinal outcomes to better understand how trauma-informed systems sustain change over time. There is also a need for mixed-method designs that integrate quantitative measures of effectiveness with qualitative accounts of lived experience. Such approaches can capture the depth of human transformation that numbers alone cannot describe (Isobel & Edwards, 2017).

Cross-cultural research remains a priority. Studies should examine how trauma-informed principles are interpreted and practiced in different cultural and socioeconomic contexts (Kim et al., 2023; Berring et al., 2024). Collaboration with local practitioners can reveal creative adaptations that enrich the global understanding of trauma-informed care.

Another direction involves exploring biological correlates of trauma recovery. Advances in neuroscience show that safe and predictable environments influence neural regulation and emotional resilience (McEwen, 2021; Porges, 2022). Future interdisciplinary studies can deepen knowledge about how relational safety translates into physiological healing.

Evaluation tools also need refinement. Standardized indicators of trauma-informed practice should include both clinical and organizational outcomes. Measures of trust, safety, and empowerment can provide a fuller picture of success than symptom scales alone (Lotzin et al., 2022). Developing these tools requires collaboration among researchers, practitioners, and policy makers.

The future of trauma-informed care extends beyond mental health. The same principles can inform education, criminal justice, and community development. Schools that cultivate emotional safety enhance learning and reduce behavioral difficulties (Kim et al., 2023). Correctional programs that integrate trauma awareness show lower recidivism and greater rehabilitation (Leitch, 2022). Social policies that prioritize equity and belonging can address collective forms of trauma rooted in historical injustice (Bloom, 2019; Yehuda et al., 2023).

As trauma-informed care continues to develop, its ethical dimension becomes increasingly central. The approach challenges professionals and institutions to move from procedure to presence, from compliance to compassion, and from reaction to reflection. These shifts require courage, humility, and ongoing dialogue. Trauma-informed systems thrive when leaders view care as both a moral and relational act.

The evidence presented throughout this work supports the view that trauma-informed care represents more than a set of techniques. It is a comprehensive vision of human interaction grounded in empathy and respect. When consistently practiced, it transforms both individuals and institutions, helping them replace fear with understanding and isolation with connection.

Future progress depends on collaboration among disciplines and across cultures. The continued exchange of knowledge between researchers, practitioners, and communities will ensure that trauma-informed principles remain dynamic and relevant. By holding space for both science and compassion, trauma-informed care points toward a future where healing is not the privilege of a few but a shared human capacity.

REFERENCES

Argyriadi, A., Katsarou, D., Patelarou, A., Megari, K., Patelarou, E., Kotrotsiou, S., Giakoumidakis, K., Abdoola, S., Mantsos, E., Efthymiou, E., & Argyriadis, A. (2025). Digital Stress Scale (DSC): Development and Psychometric Validation of a Measure of Stress in the Digital Age. *International Journal of Environmental Research and Public Health*, *22*(7), 1080. DOI: 10.3390/ijerph22071080 PMID: 40724147

Beauchamp, T. L., & Childress, J. F. (2019). *Principles of biomedical ethics* (8th ed.). Oxford University Press.

Bendall, S., Eastwood, O., Cox, G., Farrelly-Rosch, A., Nicoll, H., Peters, W., Bailey, A. P., McGorry, P. D., & Scanlan, J. N. (2020). A Systematic Review and Synthesis of Trauma-Informed Care Within Outpatient and Counseling Health Settings for Young People. *Child Maltreatment*, *26*(5), 533–545. DOI: 10.1177/1077559520927468 PMID: 32536207

Berring, L. L.. (2024). Implementing trauma-informed care—Settings, definitions, models, and outcomes. *International Journal of Mental Health Nursing*, *33*, e130–e149. DOI: 10.1111/inm.13144

Bloom, S. L. (2019). *Creating sanctuary: Toward the evolution of sane societies*. Routledge.

Bloom, S. L., & Farragher, B. (2018). *Restoring sanctuary: A new operating system for trauma-informed systems of care*. Oxford University Press.

Buber, M. (1958). *I and Thou* (2nd ed.). (Smith, R. G., Trans.). Charles Scribner's Sons.

Bunting, L., Montgomery, L., & Mooney, S.. (2021). Implementing trauma-informed approaches in healthcare: A mixed-methods systematic review. *BMJ Open*, *11*, e043817. DOI: 10.1136/bmjopen-2020-043817

Champine, R. B., Johnson, M., & Green, A. (2023). Trauma-informed care: Recent advances, limitations, and future directions. *Journal of Trauma & Dissociation*, *24*(1), 1–17. DOI: 10.1080/15299732.2022.2148474 PMID: 36567526

Courtois, C. A., & Ford, J. D. (2020). *Treating complex traumatic stress disorders (Adults): Scientific foundations and therapeutic models*. Guilford Press.

D'Andrea, W., Ford, J. D., & Courtois, C. A. (2020). Integrating trauma-informed care in psychotherapy for complex PTSD. *Journal of Contemporary Psychotherapy*, *50*(2), 109–122. DOI: 10.1007/s10879-019-09449-7

De Candia, C., Hughes, M., & Hopper, E. K. (2022). Trauma-informed TF-CBT with children exposed to violence: Outcomes and challenges. *Child Abuse & Neglect, 132*, 105797. DOI: 10.1016/j.chiabu.2022.105797

Dimitros, E., Katsarou, D. V., Mantsos, E., Bara, A., Argyriadi, A., Argyriadis, A., & Goupos, T. (2025). Perceptions of primary and secondary school principals on the support, educational forms and methods of gifted students in Greece. *Journal of Research in Special Educational Needs*. Advance online publication. DOI: 10.1111/1471-3802.70045

Felitti, V. J., Anda, R. F., Nordenberg, D., Williamson, D. F., Spitz, A. M., Edwards, V., Koss, M. P., & Marks, J. S. (1998). Relationship of childhood abuse and household dysfunction to many of the leading causes of death in adults. *American Journal of Preventive Medicine, 14*(4), 245–258. DOI: 10.1016/S0749-3797(98)00017-8 PMID: 9635069

Figley, C. R. (2021). Compassion fatigue and secondary trauma: Implications for mental health professionals. *Journal of Clinical Psychology, 77*(11), 2433–2445. DOI: 10.1002/jclp.23121

Horesh, D., & Brown, A. D. (2020). Traumatic stress in the age of COVID-19: A call to close critical gaps and adapt to new realities. *Psychological Trauma: Theory, Research, Practice, and Policy, 12*(4), 331–335. DOI: 10.1037/tra0000592 PMID: 32271070

Hughes, K., Ford, K., & Bellis, M. A.. (2021). Health impacts of adverse childhood experiences: A systematic review and meta-analysis. *The Lancet. Public Health, 6*(11), e848–e858. DOI: 10.1016/S2468-2667(21)00232-2 PMID: 34756168

Isobel, S., & Edwards, C. (2017). Using trauma informed care as a framework to promote the positive mental health of people with intellectual disability. *Journal of Intellectual Disabilities, 21*(3), 228–248. DOI: 10.1177/1744629517716738

Isobel, S., Goodyear, M., Furness, T., & Foster, K. (2021). Individual and organizational change: Trauma-informed care implementation in mental health services. *Issues in Mental Health Nursing, 42*(9), 821–832. DOI: 10.1080/01612840.2021.1962485

Johnson, L. M., West, C., & Lange, B. (2021). Trauma-informed cognitive-behavioral therapy: Clinical outcomes in adult survivors of abuse. *Psychotherapy Research, 31*(8), 1094–1108. DOI: 10.1080/10503307.2020.1865078

Khalifeh, H., Dean, K., & Osborn, D. (2022). Reducing coercion through trauma-informed psychiatric care: A multicenter study. *European Psychiatry : the Journal of the Association of European Psychiatrists, 65*(1), e21. DOI: 10.1192/j.eurpsy.2022.21 PMID: 35189997

Kim, J., Lee, H., & Park, S. (2023). Trauma-informed approaches in school-based mental health programs: A meta-analysis. *School Psychology International, 44*(3), 235–256. DOI: 10.1177/01430343221149983

Knight, C. (2021). Trauma-informed practice and care: Implications for social work. *Clinical Social Work Journal, 49*(4), 433–445. DOI: 10.1007/s10615-021-00792-z

Leitch, L. (2022). The evolution of trauma-informed care: Moving toward relational safety. *Frontiers in Psychology, 13*, 853730. DOI: 10.3389/fpsyg.2022.853730

Lotzin, A., Buth, S., & Sehner, S.. (2022). A systematic review and meta-analysis on the effects of trauma-informed care. *European Journal of Psychotraumatology, 13*(2), 2067891. DOI: 10.1080/20008198.2022.2067891 PMID: 38872598

McEwen, B. S. (2021). Neurobiology of stress and resilience: Implications for trauma recovery. *Nature Reviews. Neuroscience, 22*(7), 420–433. DOI: 10.1038/s41583-021-00495-9

Menschner, C., & Maul, A. (2023). Building a trauma-informed workforce: Evaluation of professional training outcomes. *The Journal of Behavioral Health Services & Research, 50*(2), 210–225. DOI: 10.1007/s11414-022-09821-0

Porges, S. W. (2022). Polyvagal theory and the biology of safety. *Frontiers in Integrative Neuroscience, 16*, 871227. DOI: 10.3389/fnint.2022.871227 PMID: 35645742

SAMHSA. (2014). *SAMHSA's concept of trauma and guidance for a trauma-informed approach.* U.S. Department of Health and Human Services.

Schwarz, L. E., Corrigan, F. M., & Hull, A. M. (2021). Trauma-focused psychotherapies: Mechanisms of change and outcome evidence. *Journal of Contemporary Psychotherapy, 51*(2), 119–130. DOI: 10.1007/s10879-020-09481-6

Sweeney, A., Clement, S., Filson, B., & Kennedy, A. (2018). Trauma-informed mental healthcare in the UK: What is it and how can we further its development? *Mental Health Review (Brighton), 23*(3), 131–144. DOI: 10.1108/MHRJ-01-2018-0008

van der Kolk, B. A. (2014). *The body keeps the score: Brain, mind, and body in the healing of trauma.* Viking Press.

Yehuda, R., Lehrner, A., & Bierer, L. M. (2023). Cultural and epigenetic influences in trauma response. *Current Opinion in Psychology*, *48*, 101481. DOI: 10.1016/j.copsyc.2022.101481

Chapter 2
A Review on Psychological Health and Wellbeing Affecting Factors With Special Reference to Practices of Forgiveness

Chitralekha Thapliyal
http://orcid.org/0009-0006-8792-8830
Department of Humanities and Social Sciences, Graphic Era (Deemed to be) University, Dehradun, India

Ajay Kumar Singh
http://orcid.org/0000-0003-0429-0925
Department of Humanities and Social Sciences, Graphic Era (Deemed to be) University, Dehradun, India

Ravindra Singh
http://orcid.org/0000-0003-3062-1812
PG Department of Psychology, Magadh University, Bodh Gaya, India

ABSTRACT

Psychological health of the people is highly essential to achieve their desired tasks. While the practice of forgiveness enables individuals to focus on inner peace, mindfulness, quality of life, and satisfaction with life. This chapter, therefore, assesses how negatively reinforced feelings can affect physiological wellbeing and health of youth? It is based on previous studies which explored the association of forgiveness

DOI: 10.4018/979-8-3373-6294-6.ch002

with psychological well-being of youths. It highlights the impact of social, economic, environmental, biological, lifestyle and technological fields on psychological health. It discovers the implications of forgiveness on psychological health of youths. Social support, social networks and environmental quality have a positive implication on psychological health. Excessive technological addiction, inappropriate diet patterns and biological characteristics have a negative impact on psychological health. Forgiveness practice has a positive impact on the learning process, psychological wellbeing, social wellbeing and psychological health of people.

1. INTRODUCTION

Psychological health is an essential driver to increase the physical and psychological wellbeing of people. Psychological wellbeing is an appropriate measurement of mental health (Tang et al., 2019). Further, mental health is also a key driver to enhance physical health. Mental health includes mental illness and psychological wellbeing (Tang et al., 2019). Appropriate mental health work as a better resource of interaction in families and societies (Gautam et al., 2024). Psychological health can be defined as the happiness of people and their active involvement in society. It also improves the social value of the people in the society (Gautam et al., 2024). Psychological health helps people to achieve their different tasks in social and economic and psychological fields. Appropriate psychological health maintains the efficiency and productivity of people. Appropriate psychological health of people increases their social communication in society. While mental disorders reduce the social communication of an individual with others. Mental disorder is identified in several forms like anxiety disorder, depressive disorder, etc. Mental disorders bring negative thoughts among the people and reduce their psychological behaviour and wellbeing (Gautam et al., 2024).

Mental health is associated with physical health and behaviour of people (Gautam et al., 2024). Negative thoughts hamper the thinking capacity and learning ability of a person. Thus, mental disorders reduce the productivity and efficiency of people. Mental disorders also reduce psychological behaviour and abilities of people (Gautam et al., 2024). Furthermore, positive mental health enhances the level of happiness of people (Gautam et al., 2024). Psychological health of an individual depends on multiple activities in psychological, social, environmental and economic dimensions, and food and nutritional security (Myers, 2020; Cedillo et al., 2023). For instance, the income of people helps to reduce their mental stress. While lack of job opportunities reduces the psychological health of people. Social communication among the people enhances their psychological health. Therefore, social development may be a crucial driver to improve the psychological health of people. Environmental quality in terms of clean air, clean water and clean food helps to improve psychological health of Individuals. Food insecurity is caused to increase psychological distress (Myers, 2020). Conversely, environmental degradation has negative implications on the psychological health of people. Thereupon, food and nutritional security help to maintain the psychological health of people (Myers, 2019; Cedillo et al., 2023). Existing theoretical literature notified various indicators in areas of social, economic, environmental and technological fields in different countries. Most scholars examined the factors affecting psychological and mental health of people using primary data (Wind et al., 2013; Tang et al., 2019; Tikka et al., 2020; Myers, 2020; Tater & John, 2024). These studies applied psychometric tools and techniques developed by leading psychologists.

Most specifically, psychological health and psychological behaviour are also determined by the various activities like the ability of forgiveness of an individual (Griffin et al., 2015; Bechara et al., 2024). However, forgiveness is a subjective matter of individuals to increase their mental happiness (Gunjan & Rana, 2023). While avoiding the practices of forgiveness would create more problems for an individual for a longer period of time. Forgiveness is a crucial driver to mediate the association between wisdom and psychological wellbeing among the people (Brudek et al., 2023). The phenomenon of forgiveness helps an individual to learn, and adopt practical skills to overcome a negative emotional state. Forgiveness is the intentional, individual internal process of letting go of sentiments and ideas of bitterness, anger, and the need for revenge and retaliation against the transgressor (Kim et al., 2022).

Furthermore, forgiveness is positively related to resilience and helps people to increase their psychological health (Lijo, 2018) and psychological wellbeing. One of the key ideas in the analysis of the processes of adaptation and resistance to unfavourable environmental impacts is psychological resilience (Cleverley & Kidd, 2011; Kravchuk, 2021). Kravchuk (2021) argued that resilience and grit are substantially associated when there is a positive attitude towards the offender, as opposed to when there is no negative sentiment towards them. It is also discovered that self-forgiveness lowers the likelihood of suicidal thoughts and post-traumatic stress disorder (Lijo, 2018). Çelik & Ertürk (2022) conducted research on psycho-education on forgiveness. It is observed that high school students who participate in forgiveness psycho-education programmes have higher levels of forgiveness and life happiness. Also, the students can assess their progress, ability, and experience, and learning practices of forgiveness. Thereupon, it also enhances the involvement of students with several social groups for sharing their problems and they can also get alternatives for resolving their issues. Hence, it may be a proactive option for individuals to pursue a practice of forgiveness in long-time.

Forgiveness and vengeance are social tendencies, and both provide primitive solutions to solve human problems in mental and psychological fields. Although these two characteristics of human nature are fixed. Forgiveness is necessary for making a peaceful world (McCullough, 2008). Research has found that students who react with rage or bitterness are poor learners and have lower scores of GPAs than those who are identified to have low anger (Freedman, 2018). Fitzgibbons (1998) also found that anger is ingrained in young children and is felt daily in the home, at school, in the community, and at work place. Moreover, classroom teaching can facilitate forgiveness programs to help kids who have experienced poverty and violence feel less angry. Therefore, positive psychological behaviour with children plays a key role to increase their psychological and mental ability to adopt better practices of forgiveness. Most learning is surrounded by a strong emotional context, which can either promote or impede it. Hence, an appropriate surrounding environment is also making easier ways for children to pursue positive psychology and adopt a better learning for forgiveness.

Further, it also enhances psychological wellbeing and psychological health of children. One good example is helping out of empathy as it enables us to develop compassion for the well-being of strangers and then take action to advance their needs in some way (McCullough, 2000). Willingness to sacrifice, or the disposition to put aside one's own needs to further enhance the well-being and improve prosocial activity (Van Lange et al., 1997). Emotions act as the seed for psychological health problems also these are the negative emotions that directly harm mental and physiological health of people. Therefore, any individual can opt the path of forgiveness to deal with these emotions. While forgiveness is not a mental-emotional process but rather an amalgamation of both psychological and physiological processes (Worthington, 2007). Further, psychological and physiological processes have an impact on psychological health and well-being of individuals for the long-term. Previous literature claimed that practices of forgiveness are helpful for youth to increase their psychological and mental wellbeing. However, past literature could not develop a conceptual model to examine the association of forgiveness with psychological wellbeing of youth. Therefore, academician could not find the answer following research questions:

- How forgiveness helps to increase the psychological health of youths?
- What may be consequences of mental disorder among the youths?
- How is forgiveness associated with the psychological health of youths?
- What are the key drivers for improving psychological health?
- What may be consequences of positive and negative implications of forgiveness among the youths?

This chapter, therefore, has achieved the following objectives as per the relevance to the above- mentioned research questions:

- To explore the psychological health affecting factors.
- To assess the impact of forgiveness on psychological wellbeing.
- To explain the relationship between forgiveness and social behaviour.

This research is based on previous literature. Published articles are taken from Scopus database. While most relevant studies pertinent to this research are reviewed. Content-based analytical tools are used for select the most suitable published research article. It used an indicators-based approach to analyse the association of forgiveness with psychological health of youths. Tabulation presentation is formulated to explore the conceptual framework of the indicators.

2. IMPLICATIONS OF FORGIVENESS

2.1. Forgiveness and Learning

Forgiveness is an utmost required human quality that refers to abandoning negative emotionality, grudges, and retaliation in the face of perceived transgressions (Worthington & Wade, 2020; Tiwari et al., 2022; Thapliyal et al., 2025). The previous ancient literature sets an example of forgiving practices and messages (Hunter, 2007, Tripathi & Mullet, 2010; van Oosten, 2008). The notion of forgiveness was always present in the field of positive psychology to explain human potential and positive aspects of human behaviour (Gable & Haidt, 2005). Despite the availability of various psychological therapies and other assistance, forgiveness has made great success in understanding, explaining, and treating people with emotional overburden (Gable & Haidt, 2005). In the recent advancement of positive psychology, forgiveness was a neglected part of the learning program that led to happiness and contentment. Moreover, forgiveness training and practice is identified in the past. It was always present since ancient times and deep rooted in history (Hunter, 2007; van Oosten, 2008; Worthington, 2001).

Theoretical literature argued that learning forgiveness creates happiness for the people (Thapliyal et al., 2025). It also improves adjustment capacity to deal with negative emotional experiences, such as fragmented interpersonal relationships, and both the physical and psychological problems. It is positively related with health and well-being, and negatively with anxiety, suicidal behaviors, and depression (Epstein et al., 1998; Pandey et al., 2020; Parihar et al., 2020). Available research is also reporting many positive outcomes of practising forgiveness at the individual, interpersonal and organizational levels (Ahirwar et al., 2019; Pandey et al., 2020; Parihar et al., 2020; Tiwari et al., 2022; Toussaint et al., 2020). Ahirwar et al. (2019) examined the attributes and consequences of forgiveness among the children using qualitative data. Thus, keeping forgiveness in mind may be beneficial when the nature of transgression is severe and immoral.

Previous studies are also reposted the existence of significant gender differences in forgiveness. Bullying in schools has gained global recognition in recent years as a major issue affecting children everywhere. Numerous studies have also shown that victims of school bullying suffer from stress, anxiety, and depression and that can sometimes lead to suicide. Additionally, bullying is hard to stop; even the most effective interventions have a limited impact. Thus, it is essential to examine other possible coping mechanisms to deal with bullying. It is suggested by the researchers that practicing forgiveness can significantly act as an effective coping tool.

2.2. Forgiveness and Psychological health

Ensuring safe surroundings is an important part for every parent, educator, and psychological health expert's work (Mcloughlin et al., 2002). Physical and sexual assault, illicit drug usage, self-harm, bullying, gang-related crime, and teenage pregnancy are dangerous for increasing mental disability (Kagan, 1991). Research has shown that forgiveness acts as an effective coping method for adults to deal with the above-mentioned issues in their life. However, some incidents can be controlled or managed through forgiveness by adults. As indicated by the prevalence of school violence, adolescents require beneficial coping mechanisms to overcome anger produced by personal injury (Freedman, 2007). Physical abuse is also caused to increase mental disorder and depression among the students (Ammerman et al., 1986). Griffin et al. (2015) also pointed out that forgiveness is a coping mechanism to increase psychological health of victims and perpetrators. Kagan (1991) identified five distinct groups that increase risk among the adolescents (Table 1). Firstly, academic failure is caused to increase anger and antisocial prevalence among adolescents. Secondly, negative environments also increase risk of anger, teenage pregnancy, drug addiction, and disobeying authority among the youth. Thirdly, low-esteem and desire to be part of the social violence of adolescents may also increase due to being susceptible to peer pressure. Fourthly, often involved in delinquent behaviour may also be harmful for youth to be perceived as brave. Fifthly, the youths may be engaged in stealing, drug use and teenage pregnancy due to the existence of robbery and addiction of drugs in the society.

Table 1. Five distinct groups that increase risk among the adolescents

At-risk adolescent	Predicted features and behaviour
Chronic school/academic failure	Anger issue and antisocial, drug use
Negative environment (anger, abuse, and neglect)	Risk of anger issues, adolescent pregnancy, drug use, and disobeying authority figure.
Susceptible to peer pressure	Low self-esteem, desire to be a part of a group
Desire to be perceived as brave	Often involved in delinquent behaviour.
Existence of robbery, illegal sexual activities, and / addiction of drugs in the society	Stealing, drug use and teenage pregnancy

Source: Adopted from Kagan (1991)' study.

Forgiveness is conceptualized as a developmental concept in theoretical literature (Enright & HDSG, 1994). According to Kagan (1991), the level of success while conducting interventions involving such adolescents will differ depending on their challenging psychological features. These psychological features include multiple activities that ensure the psychological health of adolescents. When children do not feel loved and affection by parents they may feel rage, embarrassment, guilt, and/or betrayal. This type of behaviour and attitude to parents towards their children may increase mental and psychological problems among them. Thereafter, Gambaro (2002) introduced forgiveness and Rogerian-based group therapy for the elementary school children to cope with anger caused by a terrible event. Forgiveness therapy is also positive to reduce depression, stress, and create positive thoughts in the mind of an individual (Gunjan & Rana, 2023). This forgiveness intervention helps to increase favourable attitudes of children towards educators, schools, parents, and friends. Hence, it is noticed as a significant measure to increase the mental and psychological wellbeing of children in elementary school. An eight-week forgiveness intervention is also conducted by Freedman and Knupp (2003). This intervention is helpful for adolescents to cope with the separation of parents. It also reduces participant's anxiety and develops an optimistic attitude towards their goals.

2.3. Forgiveness and Psychological Wellbeing

Forgiveness has a direct and indirect influence on mental and psychological health (Kim et al., 2022; Thapliyal et al., 2025). Forgiveness is a revolutionary tool to increase psychological wellbeing and psychological health. Practices of forgiveness are highly essential in positive psychology. It helps to minimize negative thoughts and enhance positively among the youth. Further, it also works as psychological resilience to overcome the challenges of people in social relations with others. Thus, it may be beneficial to increase the physical health of the people. Further, the relationship between forgiveness and psychological health is dependent on where a person is in the developmental process of forgiving. During the initial phases of the process (discovery and decision-making), there may be a connection between forgiveness and worse psychological health. While worse psychological health led to reduced psychological wellbeing.

2.4. Social-Emotional Learning (SEL) and Forgiveness

SEL focuses on empathy and emotion regulation. SEL provides the important attitudes and skills to the individuals for managing emotions, observing, experiencing empathy for others. SEL is helpful for an individual for making a meaningful and responsible decision maker. At its foundation, SEL is about developing self-awareness, which starts with an understanding of emotions (Zakrzewski, 2015). Emotions function in harmony with cognition in a smooth and coherent way to help in managing education, career, relationships, and life choices (Zakrzewski, 2015). Similarly, forgiveness education focuses on recognising and acknowledging children' anger. Therefore, forgiveness education is a proactive action to increase the learning abilities of the adults (Coyle & Enright, 1998). Gambaro (2002) also concluded the significant impact of forgiveness education on anger among adolescents. Gambaro et al. (2008a) explored the role of forgiveness counselling for improving the academic achievement of students. Further, it plays a crucial role for educating children to control their emotions in a healthy manner, comprehend the perspective of others, recognise the inherent goodness in all, and increase empathy and compassion. According to research, earlier unpleasant treatment from others may contribute to increased emotional or behavioural dysregulation as well as academic problems among the children.

Table 2. Enright's four-phase, 20-unit process model

Phases	Procedure
Uncovering Phase	To investigate the degree of anger that come from an offence among the students
Decision Phase	Decision making. To decide and commit to forgiveness
Work Phase	To take action. Forgive the transgressor
Deepening Phase	Self-awareness and free from the emotional prison

Source: Adopted from Enright's study.

Emotions and intellect may also increase dysregulation and poor academic performance of the students. An individual often feels anger, a sense of injustice and hostility after the transgression. These negative emotions can trigger stress and anxiety among individuals (Berry et al., 2001b). Forgiveness is an emotion-regulation method for dealing with interpersonal disputes among the students (Worthington and Wade, 2020). Forgiveness is one of the ways to cope with the stress and anxiety (Lazarus & Folkman, 1984). Enright's four-phase, 20-unit process model is significantly linked with the SEL. According to their model of forgiveness, Enright and HDSG (1994) designed an intervention that contains 20 distinct components within four phases (Table 2). Table 2 explains the four different phases of SEL.

In this model, individuals go through 20 questions for estimating their SEL. 1st phase helps a person to uncover the root of the anger, awareness about the situation and the bottled-up negative emotion that was harming them more (Table 2). In the decision phase a new insight form about the transgressor and the situation, willingness to forgive is surfacing up. The deepening phase helps a person to actualize their self-reliance and awareness. Forgiveness helps an individual to free from the victim state and the emotional turmoil (Enright & HDSG, 1991). Other than Enright's model of forgiveness, Worthington's Five stems Recall, Empathy, Altruistic, Commit, and Hold (REACH) model also helps in SEL (Worthington et al, 2006). Developing empathy in victims towards their offenders is an important technique for attaining forgiveness. Thus, encouraging empathy can promote self-awareness and facilitate forgiveness in students (Enright and HDSG, 1996). Gambaro at al. (2008a) conducted an intervention on at-risk adolescents. At-risk and trait anger adolescents suffer from psychologically, socially, and academically (Loveland et al., 2007). Results of the study show that forgiveness helps to improve attitudes towards self, school, parents, educators, and interpersonal relationships (Gambaro et al., 2008a).

2.5. Enhancing the Learning Potential, Therapies and Intervention of Forgiveness

For enhancing the learning potential, it is, thus, necessary to introduce forgiveness as an instrument way to deal with anger, resentment, and free one-self from the attachment of the transgression and from the victim state. Such programs can assist students to deal with anger issues and reduce frequency of violent behaviour. In children and adults, forgiveness counselling is a crucial intervention tool that can help to calm down individuals' emotional expression such as disgust, anger, anxiousness, and depression (Enright et al., 2007; Gambaro et al., 2008a; Reed & Enright, 2006). According to Fitzgibbons (1998) the psychotherapeutic utilization of forgiveness can significantly diminish the emotion, physical, and mental suffering. Additionally, it is also beneficial in the sense of freedom, reduced stress, resentment, and anger.

3. PSYCHOLOGICAL HEALTH AFFECTING FACTORS

The existing review indicates that psychological health is significantly associated with the indicators in the domain of social, economic, technological, environmental development, and geographical, biological and lifestyle. Family and social support are found crucial to increase psychological health in the social sector (Kawachi & Berkman, 2001; Barua et al., 2010; Reddy 2019; Acoba, 2024). Low socioeconomic status is linked with poor psychological health of people. Kawachi and Berkman (2001) argued that social networks are a crucial driver to increase psychological health. While chronic illness is caused to reduce psychological wellbeing of an individual. Other issues like love failure of youths and low strata are found accountable for increasing their mental disorder.

Food and its quality are also useful to reduce mental disorders (Cedillo et al., 2023). While lead and cadmium are associated with depressive symptoms (Buser & Scinicariello, 2017). Further, nutrition therapy can be helpful to recover from the mental stress and disorder (Rao et al., 2008). Culture influences different aspects of psychological health like perceived mental illness, prevalence of mental disorder, epidemiology and coping strategies (Hwang et al., 2007). Climate change and extreme variability in weather indicators are also causing psychological health of people (Padhy et al., 2015). Moreover, disaster is caused to increase PTSD, depression, anxiety and common mental disorders (Makwana, 2019; Negi et al., 2025). High occurrence of disasters is leading to increased mental disorder among the people (Wind et al., 2013; Negi et al., 2025). Clean environment also determines psychological health and subjective wellbeing (Belsky & Pluess, 2009). Psychological health is also adversely affected due to air pollution (Kapoor et al., 2024). Moreover, people are found susceptible to their environmental stimuli due to their genetic makeup (Belsky & Pluess, 2009; Baker et al, 2023). Higher green space is associated with high restrictiveness, mindfulness, and resilience therefore, better psychological health (Kim & Kim, 2017; Callaghan et al., 2020). High sensitivity in the environmental factors may lead to increased mental disorder (Assary et al., 2024). Higher greenery space is positive to increase psychological health (Dzhambov et al., 2019). Also, lead and cadmium are caused to increase depression symptoms.

Addiction of tobacco and liquor among the people are also increasing the mental disorder. Low health literacy is also increasing the prevalence of poor psychological health and low quality of life (Lee et al., 2015). Therefore, health literacy plays a crucial role for increasing quality of life and psychological health (Degan et al., 2018). The urban population have more mental disorders as compared to rural dwellers (Gruebner et al., 2017). Low social support for females increases their poor psychological health. It is also noted a strong relationship between demographic characteristics and psychological health. Sleep duration is correlated with psychological health (stress and depressive symptoms) and chronic diseases (osteoarthritis, cancer and diabetes etc.) (Lee et al., 2015). Internet use is also causing mental disorders and poor psychological health among youth and children (Siste et al., 2021). Physical and Psychological health of youth is also hampering due to extensive application of smartphones (Tater & John, 2024). Social media addiction is also causing psychological health among the youth (Taddi et al., 2024). A shared genetic common variant can cause MDD-AD comorbidity. An elevated polygenic person with AD is at high risk for MDD and vice versa (Andersen et al., 2017). Biological factors also determine the psychological health of people (Hyman, 2000; Kendler et al., 2011). Table 3 explains the psychological health affecting indicators are per the existing literature.

Table 3. Psychological health affecting indicators

Author(s)	Study Area	Main Objective	Psychological health promoting indicators	Major findings
Acoba (2024)	Philippines	Observe the correlation of stress with psychological health	Social support	Family support decreases stress, anxiety, and depression.
Barua et al. (2010)	Asia, Europe, Australia, North and South America	Identify the significance of socio-demographic factors and depression in the old population	Social support	Social risk factors (low strata, loss of loved one, and chronic illness) in the old population are positively related to depression.
Kawachi & Berkman (2001)	Review	Highlight the different path of social dynamics and psychological health	Social support	Social network influence psychological health. Low support for female is caused to increase their poor psychological health.
Bedaso et al. (2021)	Review	Find the relationship between social support and psychological health in pregnant women.	Social support	No antenatal care is positively correlated with anxiety, depressive symptoms, and self-harm of pregnant women.
Reddy (2019)	India	Assess the factors affecting the burden of mental disorders	Social support	Women, elderly, trauma survivors, individual with low socioeconomic status, and chronic illness patients are more susceptible to develop mental disorders.

continued on following page

Table 3. Continued

Author(s)	Study Area	Main Objective	Psychological health promoting indicators	Major findings
Hwang et al. (2007)	Review	Explore the importance of culture in a person's psychological health	Social support	Culture influences different aspects of psychological health like perceived mental illness, prevalence of mental disorder, epidemiology and coping strategies.
Andersen et al. (2017)	USA	Examine the genetic connection between alcohol dependence (AD) and major depressive disorder (MDD)	Biology	A shared genetic common variant can cause MDD-AD comorbidity. An elevated polygenic person with AD is at high risk for MDD and vice versa.
Hyman (2000)	Review	Find the significance of genes in psychological health	Biology	Genes, molecules and biological factors play a crucial role in developing psychological health. Genetic information of a person can help in treatment and therapies.
Assary et al. (2024)	England and Wales	The relationship between how an individual's genetic makeup can affect environmental factors and psychological health.	Biology and environment	Environment sensitivity is significantly connected with emotional problems.
Kendler et al. (2011)	USA	Investigate the link between environment and genetic factor for common mental disorders and mental well-being	Environment and biology	There is genetic propensity in depression disorder, anxiety disorder and panic attack also with mental well-being.
Belsky and Pluess (2009)	Review	Find the influence of temperament, perceived parenting, and gene-environment interaction on psychological health	Biology, social, and environment	People are differently susceptible to their environment stimuli because of their genetic makeup.
Baker et al. (2023)	Review	Evaluate the assessment tools for assess the impact of the environment on psychological health	Environment	Due to the uprise in the impact of environment on psychological health the tools are not sufficient to co-ordinate with each other for the global population.

continued on following page

Table 3. Continued

Author(s)	Study Area	Main Objective	Psychological health promoting indicators	Major findings
Callaghan et al. (2020)	Review	Evaluate the impact of greenery on psychological health.	Environment	Green environment is significantly related with psychological health.
Dzhambov et al. (2019)	Bulgaria	Find how green space can help in decreasing anxiety and depression symptoms by means of restorativeness and mindfulness	Environment	Higher greenery is associated with high restorativeness, mindfulness, and resilience.
Gruebner et al. (2017)	Review	Find relationship between cities and psychological health	Environment	Risk of mental disorders like schizophrenia are higher in urban areas. Low social and economic status can be linked with poor psychological health.
Kim and Kim (2017)	South Korea	Relationship of demography and environment factor on psychological health	Environment	There is a strong relationship between demographic characteristics and psychological health, and moderate relationship between green spaces and psychological health.
Makwana (2019)	Review	Find an association between disasters and psychological health	Environment	Disaster is caused to increase PTSD, depression, anxiety and common mental disorders.
Wind et al. (2013)	India	Impact of seasonal floods on psychological health	Environment	Recurrent disasters are strongly related with mental disorders and poor functioning.
Kapoor et al. (2024)	India	Observe the impact of air pollution on psychological health	Environment	Air pollution is altering brain chemistry, accelerating mental disorders, and decreasing cognition.
Padhy et al. (2015)	India	Examine relationship between climate change and psychological health	Environment	Climate change leads to increase mental disorder.

continued on following page

Table 3. Continued

Author(s)	Study Area	Main Objective	Psychological health promoting indicators	Major findings
Buser and Scinicariello (2017)	USA	Examine the relationship between the ingredients of tobacco (cadmium and lead) and depression	Lifestyle	Lead and cadmium are associated with depressive symptoms. While tobacco cessation can help in the recovery from depression.
Lakhan and Vieira (2008)	Review	Emphasize nutrition therapy (dietary aid) for the recovery of mental disorder	Lifestyle	Nutrition therapy can be helpful for recovery of mental disorder.
Degan et al. (2018)	Australia	Find the relationship between health literacy in substance use disorder patients with quality of life, and health (mental and physical)	Lifestyle	Health literacy plays a crucial role for increasing quality of life and psychological health. Low to moderate health literacy is associated with poor psychological health and low quality of life.
Lee et al. (2015)	Korea	Find relationship among duration of sleep, psychological health and chronic disease	Lifestyle	Sleep duration is correlated with psychological health (stress and depressive symptoms) and chronic diseases (osteoarthritis, cancer and diabetes etc).
Lim et al. (2016)	Review	Determine nutritional factors for increasing psychological health	Lifestyle	Niacin, and Folate are effective to increase psychological health.
Rao et al. (2008)	India	Examine the nutrition impact on mental illness.	Lifestyle	Nutrition intervention and therapy have an impact on mental illnesses like depression, anxiety, ADHD and eating disorders.
Tikka et al. (2020)	India	Examine the contribution of physical activity in psychological health	Lifestyle	Physical activity, exercise and yoga help for decreasing depression, anxiety and stress.

continued on following page

Table 3. Continued

Author(s)	Study Area	Main Objective	Psychological health promoting indicators	Major findings
Tater and John (2024)	India	Evaluate the link between smartphone addiction and psychological health	Technology addiction	Smartphone addiction is impacting negatively the physical and mental well-being of people.
Taddi et al. (2024)	India	Impact of social media use on teenagers' psychological health.	Technology addiction	Social media addiction is linked with mental problems like OCD, anxiety, depression and victimization of cyberbullying.

4. FORGIVENESS AND MENTAL WELLBEING

Table 4 summaries the findings of related literature that could be helpful to draw conclusive perspectives about the relationship of forgiveness with psychological wellbeing and psychological health. Accordingly, following major findings are provided in this chapter:

Enhanced Learning Environment: Learning environment is an essential component to resolve most issues that are leading to create barriers for psychological health and psychological wellbeing of the people. Further, the notion of forgiveness significantly adds to the learning environment. In the elementary and middle school educational setups training in forgiveness is provided and practiced, and children feel secure and attached. Such a supporting environment facilitates academic achievement and overall well-being of the students. Such encouraging findings among children's education programs, not only create a positive teaching learning environment but also add value to the entire education system. Additionally, it also increases student interaction for more meaningful social interactions.

Enhanced Psychological health and Wellbeing: Forgiveness is directly and indirectly linked with stress levels, state anxiety, and mild to moderate levels of depression. Practicing forgiveness can assist individuals to experience greater psychological wellbeing. Forgiveness can also increase learning ability and focus and increase social engagement. Considering forgiveness and its relation with psychological health outcomes, it is important to understand a few key things. (1) Inability to forgive may result in stress and interpersonal offense, which ultimately decreases psychological health. (2) Due to an unforgiveness tendency of an individual, it may cause increased levels of guilt, shame, and regret further reported as negative psychological health. (3) The global burden of poor psychological health is a potential threat to society. (4) Forgiveness treatment can be recognized as a viable mode of intervention and treatment.

Boost Interpersonal Relationships: The process of forgiveness not only fosters positive relationships but also promotes empathy, and sympathy, and increases meaningful communication. When an individual forgives someone for their past misbehaviours, it often leads to healthier interactions and in-depth association, contributing to greater social well-being.

Increased Resilience: Forgiveness is also linked with greater resilience during adverse conditions. A greater propensity for forgiveness is linked to a higher degree of psychological resilience. Individuals with a greater capacity for forgiveness tend to perform better under pressure (Kravchuk, 2021). Along with, psychological resilience has a direct and significant connection with control, toughness, and stress tolerance. Additionally, psychological resilience is found to have a negative and substantial relationship with emotional instability, shyness, anxiety, sadness, neuroticism, and anger. People reported better coping and fewer setbacks when they forgive. Furthermore, it also facilitates learning and self-growth. Moreover, ignorance of the negative emotions associated with past conflicts can redirect individuals' energy toward a constructive mindset.

Promotion of Prosocial Behavior: It is also found that forgiveness encourages prosocial behavior (cooperation, kindness, and self-compassion). Lack of forgiveness reduces generalized prosocial orientation, congruent with the findings of García-Vázquez (2020). While prosocial behavior is positively correlated with forgiveness, gratitude, and happiness.

Reduction of Negative Behaviors: One of the ongoing issues that children deal with is bullying at school. According to research, forgiveness reduces the likelihood that someone will become a transgressor by releasing them from the concept of bullying (Enright et al., 2007). Thus, letting go of an attitude is likely to engage in destructive behaviours that can hinder learning and damage social relationships.

Table 4. Implications of forgiveness on psychological health as per previous studies

Author(s)	Areas	Method	Objective(s)/research question(s)/ perspective(s)	Major findings
Lee and Enright (2009)	USA and surrounding countries	Empirical research	How fathers' anger towards their kid and their perception of unfair treatment (PUT) from a member of their family of origin are mediated and moderated by forgiveness?	Forgiveness helps to maintain social and mental wellbeing.
Worthington and Scherer (2004)	USA	Review	Reduction of health risks and promotion of health resilience can be achieved through the emotion-focused coping approach of forgiveness	It indicates a connection between moderating physiological processes and health outcomes through forgiving.
Akhtar and Barlow (2018)	USA	Meta-analysis	Importance of forgiveness therapy to promote psychological health and well-being	Forgiveness therapies may be crucial for enhancing the overall psychological health of people and groups that suffer from a variety of issues.
Enright et al. (2007)	Nothern Ireland and USA	Empirical research	Child-centered peace initiatives are rare and less studied. Student's anger is a significant and growing concern in the school environment. Extreme anger can result in violence among children. Children who grew up in violent and deprived homes displayed statistically considerably more rage.	The forgiveness intervention improved more in forgiveness and decreased clinical despair and anger.
McCullough (2001)	USA	Review	In light of modern trait theory, what are the various attributes that facilitate the process of forgiveness? How forgiveness establishes a more cohesive picture of psychological health?	It seems that a number of psychological mechanisms either promote or prevent forgiveness.
Kravchuk (2021)	Ukraine	Empirical Research	Investigations are conducted into the components of psychological resilience as well as the relationship between the propensity for forgiveness and psychological resilience.	It highlighted the key components of psychological resilience.
Lijo (2018)	India	Review	The study examines issues regarding forgiveness. Outline the challenges faced by the idea of forgiveness to give it a form, make it relevant in context, and identify its allies.	It also has been discovered that self-forgiveness lowers the likelihood of suicidal thoughts and post-traumatic stress disorder.

continued on following page

Table 4. Continued

Author(s)	Areas	Method	Objective(s)/research question(s)/ perspective(s)	Major findings
Sutton (2013)	USA	Review	Enright Developmental model	The model provides direction on how anybody can participate in the basic, psychological process of forgiveness that is shared by all people, regardless of their primary purpose being religious, moral, or psychological.
Freedman (2018)	USA	Empirical Research	Using forgiveness as an education intervention program for at-risk adolescents	Students who react with rage or bitterness are poor learners and score lower GPAs than those who are identified to have low anger.
Griffin et al. (2015)	Review	Review	Detect the association of forgiveness with psychological health	Forgiveness is noticed as coping strategy to increase psychological health.
Bechara et al. (2024)	Colombia	Empirical Research	Role of forgiveness campaign in psychological health	Forgiveness campaign is found effective to increase psychological health.

5. CONCLUSION AND POLICY IMPLICATIONS

The review results suggested that family support is highly effective to reduce stress, anxiety and depression among the youths (Acoba, 2024). Chronic illness patients are noted more susceptible (Reddy, 2019). Diversity in culture has also increased the prevalence of mental disorder (Hwang et al., 2007). Biological factors like gens, molecules also improve psychological health (Andersen et al., 2017). While loss of love and chronic illness are caused to increase depression (Barua et al., 2010). Hence, psychological health has multidimensional aspects which depend on family and social support at individual level (Kawachi & Berkman, 2001; Barua et al., 2010; Reddy 2019; Acoba, 2024). Psychological health of youth is also adversely affected due to love failure and academic stress. Existence of chronic illness also reduces the psychological health and wellbeing of people. Appropriate food availability with proper nutritional contents help to recover the mental stress. While addiction to tobacco and liquor are reducing the psychological health of people. Climate change and natural disasters hamper psychological wellbeing (Padhy et al., 2015; Makwana, 2019; Negi et al., 2025). Moreover, a clean environment and green spaces are supportive to increase psychological health (Belsky & Pluess, 2009; Callaghan et al., 2020; Dzhambov et al., 2019). The results suggested that practices of forgiveness enhance the learning environment which helps to increase psychological wellbeing. Practices of forgiveness will reduce stress and improve interpersonal relationships between people. Moreover, forgiveness develops a greater resilience capacity among the youths to minimize social challenges (Kravchuk, 2021). Forgiveness is also supportive to increase prosocial behaviour, and reduce clinical despair and anger (Enright et al., 2007; García-Vázquez, 2020). Forgiveness is reported as a coping strategy to improve psychological health.

Forgiveness is the attitude or behaviour of an individual to avoid or forget negative aspects during social discussion with other peers, friends, parents, siblings, teachers, seniors and juniors. Thus, practices of forgiveness for an individual are highly essential to improve their psychological health. There must be appropriate family support for youths to increase their psychological health. Youths should have an interpersonal relationship with their friends and relatives. Youths should adopt practices of forgiveness to increase their psychological health. Practices of positive psychology are essential to increase the psychological wellbeing of youth. Interpersonal abilities, social support, and positive behaviour are positively linked with forgiveness, and psychological and mental wellbeing (Temoshok, 2005; Worthington, 2001; Worthington, 2007). Hence, youths must improve interpersonal abilities to move out of the trap of mental disorder, depression, anxiety, and anger. Teachers should create the skills among the students for increasing practices of forgiveness. Forgiveness campaigns are essential to increase psychological health. Forgiveness intervention is also required to increase psychological health. Forgiveness therapies may be crucial for enhancing the overall psychological health of people. Moreover, youths should develop an appropriate social network to increase their psychological health and wellbeing. Appropriate medical facilities are required to enhance psychological wellbeing. Improvement in health literacy would ensure the psychological and mental health of dwellers. Extensive addiction use of technologies is creating mental stress and disorder among the youths. Hence, they should avoid the unnecessary use of digital technologies in their life to avoid mental disorders. Furthermore, youths should give up consumption of tobacco and liquor to improve their psychological health and wellbeing. Youths should take proper sleeping to reduce their psychological and mental health. Youth should adopt forgiveness practices to enhance psychological well being.

6. INNOVATION AND SIGNIFICANCE OF THIS STUDY

This chapter provides the conceptual review on psychological health and wellbeing affecting factors as giving more focus on forgiveness. It explores the significance of forgiveness in learning, psychological health, psychological wellbeing, social-emotional learning and learning potential. Thereupon, it also assesses the role of multiple variables in the areas of social, economic, technological and environmental development for improving psychological health. The findings claimed that forgiveness is helpful to increase learning environment, psychological health and wellbeing, interpersonal relationship, resilience, and prosocial behaviour, and reduce negative behaviour. Therefore, this chapter suggested practical policy implications to increase psychological health. Finally, scope of further studies is also highlighted in this chapter.

7. LIMITATION OF THIS CHAPTER AND SCOPE OF FURTHER RESEARCH

This chapter has novel contributions in the existing literature as it examines the psychological health affecting factors as giving more focus on forgiveness. Despite that, it has several limitations like it is based on review of literature. This chapter does not apply any statistical and empirical investigation for assessing the psychological health affecting factors. Therefore, existing researchers can examine the impact of highlighted variables on psychological health as developing advanced empirical models. Further research can be considered in multiple aspects like impact of forgiveness on social learning of the people. Existing researchers can develop empirical model to examine the impact of social, economic and environmental development associated variables on psychological wellbeing of the people. Psychological health and wellbeing of youth is negatively due to use of digital technologies. Thus, further research is required to minimize the impact of digital technologies on psychological health and wellbeing.

REFERENCES

Acoba, E. F. (2024). Social support and mental health: The mediating role of perceived stress. *Frontiers in Psychology, 15*(1), 1–10. DOI: 10.3389/fpsyg.2024.1330720

Ahirwar, G., Tiwari, G. K., & Rai, P. K. (2019). Exploring the nature, attributes and consequences of forgiveness in children: A qualitative study. *Psychological Thought, 12*(2), 214–231. DOI: 10.5964/psyct.v12i2.347

Akhtar, S., & Barlow, J. (2018). Forgiveness therapy for the promotion of mental well-being: A systematic review and meta-analysis. *Trauma, Violence & Abuse, 19*(1), 107–122. DOI: 10.1177/1524838016637079

Ammerman, R. T., Cassisi, J. E., Hersen, M., & Van Hasselt, V. B. (1986). Consequences of physical abuse and neglect in children. *Clinical Psychology Review, 6*(4), 291–310. DOI: 10.1016/0272-7358(86)90003-6

Andersen, A. M., Pietrzak, R. H., Kranzler, H. R., Ma, L., Zhou, H., Liu, X., Kramer, J., Kuperman, S., Edenberg, H. J., Nurnberger, J. I.Jr, Rice, J. P., Tischfield, J. A., Goate, A., Foroud, T. M., Meyers, J. L., Porjesz, B., Dick, D. M., Hesselbrock, V., Boerwinkle, E., & Han, S. (2017). Polygenic scores for major depressive disorder and risk of alcohol dependence. *JAMA Psychiatry, 74*(11), 1153. DOI: 10.1001/jamapsychiatry.2017.2269

Assary, E., Oginni, O. A., Morneau-Vaillancourt, G., Krebs, G., Peel, A. J., Palaiologou, E., Lockhart, C., Ronald, A., & Eley, T. C. (2024). Genetics of environmental sensitivity and its association with variations in emotional problems, autistic traits, and wellbeing. *Molecular Psychiatry, 29*(8), 2438–2446. DOI: 10.1038/s41380-024-02508-6

Baker, E., Barlow, C. F., Daniel, L., Morey, C., Bentley, R., & Taylor, M. P. (2023). Psychological health impacts of environmental exposures: A scoping review of evaluative instruments. *The Science of the Total Environment, 912*(1), 1–10. DOI: 10.1016/j.scitotenv.2023.169063

Barua, A., Ghosh, M. K., Kar, N., & Basilio, M. A. (2010). Socio-demographic factors of geriatric depression. *Indian Journal of Psychological Medicine, 32*(2), 87–92. DOI: 10.4103/0253-7176.78503

Bechara, A. O., Chen, Z. J., Cowden, R. G.Jr, Worthington, E. L., Toussaint, L., Rodrigquez, N., Murillo, H. G., Ho, M. Y., Mathur, M. B., & VanderWeele, T. J. (2024). Do forgiveness campaign activities improve forgiveness, mental health, and flourishing? *International Journal of Public Health, 69*(1), 1–15. DOI: 10.3389/ijph.2024.1605341

Bedaso, A., Adams, J., Peng, W., & Sibbritt, D. (2021). The relationship between social support and mental health problems during pregnancy: A systematic review and meta-analysis. *Reproductive Health, 18*(1), 1–9. DOI: 10.1186/s12978-021-01209-5

Belsky, J., & Pluess, M. (2009). Beyond diathesis stress: Differential susceptibility to environmental influences. *Psychological Bulletin, 135*(6), 885–908. DOI: 10.1037/a0017376

Berry, J. W., Worthington, E. L.Jr, Parrott, L.III, O'Connor, L. E., & Wade, N. G. (2001b). Transgression narrative test of forgivingness. *Personality and Social Psychology Bulletin, 27*(10), 1277–1290. Advance online publication. DOI: 10.1177/01461672012710004

Brudek, P., Steuden, S., & Kaleta, K. (2023). Wisdom and wellbeing polish older adults: The mediating role of forgiveness. *Frontiers in Psychology, 14*(1), 1–7. DOI: 10.3389/fpsyg.2023.1163113

Buser, M. C., & Scinicariello, F. (2017). Cadmium, lead, and depressive symptoms: Analysis of national health and nutrition examination survey 2011-2012. *The Journal of Clinical Psychiatry, 78*(5), 515–521. DOI: 10.4088/JCP.15m10383

Callaghan, A., McCombe, G., Harrold, A., McMeel, C., Mills, G., Moore-Cherry, N., & Cullen, W. (2020). The impact of green spaces on mental health in urban settings: a scoping review. *Journal of Psychological health, 30*(2), 179–193. DOI: 10.1080/09638237.2020.1755027

Cedillo, Y. E., Kelly, T., Davis, E., Durham, L., Smith, D. L.Jr, Kennedy, R. E., & Fernandez, J. R. (2023). Evaluation of food security status, psychological well-being, and stress on BMI and diet-related behaviors among a sample college students. *Public Health, 224*(1), 32–40. DOI: 10.1016/j.puhe.2023.08.015

Çelik, E., & Ertürk, K. (2022). The effect of forgiveness psychoeducation on forgiveness and life satisfaction in high school students. *Counselling & Psychotherapy Research, 22*(1), 187–196. DOI: 10.1002/capr.12418

Cleverley, K., & Kidd, S. A. (2011). Resilience and suicidality among homeless youth. *Journal of Adolescence, 34*(5), 1049–1054. DOI: 10.1016/j.adolescence.2010.11.003

Coyle, C. T., & Enright, R. D. (1998). Forgiveness education with adult learners. In T. Pourchot, & M. C. Smith (Eds.), *Adult learning and development: Perspectives from Educational Psychology*, 296(1), 1-11. DOI: 10.4324/9781410603418

Degan, T. J., Kelly, P. J., Robinson, L. D., & Deane, F. P. (2018). Health literacy in substance use disorder treatment: A latent profile analysis. *Journal of Substance Abuse Treatment, 96*(1), 46–52. DOI: 10.1016/j.jsat.2018.10.009

Dzhambov, A. M., Hartig, T., Tilov, B., Atanasova, V., Makakova, D. R., & Dimitrova, D. D. (2019). Residential greenspace is associated with mental health via intertwined capacity-building and capacity-restoring pathways. *Environmental Research, 178*(1), 1–13. DOI: 10.1016/j.envres.2019.108708

Enright, R. D., Knutson, J. A., Holter, A. C., Baskin, T., & Knutson, C. (2007). Waging peace through forgiveness in Belfast, Northern Ireland II: Educational programs for mental health improvement of children. *Journal of Research in Education, 17*(1), 63–78.

Enright, R. D.The Human Development Study Group (HDSG). (1994). Piaget on the moral development of forgiveness: Reciprocity or identity? *Human Development, 37*(2), 63–80. DOI: 10.1159/000278239

Epstein, L., Epstein, F., & Kirkilis, R. E. (1998). *Trusting you are loved: Practices for partnerships.* Partnership Foundation.

Fitzgibbons, R. (1998). *Anger and the healing power of forgiveness: A psychiatrist's view. Exploring forgiveness.* University of Wisconsin Press. DOI: 10.2307/jj.36032636.10

Freedman, S. (2007). Forgiveness education with at-risk adolescents: A case study analysis. In Malcom, W., DeCourville, N., & Belicki, K. (Eds.), *Women's reflections on the complexities offorgiveness* (pp. 91–115). Routledge.

Freedman, S. (2018). Forgiveness as an educational goal with at-risk adolescents. *Journal ofMoral Education, 47*(4), 415–431. DOI: 10.1080/03057240.2017.1399869

Freedman, S., & Knupp, A. (2003). The impact of forgiveness on adolescent adjustment to parental divorce. *Journal of Divorce & Remarriage, 39*(1/2), 135–165. DOI: 10.1300/J087v39n01_08

Gable, S. L., & Haidt, J. (2005). What (& why) is positive psychology? *Review of General Psychology, 9*(2), 103-110. . 103DOI: <ALIGNMENT.qj></ALIGNMENT>10.1037/1089-2680.9.2

Gambaro, M. E. (2002). School-based forgiveness education in the management of trait anger in early adolescents. Unpublished doctoral dissertation, University of Wisconsin-Madison.

Gambaro, M. E., Enright, R. D., Baskin, T. A., & Klatt, J. (2008a). Can school-based forgiveness counselling improve conduct and academic achievement in academically at-risk adolescents? *Journal of Research in Education, 18*(1), 16–27.

García-Vázquez, F. I., Valdés-Cuervo, A. A., Martínez-Ferrer, B., & Parra-Pérez, L. G. (2020). Forgiveness, gratitude, happiness, and prosocial bystander behavior in bullying. *Frontiers in Psychology, 10*(1), 28–37. DOI: 10.3389/fpsyg.2019.02827

Gautam, S., Jain, A., Chaudhary, J., Gautam, M., Gaur, M., & Grover, S. (2024). Concept of mental health and mental well-being, it's determinants and coping strategies. *Indian Journal of Psychiatry, 66*(2, Suppl 2), 231–244. DOI: 10.4103/indianjpsychiatry.indianjpsychiatry_707_23

Griffin, B. J., Worthington, E. L., Lavelock, C. R., Wade, N. G., & Hoyt, W. T. (2015). Forgiveness and mental health. In Toussaint, L., Worthington, E., & Williams, D. (Eds.), *Forgiveness and Health*. Springer., DOI: 10.1007/978-94-017-9993-5_6

Gruebner, O., Rapp, M. A., Adli, M., Kluge, U., Galea, S., & Heinz, A. (2017). Cities and Psychological health. *Deutsches Ärzteblatt International, 114*(1), 121–127. DOI: 10.3238/arztebl.2017.0121

Gunjan, G., & Rana, S. S. (2023). Effect of forgiveness on happiness and well-being. *Indian Journal of Positive Psychology, 14*(3), 360–363.

Hunter, A. (2007). Forgiveness: Hindu and western perspectives. *Journal of Hindu-Christian Studies, 20*(1), 11. DOI: 10.7825/2164-6279.1386

Hwang, W., Myers, H., Abekim, J., & Ting, J. (2007). A conceptual paradigm for understanding culture's impact on mental health: The cultural influences on mental health (CIMH) model. *Clinical Psychology Review, 28*(2), 211–227. DOI: 10.1016/j.cpr.2007.05.001

Hyman, S. E. (2000). The genetics of mental illness: Implications for practice. *Bulletin of the World Health Organization, 78*(4), 455–463.

Kagan, J. (1991). Etiologies of adolescents at risk. *The Journal of Adolescent Health, 12*(1), 591–596. DOI: 10.1016/1054-139X(91)90006-J

Kapoor, A. R., Patel, A., & Nair, V. P. (2024). Exploring the neurobiological mechanisms mediating the impact of air pollution on cognitive and emotional health in urban residents of New Delhi. *Studies in Psychological Science, 2*(2), 21–31. DOI: 10.56397/SPS.2024.06.03

Kawachi, I., & Berkman, L. F. (2001). Social Ties and Psychological health. *Journal of Urban Health, 78*(3), 458–467. DOI: 10.1093/jurban/78.3.458

Kendler, K. S., Myers, J. M., Maes, H. H., & Keyes, C. L. M. (2011). The relationship between the genetic and environmental influences on common internalizing psychiatric disorders and mental well-being. *Behavior Genetics*, *41*(5), 641–650. DOI: 10.1007/s10519-011-9466-1

Kim, J., & Kim, H. (2017). Demographic and environmental factors associated with mental health: A cross-sectional study. *International Journal of Environmental Research and Public Health*, *14*(4), 1–12. DOI: 10.3390/ijerph14040431

Kim, J. J., Payne, E. S., & Tracy, E. L. (2022). Indirect effects of forgiveness on psychological health through anger and hope: A parallel mediation analysis. *Journal of Religion and Health*, *61*(5), 3729–3746. DOI: 10.1007/s10943-022-01518-4

Kravchuk, S. (2021). The relationship between psychological resilience and tendency to forgiveness. *Academic Journal of Interdisciplinary Studies*, *10*(1), 11–21. DOI: 10.36941/ajis-2021-0002

Lakhan, S. E., & Vieira, K. F. (2008). Nutritional therapies for mental disorders. *Nutrition Journal*, *7*(2), 1–11. DOI: 10.1186/1475-2891-7-2

Lazarus, R. S., & Folkman, S. (1984). *Stress, Appraisal, and Coping*. Springer.

Lee, M. S., Shin, J. S., Lee, J., Lee, Y. J., Kim, M. R., Park, K. B., Shin, D., Cho, J. H., & Ha, I. H. (2015). The association between mental health, chronic disease and sleep duration in Koreans: A cross-sectional study. *BMC Public Health*, *15*(1), 1–13. DOI: 10.1186/s12889-015-2542-3

Lee, Y. R., & Enright, R. D. (2009). Fathers' forgiveness as a moderator between perceived unfair treatment by a family of origin member and anger with own children. *The Family Journal (Alexandria, Va.)*, *17*(1), 22–31. DOI: 10.1177/1066480708328474

Lijo, K. J. (2018). Forgiveness: Definitions, perspectives, contexts and correlates. *Journal of Psychology & Psychotherapy*, *8*(3), 342–350. DOI: 10.4172/2161-0487.1000342

Lim, S. Y., Kim, E. J., Kim, A., Lee, H. J., Choi, H. J., & Yang, S. J. (2016). Nutritional factors affecting mental health. *Clinical Nutrition Research*, *5*(3), 1–15. DOI: 10.7762/cnr.2016.5.3.143

Loveland, J. M., Lounsbury, J. W., Welsh, D., & Buboltz, W. C. (2007). The validity of physical aggression in predicting adolescent academic performance. *The British Journal of Educational Psychology*, *77*(1), 167–176. DOI: 10.1348/000709905X79563

Makwana, N. (2019). Disaster and its impact on mental health: A narrative review. *Journal of Family Medicine and Primary Care*, *8*(10), 1–9. DOI: 10.4103/jfmpc.jfmpc_893_19

McCullough, M. (2001). Forgiveness: Who does it and how do they do it? *Current Directions in Psychological Science*, *10*(6), 194–197. 194-197.doi.org/10.1111/1467-8721.00147. DOI: 10.1111/1467-8721.00147

McCullough, M. (2008). *Beyond revenge: The evolution of the forgiveness instinct*. John Wiley & Sons.

McCullough, M. E. (2000). Forgiveness as human strength: Theory, measurement, and links to well-being. *Journal of Social and Clinical Psychology*, *19*(1), 43–55. DOI: 10.1521/jscp.2000.19.1.43

Mcloughlin, C. S., Kubick, R. J., & Lewis, M. (2002). Best practices in promoting safe schools. In Thomas, A., & Grimes, J. (Eds.), *Best Practices in School Psychology IV* (pp. 1181–1194). NASP Publications.

Myers, C. A. (2020). Food insecurity and psychological distress: A review of the recent literature. *Current Nutrition Reports*, *9*(2), 107–118. DOI: 10.1007/s13668-020-00309-1

Negi, S., Singh, R., & Singh, A. K. (2025). Natural disaster: prevalence of post - traumatic stress and psychological outcome of Survivors in Joshimath, Uttarakhand, India. In Kurebwa, J., & Makwerere, D. (Eds.), *Managing the Health Risks of Climate Change* (pp. 107–134). IGI Global Scientific Publishing., DOI: 10.4018/979-8-3693-4183-4.ch005

Padhy, S., Sarkar, S., Panigrahi, M., & Paul, S. (2015). Psychological health effects of climate change. *Indian Journal of Occupational and Environmental Medicine*, *19*(1), 3–13. DOI: 10.4103/0019-5278.156997

Pandey, R., Tiwari, G. K., Pandey, R., Mandal, S. P., Mudgal, S., Parihar, P., & Shukla, M. (2020). The relationship between self-esteem and self-forgiveness: *Understanding the mediating role of positive and negative self-compassion*. DOI: 10.22541/au.158981530.01103201

Parihar, P., Tiwari, G. K., & Rai, P. K. (2020). Understanding the relationship between self-compassion and interdependent happiness of the married Hindu couples. *Polish Psychological Bulletin*, *51*(4), 260–272. DOI: 10.24425/ppb.2020.135458

Rao, T. S. (2008). Understanding nutrition, depression and mental illnesses. *Indian Journal of Psychiatry*, *50*(2), 77–88. DOI: 10.4103/0019-5545.42391

Reddy, V. (2019). Psychological health issues and challenges in India: A review. [IJSSME]. *International Journal of Social Sciences Management and Entrepreneurship*, *3*(2), 1–11.

Reed, G., & Enright, R. D. (2006). The effects of forgiveness therapy on depression anxiety, and post-traumatic stress for women after spousal emotional abuse. *Journal of Consulting and Clinical Psychology*, *74*(5), 920–929. DOI: 10.1037/0022-006X.74.5.920

Siste, K., Hanafi, E., Sen, L. T., Murtani, B. J., Christian, H., Limawan, A. P., Siswidiani, L. P., & Adrian, N. (2021). Implications of COVID-19 and lockdown on internet addiction among adolescents: Data from a developing country. *Frontiers in Psychiatry*, *12*(1), 1–13. DOI: 10.3389/fpsyt.2021.665675

Sutton, P. M. (2013). The Enright process model of psychological forgiveness.

Taddi, V. V., Kohli, R. K., & Puri, P. (2024). Perception, use of social media, and its impact on the mental health of Indian adolescents: A qualitative study. *World Journal of Clinical Pediatrics*, *13*(3), 1–9. DOI: 10.5409/wjcp.v13.i3.97501

Tang, Y. Y., Tang, R., & Gross, J. J. (2019). Promoting psychological well-being through an evidence-based mindfulness training program. *Frontiers in Human Neuroscience*, *13*(1), 1–5. DOI: 10.3389/fnhum.2019.00237

Tater, B., & John, K. (2024). Effects of smartphone addiction on the physical and mental well-being of Indian students. *Indian Journal of Science and Technology*, *17*(25), 2622–2634. DOI: 10.17485/IJST/v17i25.1355

Temoshok, L. R. (2005). *Forgiveness and health in persons living with HIV/AIDS. Handbook of Forgiveness*. Routledge.

Thapliyal, C., Singh, R., & Singh, A. K. (2025). Association of forgiveness with learning: for social and psychological wellbeing. In Benoit, S. (Ed.), *Cultivating Flourishing Practices and Environments by Embracing Positive Education* (pp. 335–360). IGI Global Scientific Publishing., DOI: 10.4018/979-8-3693-9466-3.ch011

Tikka, S. K., Garg, S., & Siddiqui, M. A. (2020). Prescribing physical activity in psychological health: A focused review on the latest evidence, recommendations, challenges, and relevance to India. *Indian Journal of Psychological Medicine*, *43*(6), 535–541. DOI: 10.1177/0253717620972330

Tiwari, G. K., Kashyap, A. K., Rai, P. K., Tiwari, R. P., & Pandey, R. (2022). Collective affirmation in action: Understanding the success of lockdown in India during the first wave of the COVID-19 pandemic. *Journal of Research and Health*, *12*(3), 137–150. DOI: 10.32598/JRH.12.3.1992.1

Toussaint, L. L., Worthington, E. L., Williams, D. R., & Webb, J. R. (2020). Forgiveness and physical health. In Worthington, E. L.Jr, & Wade, N. G. (Eds.), *Handbook of Forgiveness* (2nd ed., pp. 178–187).

Tripathi, A., & Mullet, E. (2010). Conceptualizations of forgiveness and forgivingness among Hindus. *The International Journal for the Psychology of Religion, 20*(4), 255–266. DOI: 10.1080/10508619.2010.507694

Van Lange, P. A., Rusbult, C. E., Drigotas, S. M., Arriaga, X. B., Witcher, B. S., & Cox, C. L. (1997). Willingness to sacrifice in close relationships. *Journal of Personality and Social Psychology, 72*(6), 1373–1395. DOI: 10.1037/0022-3514.72.6.1373

Van Oosten, K. (2008). Kamma and forgiveness with some thoughts on Cambodia. *Exchange, 37*(3), 237–262. DOI: 10.1163/157254308X311974

Wind, T. R., Joshi, P. C., Kleber, R. J., & Komproe, I. H. (2013). The impact of recurrent disasters on mental health: A study on seasonal floods in northern India. *Prehospital and Disaster Medicine, 28*(3), 279–285. DOI: 10.1017/S1049023X13000290

Worthington, E.Jr, & Wade, N. (2020). *Handbook of Forgiveness* (2nd ed.). Routledge., DOI: 10.4324/9781351123341

Worthington, E. L. (2001). *Five steps to forgiveness: The art and science of forgiving*. Crown.

Worthington, E. L.Jr., (Ed.). (2007). *Handbook of forgiveness*. Routledge. DOI: 10.4324/9780203955673

Worthington, E. L., Mazzeo, S. E., & Canter, D. E. (2006). Forgiveness-promoting approach: Helping clients REACH forgiveness through using a longer model that teaches reconciliation. In *American Psychological Association eBooks* (pp. 235–257). DOI: 10.1037/10886-010

Worthington, E. L.Jr, & Scherer, M. (2004). Forgiveness is an emotion-focused coping strategy that can reduce health risks and promote health resilience: Theory, review, and hypotheses. *Psychology & Health, 19*(1), 385–405. DOI: 10.1080/0887044042000196674

Worthington, E. L.Jr, & Wade, N. G. (Eds.). (2020). *Handbook of forgiveness* (2nd ed.).

Zakrzewski, V. (2015). Social-emotional learning: why now? Greater Good Magazine. https://greatergood.berkeley.edu/article/item/social_emotional_learning_why_now

KEY TERMS AND DEFINITIONS

Forgiveness Education: It enhances the importance of forgiveness in daily life of learner and people.

Forgiveness: It is a personal ability of a person to avoid the misbehave of someone who wishes to harm you and enhance your anger. It is a process in which an individual person avoids the practices of revenge and bitterness with someone.

Health Literacy: It increases the awareness among the people toward physical and mental illness.

Learning: It is a practice of an individual for adopting or pursuing the behaviours of others in different sectors like, education, discussion, eating, doing something, etc.

Mental Disorder: It is a measurement of mental illness in terms of anxiety, depression, mood, thinking and behaviour capacity of the people.

Positive Psychology: It enhances the positive human thoughts, feeling and behaviour which further improve psychological wellbeing health.

Psychoeducation: Learning program built for special mental health causes to deal with daily stressors and obstacles. It aims to educate about the mental problem, prevention and possible treatment if needed.

Psychological health: It includes a broad range of activities of individuals that make their life easier to maintain peace, social calm and happy and balanced life.

Psychological wellbeing: It avoids all stress, depression, anger, etc. that have adverse impact on social and psychological health of an individual.

Social-emotional Learning (SEL): It creates important attitudes and skills among the people that are required for comprehending and managing their emotions.

Unforgiveness: A person's choice not willing to forgive the offender/ offence/ event, or situation and harbour anger or rage towards the same.

Chapter 3
Balancing Stress Through Emotion Regulation and Coping Strategies

Awesh Khati
http://orcid.org/0009-0009-9090-1593
Lakshmibai National Institute of Physical Education, India

Anindita Das
http://orcid.org/0000-0002-6502-9619
Lakshmibai National Institute of Physical Education, India

Tashi Ongmu Bhutia
http://orcid.org/0009-0000-0127-5709
Sikkim Government B.Ed. College, Soreng, India

Sohom Saha
http://orcid.org/0009-0006-9438-1554
Lakshmibai National Institute of Physical Education, India

ABSTRACT

This chapter explores the complex nature of stress and how important emotion control and coping mechanisms are to preserving both physical and mental equilibrium. Stress is defined as a dynamic interplay between personal evaluation processes and outside pressures that influence emotional and behavioral reactions. The chapter distinguishes between adaptive and maladaptive regulation approaches while examining the biological, cognitive, and environmental systems that underlie stress. The impacts of stress on resilience, performance, and health in the academic, professional, and athletic spheres are mediated by coping and emotional regulation, according to evidence-based discourse. The chapter highlights multimodal thera-

DOI: 10.4018/979-8-3373-6294-6.ch003

pies like mindfulness, cognitive-behavioral therapy, and resilience training while incorporating concepts from behavioral health, psychology, and neuroscience. Future directions highlight how community-based strategies and technology-based solutions can support long-term emotional health and stress resilience in a variety of demographics.

INTRODUCTION

Stress is a complicated phenomenon that is physically grounded and psychologically interpreted. It determines how individuals respond to environmental demands. According to contemporary definitions, stress is the dynamic interaction between an external demand, known as a stressor, and an individual's assessment of and coping strategies in response to that stressor, which culminates in coordinated reactions at the physiological, emotional, cognitive, and behavioral levels (McEwen, 2012). The disciplines of population and health sciences should view stress as a complicated process that encompasses a variety of dimensions rather than as a single entity. These dimensions include the type and timing of stressors, subjective appraisal, and physiological reactivity and recovery, each of which carries different consequences for functioning and health (Epel et al., 2018). Coping strategies and emotion control are two factors that play a significant role in this transactional framework of stress. The term "emotion regulation" refers to the methods that people employ to govern the emotions they experience, the timing of those emotions, and the manner in which they are felt and expressed. From a stress perspective, emotion regulation strategies, such as cognitive reappraisal, attentional deployment, and expressive suppression, influence the perceived consequences of stressors and modify physiological responses (Gross, 2015). Coping involves both emotion-focused and problem-focused strategies for addressing stressors and the emotional repercussions that accompany them. The degree to which the efficacy of these strategies influences exposure to stress results in negative outcomes.

When one takes into consideration the subsequent impacts of stress, it becomes apparent how important it is to regulate one's emotions and to cope. It is an adaptive process for the body to activate the cardiovascular, brain, and metabolic systems in order to take quick action in the face of a threat or challenge, as acute stress reactions do (Godoy et al., 2018). Nevertheless, the continuous activation of stress systems, particularly when recovery is insufficient, results in the accumulation of "wear and tear" on a variety of physiological systems (i.e., allostatic load), which increases the risk of cardiometabolic diseases, immune dysfunction, mood and anxiety disorders, and cognitive decline (Juster & Misiak, 2023). Studies in the field of population science have provided consistent evidence of a correlation between chronic psychosocial stressors, including social adversity and job strain, and mental and physical health outcomes. These studies have demonstrated the importance of understanding and addressing stress and coping mechanisms from a public health perspective (Niedhammer et al., 2021).

Because individuals differ in their emotional control, appraisal, life experience, and social environment, the same exposure to stressors can produce a range of different outcomes for different people. For example, the regular use of adaptive regulation methods such as cognitive reappraisal forecasts resulted in better emotional and physiological outcomes, while the regular use of expressive suppression was generally associated with lower mental health indicators. In the same way, two individuals who are facing similar stressors might display significantly different patterns of adaptation or maladaptation as a result of the influence of socioeconomic resources, social support, health behaviors (such as sleep, diet, and exercise), and early-life experiences, all of which have an impact on baseline regulatory capacity and physiological set points. Two practical implications arise from this integrated approach. In order to accurately quantify stress, a holistic approach must be taken. Epidemiological and clinical research should incorporate exposure indices (chronic strains, life events), subjective assessments (perceived stress scales), and physiological indicators (HPA-axis activity, autonomic indices, composite allostatic load measures), since each one represents a distinct route by which stress is connected to health (Epel et al., 2018). Secondly, interventions can operate on various levels to mitigate stressor exposure (for example, workplace design and social policy), improve coping and emotional regulation (for example, skills training and cognitive therapy), and address physiological dysregulation (for example, exercise, sleep, and pharmacotherapy). A multifaceted approach will likely be necessary in order to reduce the long-term effects of allostasis. The contemporary definitions of stress perceive it as a contextual and temporal process that includes the components of evaluation, control, and physiological response. The mechanisms of emotion regulation and coping have an impact on the transition of stressors into subjective experiences and physiological reactions. The ways in which these processes occur are critical to the comprehension of the influence of stress on health, performance, and well-being. Clinical therapy and public health campaigns need to have a thorough understanding of these mechanisms and the situations that cause them to become maladaptive.

COMPREHENDING STRESS

Biological and Psychological Underpinnings

The central nervous system, the endocrine system, the autonomic system, and the immune system all work together to coordinate stress responses. The hypothalamic-pituitary-adrenal (HPA) axis and the sympathetic-adrenomedullary (SAM) axis are the two primary effector systems. Epinephrine and norepinephrine are two catecholaminergic responses that are rapidly generated by the SAM system, which primes the organism for immediate action. In contrast, glucocorticoids, such as cortisol, are released by the HPA axis with a delay; these glucocorticoids are responsible for metabolic and behavioral adaptations that last for an extended period (Godoy et al., 2018). The brain regions responsible for detecting threats and directing reactions include the amygdala, prefrontal cortex, hippocampus, hypothalamus, and brainstem autonomic nuclei. The interactions between these regions determine the strength, timing, and termination of stress responses (Herman et al., 2020).

Neuroplasticity connects repeated exposure to stress to alterations in brain activity (McEwen, 2012). The hippocampus, prefrontal cortex, and amygdala are the locations where the consistent rise in glucocorticoids and catecholamines causes the reorganization of synapses and circuits to take place. These modifications affect memory, executive control, and the ability to regulate one's emotions. These alterations in the brain explain why the probability that individuals may acquire mood and anxiety disorders, in addition to cognitive impairment, increases when stress is sustained over a long period of time. "Allostatic load" is a term that refers to a complete index of dysregulation that encompasses immunological, cardiometabolic, and neuroendocrine components and has an effect on the risk of stress-related illnesses (Juster & Misiak, 2023). Continuous activation at the systems level is the cause of this effect. According to appraisal theory, stress arises when an individual perceives that the demands of a certain situation outweigh the coping options that are available to them. Cognitive appraisals, which consist of original evaluations of a situation as harmful or demanding as well as subsequent evaluations of possible coping strategies, have a significant impact on emotional and physiological reactions. These assessments, as well as the subsequent physiological responses that ensue, are affected by processes of emotion regulation. Reappraisal, for example, could decrease subjective discomfort and lessen the responsiveness of the hypothalamic-pituitary-adrenal axis in comparison to suppression. Individual differences in emotion regulation, self-efficacy, and prior experiences (which might include early trauma) result in significant heterogeneity in the ways that people react to stress and recover from it.

Categories of Stress: Acute Versus Chronic

An appropriate typology distinguishes between acute stresses that are triggered by events and chronic strains that are persistent, in addition to recognizing everyday irritations and lifetime exposures that accumulate over time. Short-term adaptive reactions include the rapid activation of the sympathetic-adrenal-medullary (SAM) system, a raised heart rate, high blood pressure, and glucose mobilization, which enhance survival and immediate performance. These are the kinds of reactions that acute stresses evoke (Godoy et al., 2018). When correctly managed, acute stress can improve focus and increase the likelihood that memories of critical events will be consolidated. In contrast to acute stress, which is defined as exposure to stressors that is repeated or protracted in duration and is not followed by enough recovery time, chronic stress qualitatively differs because it is associated with continuous or dysregulated physiological activation, a reduction in the diurnal cycles of hormones, a reduction in the amount of recovery time, and an increase in the overall allostatic load. There is a substantial correlation between the increased allostatic load and the elevated risks of cardiovascular disease, metabolic syndrome, depression, and other unfavorable outcomes associated with chronic psychosocial stresses such as caregiving burden, job pressure, and socioeconomic deprivation (Niedhammer et al., 2021). The significance of taking both the chronology and the frequency of an event into consideration when conducting an assessment is emphasized by the fact that empirical research has also revealed intermediate forms of recurring acute stressors whose cumulative impact results in chronic dysregulation (Yuen et al., 2009).

Responses to Stress: Combat, Evasion, and Immobilization

In the face of threats, organisms display a preserved protection cascade that includes both behavioral and autonomic responses. These responses include alertness, active defense (fight or flight), freezing (alert immobility), and other, more severe states of immobility that occur when the threat cannot be avoided (Kozlowska et al., 2015). Every phase has a unique neurological and autonomic profile. Active reactions are characterized by the predominance of the sympathetic nervous system and mobilization, whereas freezing is accompanied by an interplay between the parasympathetic and sympathetic nervous systems, as well as heightened sensory awareness (Herman et al., 2020). These elementary patterns are modified by cognition, appraisal, and previous experiences in humans, which is significant. Psychological factors can prolong maladaptive freeze or tonic immobility patterns or allow rapid disengagement and recovery.

The immediate repercussions are those that have clinical implications. When defensive cascade states are prolonged or are unable to be resolved, such as in the case of posttraumatic stress disorder or sustained high-demand conditions, they result in dysregulation of the autonomic nervous system and the hypothalamic-pituitary-adrenal (HPA) axis. This dysregulation contributes to long-term health difficulties and impedes the ability to regulate emotions and make decisions (McEwen, 2012). Therapeutic techniques that are centered on the control of the defensive cascade (biofeedback, somatic therapies, cognitive reappraisal) strive to reestablish adaptive transitions between states and to promote physiological recuperation.

Integrative Viewpoint and Ramifications for Health and Performance

Integrating biological systems, psychological processes, and contextual exposures is essential to understanding stress. The most reliable inferences pertaining to the relationship between stress and health can be drawn from measurement strategies that incorporate subjective evaluation (perceived stress), behavioral assessments (coping and regulation), and physiological indicators (cortisol, heart rate variability, composite allostatic load indices). Interventions should be multimodal, minimizing exposure when feasible (organizational change, policy), enhancing regulatory capacity (skills training, psychotherapy), and addressing physiological dysregulation (exercise, sleep hygiene, pharmacological treatment) to mitigate cumulative allostatic effects (Juster & Misiak, 2023). When it comes to real-world situations, which range from athletic performance to well-being in the workplace, the most important takeaway is that short, appropriately timed stress can enhance performance, provided that regulation and recovery are maintained. On the other hand, chronic or uncontrolled stress deteriorates performance, health, and well-being as a result of multisystem dysregulation. Consequently, both individual and organizational interventions should place a high priority on encouraging adaptive emotion regulation and ensuring that there are many opportunities for recovery (Gross, 2015).

EMOTION REGULATION AND COPING STRATEGIES

Definition and Theoretical Perspectives

The term "emotion regulation" refers to the methods that individuals employ in order to modify the nature, intensity, and expression of their emotions so that they can accomplish their personal and social objectives. It includes ways to boost, reduce, or maintain emotional states in response to either internal or external stimuli. The emotion regulation process model continues to be a prevailing framework. It consists of five stages: situation selection, situation alteration, attentional deployment, cognitive change, and response modulation. This paradigm concentrates on the temporal aspects of emotion regulation, allowing individuals to intervene at a variety of moments in the process of generating emotions. The extended process model incorporates neurobiological and environmental components, stressing the reciprocal interactions that exist between emotional experiences and emotion regulation (Sheppes et al., 2015). Developmental theories highlight the fact that socialization and cognitive development, especially throughout early infancy and adolescence, play a significant role in the growth of emotion regulation (Compas et al., 2017).

Cognitive, Behavioral, and Physiological Aspects

Emotion regulation functions within the domains of behavioral, cognitive, and physiological processes. Strategies such as reappraisal entail recontextualizing a situation in order to change its emotional impact from a cognitive perspective. For example, a public speaking event could be seen as an opportunity instead of a danger (McRae & Gross, 2020). When they are in the midst of an argument, for example, individuals may use expressive suppression to prevent themselves from becoming overcome with emotion by concealing their feelings of rage (Webb et al., 2012). Mindfulness and controlled breathing are two examples of techniques that can be used to manage emotions, which can have a physiological impact on autonomic responses, such as cortisol levels and heart rate. The domains are all interrelated; for example, cognitive reappraisal can decrease physiological arousal, which in turn can lead to adaptive behavioral responses such as calm communication (Troy et al., 2010).

Adaptive vs. Maladaptive Emotion Regulation

Emotional regulation that is adaptive contributes to improvements in psychological well-being and social functioning, but maladaptive techniques can intensify one's distress. Adaptive techniques, such as mindfulness and reappraisal, have been linked to lower levels of anxiety and depression (Aldao et al., 2010). The ability to maintain composure is encouraged when a failure is reframed as a chance to gain knowledge. Maladaptive behaviors, on the other hand, are associated with psychopathology, particularly mood disorders. Examples of maladaptive behaviors include excessive rumination and repression (Joormann & Stanton, 2016). The act of ruminating, which is defined by the persistence of disagreeable thoughts, exacerbates emotional pain. On the other hand, repression can hinder the development of social interactions by limiting emotional authenticity. The efficacy of a tactic is dependent on the circumstances; in formal situations, suppression may be beneficial, but it may be detrimental to personal connections (Sheppes et al., 2014).

COPING STRATEGIES AND APPROACHES

Problem-Focused vs. Emotion-Focused Coping

Coping involves behavioral and cognitive strategies to deal with pressures that are too great for an individual to manage (Folkman & Moskowitz, 2004). Making a study schedule in order to improve poor academic performance is an example of problem-focused coping, which directly addresses the stressor by taking action, such as solving the problem or acquiring knowledge. When the stressor is something that can be controlled, this method has been proven to be beneficial (Carver & Vargas, 2012). Coping with emotions addresses the feelings that stress provokes in people through the use of tactics that include seeking assistance from friends and family or seeing the problem from a new perspective, such as maintaining a journal to work through loss. Emotion-focused coping is frequently employed in conditions that are beyond the control of the individual, such as dealing with a chronic illness. The two approaches are highly effective when used in conjunction with one another. The degree of effectiveness they demonstrate is contingent on the nature of the stressor as well as the resources that are available to the individual (Compas et al., 2017).

Avoidance, Resilience, and Acceptance-Based Coping

Preventing Avoidance of the stressor is the goal of coping strategies such as distraction or denial; for example, avoiding a challenging conversation. While avoidance may provide short-term respite, it is frequently maladaptive, exacerbating long-term stress and mental health problems (Hofmann et al., 2012). Coping mechanisms, such as positive reframing and social support, which promote adaptation and optimism, can contribute to an increase in resilience, which is the ability to recover from adversity (Southwick & Charney, 2012). Acceptance-based coping, which is based on mindfulness and acceptance and commitment therapy (ACT), consists of the embracement of stress without making urgent efforts to alter it. Emotional suffering can be reduced, and the quality of life can be enhanced by coming to terms with a terminal diagnosis. Long-term well-being is promoted, and psychological flexibility is enhanced by these methods (Kashdan & Rottenberg, 2010).

Cultural and Individual Differences in Coping

Coping strategies differ from one another due to variations in both cultural and individual situations. Emotional restraint is one of many emotion-focused coping methods that people in collectivist cultures, particularly in East Asia, regularly adopt to preserve social peace (Wong et al., 2006). Individualistic cultures, on the other hand, such as those in North America, promote problem-focused coping, which emphasizes autonomy and direct action (Chun et al., 2006). Gender differences are apparent in the coping methods that are utilized by men and women. Women are more likely to utilize emotion-focused coping strategies, such as asking for aid, while males are more likely to choose problem-focused procedures. However, these tendencies are not applicable in all situations. Individuals with personality qualities such as neuroticism and conscientiousness have a significant impact on their coping preferences; those who are more prone to neuroticism tend to choose avoidance, while those who are more conscientious are more likely to favor problem-focused strategies (Carver & Connor-Smith, 2010). Because low resources may necessitate the adoption of emotion-focused tactics, socioeconomic status has an impact on the coping mechanisms that individuals employ (Wadsworth, 2015).

THE INTERPLAY OF STRESS, EMOTION REGULATION, AND COPING

How Stress Influences Emotional Control

Stress has a substantial effect on the regulation of emotions and is described as a perceived threat to a person's well-being that is greater than the resources that are accessible to them. The prefrontal cortex, which regulates executive functions such as emotional regulation, performs less effectively when an individual is experiencing stress due to the heightened activity of the amygdala, which leads to more reactive emotions (McEwen, 2012). When an individual is under a great deal of stress at work, for instance, they may find it difficult to employ cognitive reappraisal, which is a technique that may be used to alter the way stressors are perceived to reduce the emotional effects they have. They may experience increased levels of anger or anxiety as a result of this (Troy et al., 2010). Chronic stress exacerbates inadequacies in emotion regulation by draining cognitive resources, hence increasing the likelihood of maladaptive responses, such as suppression (Sheppes et al., 2014). On the other hand, the ability to skillfully regulate emotions can alleviate stress responses. Mindfulness techniques, for example, decrease the activity of the amygdala, hence improving emotional regulation in situations involving high stress.

Coping as a Mediator of Stress and Outcomes

The relationship between stress and its psychological or behavioral consequences is influenced by the coping mechanisms employed. Planning and looking for solutions are two components of problem-focused coping, which directly tackle stress and are effective when control is attainable, such as when problems at work are handled (Carver & Vargas, 2012). In conditions that are beyond one's control, such as the treatment of a chronic illness, emotion-focused coping, which includes seeking social support or cognitive reframing, is beneficial since it reduces emotional suffering. Adolescents who employed adaptive coping strategies, such as problem-solving, had lower levels of stress-related psychopathology than their peers who employed avoidance tactics. Maladaptive methods, such as avoidance, can intensify stress reactions, hence raising the likelihood of anxiety or depression, and the efficacy of coping techniques is dependent on the nature of the stressor and the resources that are accessible to the individual (Hofmann et al., 2012).

Cyclical Dynamics of Stress and Adaptation

Adaptation is influenced by a cyclical feedback loop that is composed of stress, emotional control, and coping. Coping methods, which are subsequently impacted by future stress experiences, are the mechanisms that individuals employ to navigate the emotional reactions that stress induces. If a person can use reappraisal to see their job loss as an opportunity, this could potentially lower stress and encourage adaptive coping mechanisms, like as networking, which in turn can help lessen misery. Maladaptive cycles arise when inadequate regulation, such as rumination, enhances stress, which in turn leads to avoidance coping and poor adaptability (Joormann & Stanton, 2016). Adaptive cycles gradually improve resilience, but maladaptive cycles increase the likelihood of mental health problems. Longitudinal research has shown that individuals who make use of flexible emotion regulation methods, such as switching between reappraisal and acceptance, have better adaptation to long-lasting stressors (Sheppes et al., 2015). The significance of establishing adaptive coping and control techniques is brought to light by this dynamic interaction.

IMPACT ON MENTAL AND PHYSICAL HEALTH

Stress, Emotion Regulation, and Anxiety/Depression

Particularly in the case of anxiety and depression, stress and emotional control have a substantial impact on mental health. As a result of its ability to intensify negative affect and reduce cognitive flexibility, chronic stress disturbs emotional regulation, which in turn increases the likelihood of mood disorders. There is a greater likelihood that those who rely on bad behaviors, such as ruminating, may experience depression since repeatedly contemplating unpleasant thoughts exacerbates emotional discomfort. On the other hand, methods that are adaptive in nature, such as reappraisal, are linked to a reduction in the symptoms of anxiety and depression (Aldao et al., 2010). In high-stress situations, including public speaking, reappraisal dramatically lowers anxiety, according to a meta-analysis by (Webb et al., 2012). Insufficient emotion regulation affects the relationship between stress and psychopathology. Suppression, for example, increases social anxiety by restricting emotional expression and diminishing interpersonal support.

Physiological Effects: Immunity, Sleep, and Recovery

Emotional and stress management have an impact on physical health, including recuperation, immunity, and sleep. Elevated cortisol levels, which are a result of stress that persists over an extended period of time, reduce the efficiency of the immune system, increasing the likelihood that individuals will fall ill (Segerstrom & Miller, 2004). According to research that was conducted on the effects of meditation treatment, mindfulness, and other emotion regulation techniques can be beneficial in this regard by lowering cortisol levels and strengthening the immune system. Stress can interfere with sleep through the promotion of intrusive thoughts and heightened arousal, resulting in insomnia or poorer overall sleep quality. As opposed to maladaptive strategies, such as rumination, which worsen sleep disruptions, cognitive reappraisal is a beneficial emotion management strategy that enhances sleep quality by decreasing pre-sleep arousal (Palmer & Alfano, 2017). Relaxation strategies assist with physiological recovery, but avoidance hinders recovery, and adaptive coping strategies have an impact on stress recovery (Wadsworth, 2015).

Long-Term Health Consequences

The continued effects of stress and poor emotional regulation can include the development of continuing problems with both mental and physical health. Prolonged stress and the use of poor coping mechanisms, such as suppression or rumination, are associated with an increased likelihood of developing anxiety disorders, depression, and cardiovascular illnesses. A protracted period of suppression is correlated with elevated blood pressure and an increased danger of cardiovascular disease, both of which can be ascribed to continuous physiological processes. The chance of developing diseases associated with aging is increased as a result of the acceleration of cellular aging, which occurs through telomere attrition, which is brought about by chronic stress, which is intensified by inadequate coping mechanisms such as avoidance. On the other hand, resilience is enhanced and the likelihood of developing chronic diseases is decreased by the adoption of adaptive emotion regulation and coping techniques, such as mindfulness and problem-focused methods (Southwick & Charney, 2012). According to longitudinal research, those persons who have high emotional regulation abilities are less likely to develop mental health issues and are more likely to have better physical health outcomes over time (Compas et al., 2017).

APPLICATIONS IN DAILY LIFE AND PERFORMANCE

Academic and Workplace Stress Management

Stress at school and work can harm performance, mental health, and overall health, but there are effective strategies to manage stress and emotions that can be beneficial. Stressors that students are likely to encounter in academic settings include deadlines, examinations, and social commitments. These factors have the potential to cause students to experience anxiety and burnout. When students reframe tests as opportunities for progress, they are utilizing a technique called cognitive reappraisal, which helps to reduce stress and increase academic accomplishment (Troy et al., 2010). By actively addressing stressors, problem-focused coping, which includes activities such as developing study plans and seeking out tutoring, improves performance (Carver & Vargas, 2012). Employees encounter a variety of pressures in the workplace, such as having too much work to complete or getting into arguments with coworkers. Mindfulness and mentorship are two examples of emotion-focused coping techniques that can be helpful in dealing with emotional discomfort. However, tactics that focus on the problem, such as time management and negotiating, might be of assistance in getting more accomplished (Folkman & Moskowitz, 2004). In order to reduce burnout and increase job satisfaction, organizations are starting to adopt stress management programs, such as wellness workshops and flexible work hours, which have proven to be helpful.

Sports and High-Performance Contexts

For athletes and individuals who compete at a high level, stress management is an important skill that can help them improve their performance while they are under pressure. Athletes face substantial demands, including performance expectations and competitive anxiety. Athletes can maintain their focus and reduce their fear with the help of emotion regulation techniques such as self-talk and imagery (Webb et al., 2012). For example, it is possible to improve self-confidence and emotional regulation during important events by imagining a successful performance. In contrast to emotion-focused coping, which uses techniques such as relaxation breathing to mitigate the anxiety that arises before a competition, problem-focused coping tackles stresses that are relevant to performance; this can be accomplished by means such as refining techniques via practice (Southwick & Charney, 2012).

Athletes who utilize adaptive emotion regulation strategies, such as reappraisal, show signs of improved performance and a quicker recovery from failures. An example of an equivalent strategy employed in high-performance environments, such as those in the military or performing arts, is mindfulness training. It has been demonstrated that mindfulness training enhances focus and emotional resilience in stressful situations (Jha et al., 2010).

Stress Management in Social and Interpersonal Settings

Individuals must develop individualized strategies for coping and emotion regulation in response to the unique stressors that social and interpersonal settings present, such as social overload, rejection, or conflicts. The ability to manage one's emotions effectively, such as by employing expressive suppression during formal social interactions, fosters harmony; nevertheless, excessive use of this technique may put relationships in jeopardy by lowering emotional authenticity (English et al., 2012). Interpersonal connections can be improved and stress can be reduced by employing adaptive techniques such as perspective-taking and seeking out social support. For example, having a conversation about an issue with a trustworthy friend is beneficial because it helps to alleviate emotional distress and facilitates resolution. It is possible to actively address interpersonal pressures by employing coping mechanisms such as attentive listening and forceful communication, and to decrease aggravation through acceptance-based ways, such as understanding immutable social dynamics . The strategies that are used are influenced by cultural factors; collectivist societies may place greater importance on repression to maintain social cohesion, while individualistic cultures favor direct problem-solving (Wong et al., 2006).

EVIDENCE-BASED TECHNIQUES FOR STRESS BALANCE

Cognitive-Behavioral Interventions

Cognitive-behavioral interventions (CBIs) are acknowledged for their ability to successfully alleviate stress by targeting maladaptive cognitive processes and behaviors. Patients are able to identify and restructure negative beliefs, such as the belief that failure is a disaster, into more balanced perspectives through the use of cognitive behavioral therapy (CBT), which reduces stress and anxiety. Individuals who engage in cognitive restructuring strategies are taught to challenge erroneous thoughts. In contrast, behavioral activation encourages people to take part in stress-relieving activities, such as exercise or hobbies. According to meta-analyses, cognitive-behavioral treatment (CBT) has been shown to significantly reduce stress-related symptoms such as anxiety and depression in a variety of populations (Hofmann et al., 2012). Stress inoculation training, which is a form of short-term cognitive behavioral therapy, is one example of a CBT-based therapy that might improve coping mechanisms in professional situations by preparing individuals to deal with anticipated stressors.

Mindfulness and Relaxation Techniques

Mindfulness and relaxation methods enhance stress regulation by lowering physiological and emotional arousal. Mindfulness-based stress reduction (MBSR) is an approach that includes exercises such as meditation and body scans, which work to promote awareness and acceptance of sensations in the present moment, hence reducing stress reactivity. Mindfulness-Based Stress Reduction (MBSR) decreases cortisol levels and improves emotional regulation, particularly among high-stress populations like as healthcare professionals. Diaphragmatic breathing and progressive muscle relaxation (PMR) reduce physiological stress responses, such as an elevated heart rate, by activating the parasympathetic nervous system (Gross, 2015). These approaches are easy to access, affordable, and adaptable for daily use, making them highly applicable for stress management in a wide range of situations (Palmer & Alfano, 2017).

Social Support, Resilience Training, and Lifestyle Approaches

It is imperative to employ tactics such as resilience training, lifestyle modifications, and social support in the management of stress. Social support, which includes both emotional forms, such as confiding in friends, and instrumental ones, such as receiving practical aid, reduces stress by creating a sense of comfort and belonging. Resilience training programs, especially those that are based on acceptance and commitment therapy (ACT), teach people to embrace obstacles and focus on value-oriented actions, which increases psychological flexibility. Consistent physical activity, a well-rounded diet, and getting enough sleep are examples of lifestyle strategies that can also mitigate the negative effects of stress. Physical activity reduces cortisol levels and improves mood; sleep, on the other hand, enhances emotional regulation and cognitive function. The combination of these treatments results in the establishment of a holistic paradigm for stress management, and evidence indicates that these treatments have cumulative benefits for both mental and physical health (Southwick & Charney, 2012).

FUTURE DIRECTIONS AND CHALLENGES

Advances in Neuroscience and Emotion Research

The development of therapies that are more focused is being made easier by the advancements in neuroscience that are increasing our understanding of stress and emotional regulation. Neuroimaging research has shed light on the effects of stress on brain regions, including the prefrontal cortex and amygdala, guiding techniques to enhance emotional regulation (McEwen, 2012). It has been demonstrated that real-time neurofeedback, which gives users the ability to control their brain activity, has the potential to improve emotion regulation in anxiety disorders. According to research conducted on neuroplasticity, the application of adaptive techniques, such as reappraisal, on a regular basis strengthens the brain networks associated with resilience (Davidson & McEwen, 2012). Nevertheless, there are still challenges to be faced, such as the translation of neuroscientific findings into practical therapies and the management of individual variances in brain responses to stress (Sheppes et al., 2015).

Role of Technology in Stress and Coping

New, scalable, and easily available techniques for managing stress are being developed through the use of technology. mobile applications providing mindfulness or cognitive-behavioral treatment, such as Headspace or Moodpath, effectively diminish stress and enhance emotional control (Flett et al., 2019) . Wearable devices like smartwatches monitor physiological markers, such as heart rate variability, to provide instant input on stress levels. This allows for the implementation of quick coping strategies. Clinical settings have demonstrated that virtual reality (VR) therapies, which include immersive, relaxing environments, are proving to be effective for stress reduction (Anderson et al., 2017). Ensuring that individuals from all socioeconomic strata have access to technology-based medicines, addressing the privacy concerns that they raise, and proving that these therapies are successful over the long term are all challenges (Torous et al., 2020).

Building Sustainable Resilience in Changing Environments

It is an essential task to establish long-term resilience in ecosystems that are undergoing rapid change as a result of factors such as climate change, technological upheaval, or global health crises. The ability to cope and manage one's emotions flexibly must be developed over a wide range of situations and populations in order to achieve resilience. In particular areas that are marginalized, community-based programs that include resilience training and social support may improve collective coping (Southwick & Charney, 2012). Systemic obstacles, such as limited access to mental health resources and economic inequalities, hamper the development of sustainable resilience. Future projects should focus on scalable interventions, such as online resilience training, and culturally sensitive tactics that take into consideration various coping choices (Wong et al., 2006). The combination of neuroscience, technology, and community-oriented solutions for coping with stress over an extended period of time requires interdisciplinary collaboration in order to address these challenges.

CONCLUSION

When stress, emotion regulation, and coping are examined, it becomes clear that stress is a multifaceted occurrence influenced by external factors, personal evaluation, and physiological responses. When short and effectively managed, acute stress can be beneficial, as it enhances alertness, memory, and performance. In contrast, prolonged stress negatively impacts health due to the buildup of allostatic load, which disrupts both mental and physical systems. Within this process, the regulation of emotion functions as a critical mediator. The use of adaptive strategies, such as cognitive reappraisal and mindfulness, is consistently linked with resilience and positive psychological outcomes, while maladaptive strategies, such as rumination and suppression, are associated with anxiety, depression, and reduced social functioning. Ultimately, the way an individual manages stressors determines their adaptability. When stressors are manageable, problem-focused coping increases control over the situation; when stressors are uncontrollable, emotion-focused coping provides necessary relief. Stress responses are therefore flexible and shaped by regulatory abilities, coping methods, and contextual factors such as culture, personality, and available resources.

These insights have practical applications across educational, occupational, therapeutic, and social domains. In academic settings, reappraisal and problem-solving techniques help reduce performance anxiety and foster resilience. In organizations, structured interventions such as resilience seminars, mindfulness training, and flexible work arrangements decrease burnout and enhance productivity. In athletic and high-performance environments, adaptive regulation strategies such as relaxation, self-talk, and visualization improve focus and assist in recovery from setbacks. Clinical contexts benefit from multimodal approaches: mindfulness-based programs help lower physiological arousal, cognitive-behavioral therapy addresses maladaptive thought patterns, and resilience training builds lasting adaptability. Technological tools such as mobile applications, wearable devices, and virtual reality further expand access to stress management by providing real-time feedback and scalable interventions. Nevertheless, these innovations must remain culturally sensitive and equitable, as accessibility, inclusivity, and relevance across diverse populations remain ongoing challenges. At the societal level, factors such as occupational strain, limited access to mental health resources, and socioeconomic inequality also shape stress outcomes. Policies that support community-based programs, educational initiatives, and workplace reforms can help alleviate chronic stress and strengthen individual coping capacity. For maximum effectiveness, a comprehensive framework for resilience must combine personal skill development with systemic reforms, creating environments that promote adaptive coping.

Although stress cannot be completely eliminated, its consequences can be managed and, in many cases, transformed into opportunities for growth and resilience. When stress is left unchecked, it can be harmful, but when managed effectively, it can serve as a catalyst for personal and collective strength. Those who apply flexible strategies—shifting between reappraisal, acceptance, and problem-solving depending on the situation—demonstrate greater mental well-being, physical recovery, and long-term adaptability. The integration of neuroscience, psychology, and technology is vital to advancing stress management, with innovative approaches such as digital platforms and neurofeedback offering scalable and personalized solutions. At the same time, addressing global challenges such as climate change, economic instability, and public health crises requires multidisciplinary collaboration and culturally informed practices. Coping with stress and regulating emotions is not about eliminating difficulties but about cultivating the ability to face them with clarity, resilience, and purpose. When supported by science, practice, and systemic change, stress can shift from being a pathway to vulnerability into an opportunity for resilience and thriving, ultimately enhancing health, performance, and well-being throughout the lifespan.

REFERENCES

Aldao, A., Nolen-Hoeksema, S., & Schweizer, S. (2010). Emotion-regulation strategies across psychopathology: A meta-analytic review. *Clinical Psychology Review*, *30*(2), 217–237. DOI: 10.1016/j.cpr.2009.11.004 PMID: 20015584

Anderson, A. P., Mayer, M. D., Fellows, A. M., Cowan, D. R., Hegel, M. T., & Buckey, J. C. (2017). Relaxation with Immersive Natural Scenes Presented Using Virtual Reality. *Aerospace Medicine and Human Performance*, *88*(6), 520–526. DOI: 10.3357/AMHP.4747.2017 PMID: 28539139

Carver, C. S., & Connor-Smith, J. (2010). Personality and Coping. *Annual Review of Psychology*, *61*(1), 679–704. DOI: 10.1146/annurev.psych.093008.100352 PMID: 19572784

Carver, C. S., & Vargas, S. (2012). Stress, Coping, and Health. In Friedman, H. S. (Ed.), *The Oxford Handbook of Health Psychology* (1st ed., pp. 163–188). Oxford University Press., DOI: 10.1093/oxfordhb/9780195342819.013.0008

Chun, C.-A., Moos, R. H., & Cronkite, R. C. (2006). Culture: A Fundamental Context for the Stress and Coping Paradigm. In Wong, P. T. P., & Wong, L. C. J. (Eds.), *Handbook of Multicultural Perspectives on Stress and Coping* (pp. 29–53). Springer US., DOI: 10.1007/0-387-26238-5_2

Compas, B. E., Jaser, S. S., Bettis, A. H., Watson, K. H., Gruhn, M. A., Dunbar, J. P., Williams, E., & Thigpen, J. C. (2017). Coping, emotion regulation, and psychopathology in childhood and adolescence: A meta-analysis and narrative review. *Psychological Bulletin*, *143*(9), 939–991. DOI: 10.1037/bul0000110 PMID: 28616996

Davidson, R. J., & McEwen, B. S. (2012). Social influences on neuroplasticity: Stress and interventions to promote well-being. *Nature Neuroscience*, *15*(5), 689–695. DOI: 10.1038/nn.3093 PMID: 22534579

English, T., John, O. P., Srivastava, S., & Gross, J. J. (2012). Emotion regulation and peer-rated social functioning: A 4-year longitudinal study. *Journal of Research in Personality*, *46*(6), 780–784. DOI: 10.1016/j.jrp.2012.09.006 PMID: 23471162

Epel, E. S., Crosswell, A. D., Mayer, S. E., Prather, A. A., Slavich, G. M., Puterman, E., & Mendes, W. B. (2018). More than a feeling: A unified view of stress measurement for population science. *Frontiers in Neuroendocrinology*, *49*, 146–169. DOI: 10.1016/j.yfrne.2018.03.001 PMID: 29551356

Flett, J. A. M., Hayne, H., Riordan, B. C., Thompson, L. M., & Conner, T. S. (2019). Mobile Mindfulness Meditation: A Randomised Controlled Trial of the Effect of Two Popular Apps on Mental Health. *Mindfulness, 10*(5), 863–876. DOI: 10.1007/s12671-018-1050-9

Folkman, S., & Moskowitz, J. T. (2004). Coping: Pitfalls and Promise. *Annual Review of Psychology, 55*(1), 745–774. DOI: 10.1146/annurev.psych.55.090902.141456 PMID: 14744233

Godoy, L. D., Rossignoli, M. T., Delfino-Pereira, P., Garcia-Cairasco, N., & De Lima Umeoka, E. H. (2018). A Comprehensive Overview on Stress Neurobiology: Basic Concepts and Clinical Implications. *Frontiers in Behavioral Neuroscience, 12*, 127. DOI: 10.3389/fnbeh.2018.00127 PMID: 30034327

Gross, J. J. (2015). Emotion Regulation: Current Status and Future Prospects. *Psychological Inquiry, 26*(1), 1–26. DOI: 10.1080/1047840X.2014.940781

Herman, J. P., Nawreen, N., Smail, M. A., & Cotella, E. M. (2020). Brain mechanisms of HPA axis regulation: Neurocircuitry and feedback in context Richard Kvetnansky lecture. *Stress (Amsterdam, Netherlands), 23*(6), 617–632. DOI: 10.1080/10253890.2020.1859475 PMID: 33345670

Hofmann, S. G., Asnaani, A., Vonk, I. J. J., Sawyer, A. T., & Fang, A. (2012). The Efficacy of Cognitive Behavioral Therapy: A Review of Meta-analyses. *Cognitive Therapy and Research, 36*(5), 427–440. DOI: 10.1007/s10608-012-9476-1 PMID: 23459093

Jha, A. P., Stanley, E. A., Kiyonaga, A., Wong, L., & Gelfand, L. (2010). Examining the protective effects of mindfulness training on working memory capacity and affective experience. *Emotion (Washington, D.C.), 10*(1), 54–64. DOI: 10.1037/a0018438 PMID: 20141302

Joormann, J., & Stanton, C. H. (2016). Examining emotion regulation in depression: A review and future directions. *Behaviour Research and Therapy, 86*, 35–49. DOI: 10.1016/j.brat.2016.07.007 PMID: 27492851

Juster, R.-P., & Misiak, B. (2023). Advancing the allostatic load model: From theory to therapy. *Psychoneuroendocrinology, 154*, 106289. DOI: 10.1016/j.psyneuen.2023.106289 PMID: 37202225

Kashdan, T. B., & Rottenberg, J. (2010). Psychological flexibility as a fundamental aspect of health. *Clinical Psychology Review, 30*(7), 865–878. DOI: 10.1016/j.cpr.2010.03.001 PMID: 21151705

Kozlowska, K., Walker, P., McLean, L., & Carrive, P. (2015). Fear and the Defense Cascade: Clinical Implications and Management. *Harvard Review of Psychiatry*, *23*(4), 263–287. DOI: 10.1097/HRP.0000000000000065 PMID: 26062169

McEwen, B. S. (2012). Brain on stress: How the social environment gets under the skin. *Proceedings of the National Academy of Sciences of the United States of America*, *109*(supplement_2), 17180–17185. DOI: 10.1073/pnas.1121254109 PMID: 23045648

McRae, K., & Gross, J. J. (2020). Emotion regulation. *Emotion (Washington, D.C.)*, *20*(1), 1–9. DOI: 10.1037/emo0000703 PMID: 31961170

Niedhammer, I., Bertrais, S., & Witt, K. (2021). Psychosocial work exposures and health outcomes: A meta-review of 72 literature reviews with meta-analysis. *Scandinavian Journal of Work, Environment & Health*, *47*(7), 489–508. DOI: 10.5271/sjweh.3968 PMID: 34042163

Palmer, C. A., & Alfano, C. A. (2017). Sleep and emotion regulation: An organizing, integrative review. *Sleep Medicine Reviews*, *31*, 6–16. DOI: 10.1016/j.smrv.2015.12.006 PMID: 26899742

Segerstrom, S. C., & Miller, G. E. (2004). Psychological Stress and the Human Immune System: A Meta-Analytic Study of 30 Years of Inquiry. *Psychological Bulletin*, *130*(4), 601–630. DOI: 10.1037/0033-2909.130.4.601 PMID: 15250815

Sheppes, G., Scheibe, S., Suri, G., Radu, P., Blechert, J., & Gross, J. J. (2014). Emotion regulation choice: A conceptual framework and supporting evidence. *Journal of Experimental Psychology. General*, *143*(1), 163–181. DOI: 10.1037/a0030831 PMID: 23163767

Sheppes, G., Suri, G., & Gross, J. J. (2015). Emotion Regulation and Psychopathology. *Annual Review of Clinical Psychology*, *11*(1), 379–405. DOI: 10.1146/annurev-clinpsy-032814-112739 PMID: 25581242

Southwick, S. M., & Charney, D. S. (2012). The Science of Resilience: Implications for the Prevention and Treatment of Depression. *Science*, *338*(6103), 79–82. DOI: 10.1126/science.1222942 PMID: 23042887

Torous, J., Jän Myrick, K., Rauseo-Ricupero, N., & Firth, J. (2020). Digital Mental Health and COVID-19: Using Technology Today to Accelerate the Curve on Access and Quality Tomorrow. *JMIR Mental Health*, *7*(3), e18848. DOI: 10.2196/18848 PMID: 32213476

Troy, A. S., Wilhelm, F. H., Shallcross, A. J., & Mauss, I. B. (2010). Seeing the silver lining: Cognitive reappraisal ability moderates the relationship between stress and depressive symptoms. *Emotion (Washington, D.C.)*, *10*(6), 783–795. DOI: 10.1037/a0020262 PMID: 21058843

Wadsworth, M. E. (2015). Development of Maladaptive Coping: A Functional Adaptation to Chronic, Uncontrollable Stress. *Child Development Perspectives*, *9*(2), 96–100. DOI: 10.1111/cdep.12112 PMID: 26019717

Webb, T. L., Miles, E., & Sheeran, P. (2012). Dealing with feeling: A meta-analysis of the effectiveness of strategies derived from the process model of emotion regulation. *Psychological Bulletin*, *138*(4), 775–808. DOI: 10.1037/a0027600 PMID: 22582737

Wong, P. T. P., Wong, L. C. J., & Scott, C. (2006). Beyond Stress and Coping: The Positive Psychology of Transformation. In Wong, P. T. P., & Wong, L. C. J. (Eds.), *Handbook of Multicultural Perspectives on Stress and Coping* (pp. 1–26). Springer US., DOI: 10.1007/0-387-26238-5_1

Yuen, E. Y., Liu, W., Karatsoreos, I. N., Feng, J., McEwen, B. S., & Yan, Z. (2009). Acute stress enhances glutamatergic transmission in prefrontal cortex and facilitates working memory. *Proceedings of the National Academy of Sciences of the United States of America*, *106*(33), 14075–14079. DOI: 10.1073/pnas.0906791106 PMID: 19666502

Chapter 4
Resilience of Parents Raising Children With Intellectual Disabilities

Dimitra V. Katsarou
http://orcid.org/0000-0001-8690-0314
University of the Aegean, Greece

Maria Sofologi
http://orcid.org/0000-0003-0380-2220
University of Ioannina, Greece

Evangelos Mantsos
http://orcid.org/0009-0002-8490-2660
University of Western Macedonia, Greece

Georgios A. Kougioumtzis
http://orcid.org/0000-0002-2362-2094
National and Kapodistrian University of Athens, Greece

Efthymia Efthymiou
http://orcid.org/0000-0003-0411-1720
Zayed University, UAE

Asterios Patsiaouras
http://orcid.org/0009-0005-3398-2885
University of Thessaly, Greece

ABSTRACT

This chapter explores the dynamic process of resilience among parents raising children with intellectual disabilities (ID), emphasizing the interplay between stress, adaptation, and growth. It examines how chronic caregiving demands, systemic barriers, and social stigma affect parental well-being, while highlighting the coping mechanisms—problem-focused, emotion-focused, and meaning-focused—that sustain psychological balance. Integrating ecological and family resilience frameworks, the chapter identifies key protective factors such as parental self-efficacy, social support, optimism, family cohesion, and cultural or spiritual beliefs. It argues that resilience is a relational and systemic process fostered through supportive family dynamics, inclusive policies, and community engagement. Ultimately, the chapter

DOI: 10.4018/979-8-3373-6294-6.ch004

reframes parental resilience as both a personal strength and a societal responsibility, essential for promoting well-being and inclusion in families of children with intellectual disabilities.

INTRODUCTION

Raising a child with an intellectual disability (ID) presents a complex and emotionally layered experience that reshapes the lives of parents and families. Parents often encounter significant caregiving demands, chronic uncertainty about their child's development, and an ongoing need to navigate health, education, and social service systems. These challenges can create substantial psychological and emotional strain, sometimes leading to elevated levels of stress, anxiety, and even depression compared to parents of typically developing children (Hastings & Taunt, 2002; Lloyd & Hastings, 2008).

Despite these pressures, a substantial body of research underscores the capacity of many parents to adapt, recover, and even grow through adversity. This adaptive capacity, broadly termed resilience, refers to the dynamic process by which individuals maintain or regain psychological well-being in the face of chronic stressors or trauma (Masten, 2014; Rutter, 2012). In the context of parenting a child with ID, resilience is not a denial of difficulty but an acknowledgment that strength and struggle often coexist. Parents who exhibit resilience demonstrate psychological flexibility, effective coping strategies, and a capacity to find meaning within their caregiving experiences.

This chapter explores resilience as it pertains to parents of children with intellectual disabilities. It examines the multifaceted nature of parental stress, the mechanisms that foster positive adaptation, and the protective factors that buffer against psychological strain. It also reviews theoretical developments that have shaped the study of resilience, from ecological and systems-based frameworks to contemporary models of family resilience (Katsarou et al., 2024; Katsarou et al., 2025a, b). The aim is to provide a comprehensive understanding of how parents navigate the demands of caregiving while maintaining emotional well-being and fostering family stability.

CONCEPTUALIZING RESILIENCE

Resilience has evolved from a static personality trait to a dynamic, process-oriented construct. Early conceptualizations viewed resilience as a fixed quality that some individuals possessed inherently, distinguishing the "hardy" from the "vulnerable." However, contemporary theories position resilience as a fluid process of adaptation that unfolds over time and across contexts (Masten, 2018). This shift emphasizes interactional factors—how individuals mobilize personal, social, and environmental resources to manage adversity.

In the case of parents of children with intellectual disabilities, resilience emerges through continuous cycles of adjustment and redefinition. Parents often describe a trajectory that includes initial distress, gradual acceptance, and eventual transformation of meaning. This process aligns with Walsh's (2016) Family Resilience Framework, which defines resilience as a relational process encompassing belief systems, organizational patterns, and communication practices that foster adaptation and growth within families facing challenges.

Furthermore, resilience in this context must be understood within the broader ecological systems that influence parental experience. Bronfenbrenner's (1979) ecological systems theory remains a valuable lens for understanding how individual and family resilience interacts with mesosystemic (e.g., schools, healthcare), exosystemic (e.g., community resources), and macrosystemic (e.g., cultural attitudes and policies) factors. For instance, supportive community networks or inclusive education policies can enhance resilience by reducing external stressors and promoting empowerment.

Resilience, therefore, is best conceptualized not as an endpoint but as an ongoing adaptive process that allows parents to manage stress while maintaining emotional stability and nurturing relationships within the family system.

PARENTING STRESS IN THE CONTEXT OF INTELLECTUAL DISABILITY

Parents of children with intellectual disabilities experience unique and enduring stressors that can influence their emotional and physical well-being. These stressors stem from multiple sources: the child's behavioral and developmental needs, the demands of navigating healthcare and education systems, and the social stigma often associated with disability. Research consistently shows that behavioral and emotional challenges in children with ID are among the strongest predictors of parental stress (Totsika et al., 2011).

Beyond behavioral issues, parents frequently confront systemic barriers such as limited access to specialized services, financial strain, and societal misconceptions about disability. These external pressures can lead to chronic stress, defined as persistent physiological and psychological tension resulting from long-term caregiving demands. Chronic stress not only impacts mental health but can also affect physical health outcomes, including fatigue, sleep disturbances, and immune system dysfunction (Emerson et al., 2010).

Emotional stress is compounded by anticipatory grief—a recurrent sense of loss or uncertainty about the child's future functioning, independence, or social inclusion. While some parents report feelings of helplessness or guilt, others describe a process of meaning reconstruction that helps them reconcile expectations with reality. This adaptation process aligns with the theory of chronic sorrow (Olshansky, 1962), which posits that parents of children with disabilities may experience intermittent waves of grief throughout the child's life, interspersed with periods of acceptance and stability. Importantly, not all stress results in negative outcomes. For many parents, the experience of raising a child with ID fosters increased emotional depth, empathy, and patience—qualities that contribute to what researchers term post-traumatic growth (Tedeschi & Calhoun, 2004). These dual outcomes highlight that stress and growth can coexist, forming part of the same adaptive continuum rather than being mutually exclusive.

COPING MECHANISMS AND ADAPTIVE STRATEGIES

Coping mechanisms are central to understanding how parents manage the demands associated with raising a child with intellectual disabilities. Coping refers to the cognitive and behavioral efforts individuals employ to handle internal and external stressors that exceed their perceived resources (Lazarus & Folkman, 1984). In this context, parents draw upon a wide range of strategies to regulate their emotions, maintain family stability, and preserve psychological well-being.

Research commonly distinguishes among three major coping styles: problem-focused coping, emotion-focused coping, and meaning-focused coping. Coping mechanisms are central to understanding how parents of children with intellectual disabilities (ID) navigate the ongoing demands of caregiving. Coping refers to the dynamic cognitive and behavioral efforts that individuals employ to manage internal and external stressors perceived as exceeding their resources (Lazarus & Folkman, 1984). For parents in this context, coping is not a one-time reaction but an ongoing process of adjustment, reappraisal, and adaptation across the life course of their child. Scholars have identified several coping styles that influence resilience outcomes, including problem-focused, emotion-focused, and meaning-focused strategies.

Problem-Focused Coping

Problem-focused coping involves practical, goal-oriented strategies aimed at altering or managing the stressor itself. For parents of children with ID, this often entails seeking information, consulting professionals, engaging with advocacy networks, and securing necessary educational or healthcare services (Hastings et al., 2005). It may also include active problem-solving within the home environment—developing behavior management routines, implementing structured learning systems, or coordinating multidisciplinary care.

Parents who adopt problem-focused approaches tend to experience a greater sense of mastery and control, as they perceive themselves as active agents rather than passive recipients of circumstance. This sense of control directly contributes to psychological resilience, as perceived competence mediates the impact of chronic stress on emotional well-being (Bandura, 1997). Moreover, problem-focused coping encourages engagement with systems of support, such as teachers, therapists, and community programs, which strengthens social capital and resource access. However, problem-focused coping is most effective when stressors are modifiable. In situations where challenges are uncontrollable—such as the permanence of a diagnosis—overreliance on this strategy can lead to frustration or burnout. Therefore, successful parents often complement it with emotion- and meaning-focused coping, demonstrating cognitive flexibility and adaptive balance.

Emotion-Focused Coping

While problem-focused strategies address external demands, emotion-focused coping targets the internal emotional responses to stress. This form of coping includes behaviors and cognitive processes aimed at regulating distress, maintaining emotional stability, and preserving psychological equilibrium (Folkman & Moskowitz, 2000). Common techniques include acceptance, cognitive reframing, and emotional expression. Acceptance, in particular, plays a transformative role for parents of children with intellectual disabilities. It involves acknowledging the enduring nature of caregiving challenges while redirecting emotional energy from resistance to adaptation. Acceptance does not imply resignation but reflects a mindful recognition of reality that enables constructive engagement with it (Jones & Passey, 2004).

Reframing, another vital element, allows parents to reinterpret challenging experiences in a more positive or manageable light—for instance, perceiving their child's differences as opportunities for learning rather than as limitations. Emotional expression, through talking, journaling, or participating in support groups, also serves to release tension and validate emotional experiences. Emotion-focused coping has been linked to reductions in anxiety and depression, and to improvements in marital satisfaction and parental confidence (Lickenbrock et al., 2011). Importantly, effective emotion regulation allows parents to maintain consistent caregiving behaviors even during periods of heightened stress. Yet, emotion-focused coping alone is insufficient if it becomes avoidance-based (e.g., denial or suppression). Optimal resilience arises when emotional regulation coexists with active engagement in problem-solving and meaning construction.

Meaning-Focused Coping

Meaning-focused coping refers to the cognitive processes through which individuals find purpose, coherence, or positive significance in adverse experiences. For parents of children with ID, meaning-making often entails viewing caregiving not solely as a burden but as a profound opportunity for personal and spiritual growth.

This form of coping aligns closely with the positive psychology movement, which emphasizes hope, gratitude, and optimism as key mechanisms for resilience (Seligman, 2011). Many parents describe caregiving as a transformative journey that fosters deeper empathy, patience, and appreciation for small milestones. They may attribute meaning through spiritual frameworks ("this experience has deepened my faith"), moral narratives ("I have learned compassion and strength"), or relational connections ("my family has become closer through this experience").

Research on post-traumatic growth supports these narratives, suggesting that positive reinterpretation of adversity can lead to enhanced well-being and life satisfaction (Tedeschi & Calhoun, 2004). Meaning-focused coping enables parents to construct a coherent life story that integrates the challenges of disability into a broader identity of resilience, rather than fragmentation or despair. Practitioners can foster meaning-making by encouraging reflective dialogue, mindfulness, or narrative expression—approaches that help parents articulate purpose and derive strength from their lived experiences.

Flexibility and Integration in Coping

A key insight from resilience research is that no single coping strategy guarantees positive outcomes. Instead, coping flexibility—the capacity to modify coping strategies in response to situational demands—emerges as the most powerful predictor of sustained resilience (Bonanno, 2004). Resilient parents fluidly shift between problem-solving, emotion regulation, and meaning-making depending on context and stressor controllability.

For instance, during acute crises (e.g., a medical emergency), problem-focused action may dominate. In chronic, uncontrollable circumstances (e.g., navigating lifelong dependency), emotion- or meaning-focused coping may take precedence. This adaptive oscillation prevents emotional exhaustion and fosters balance. Moreover, cultural and contextual factors shape how coping strategies are enacted. In collectivist societies, for example, emotion-focused coping may involve communal sharing and spiritual rituals, while in individualistic cultures, problem-solving may center on advocacy and self-determination. Social support availability, parental temperament, and family cohesion also mediate coping effectiveness (McConnell & Savage, 2015). Ultimately, resilient parents exhibit a dynamic integration of coping approaches—engaging both mind and heart, cognition and emotion—to sustain well-being and nurture their children with compassion and competence.

PROTECTIVE FACTORS PROMOTING PARENTAL RESILIENCE

Protective factors are the psychological, relational, and contextual resources that buffer parents against the adverse effects of chronic stress and facilitate adaptation. They do not eliminate stressors but moderate their impact, allowing parents to maintain emotional equilibrium and positive functioning despite adversity. In the context of raising a child with intellectual disabilities (ID), protective factors operate across multiple ecological levels—individual, familial, and societal—and interact dynamically to support long-term resilience (Masten, 2018). These factors often act synergistically, meaning that the presence of one (e.g., social support) amplifies the benefits of others (e.g., parental self-efficacy or optimism).

Parental Self-Efficacy

One of the most consistently identified protective factors is parental self-efficacy—a parent's belief in their competence to influence their child's development, manage behaviors, and meet caregiving demands effectively. Rooted in Bandura's (1997) theory of self-efficacy, this construct emphasizes the role of perceived control in human motivation and resilience. Parents with high self-efficacy are more likely to engage in problem-solving, seek appropriate interventions, and maintain constructive partnerships with professionals (Hastings & Brown, 2002).

Empirical evidence shows that self-efficacy moderates the relationship between caregiving stress and psychological well-being. Parents who perceive themselves as capable report lower anxiety and depression levels, even when facing high caregiving demands (Gupta & Singhal, 2005). Moreover, self-efficacy promotes persistence and adaptability, enabling parents to remain engaged and optimistic when confronting challenges such as behavioral difficulties or service barriers.

Interventions designed to strengthen self-efficacy—such as parent training programs, coaching models, and peer mentoring—have demonstrated measurable benefits in reducing stress and improving family functioning. These programs work by offering knowledge, reinforcing mastery experiences, and reframing failures as opportunities for learning. Ultimately, self-efficacy not only enhances individual coping capacity but also acts as a catalyst for resilience across the family system.

Social Support

Social support represents one of the most powerful external buffers against the psychological strain of caregiving. It encompasses emotional, informational, and instrumental assistance provided by spouses, relatives, friends, professionals, and community organizations (Thoits, 2011). For parents of children with ID, social support mitigates isolation, enhances self-esteem, and provides both tangible help (e.g., childcare, financial aid) and intangible comfort (e.g., empathy, understanding).

Studies consistently show that perceived social support moderates the relationship between caregiving burden and psychological distress (Smith et al., 2013). Supportive networks function as a "stress filter," helping parents reappraise stressful situations as more manageable. Peer groups composed of parents in similar situations are especially valuable, as they offer validation, shared understanding, and collective problem-solving opportunities (Solomon et al., 2001).

At the community level, inclusive networks such as parent associations and disability advocacy groups serve dual roles: they provide immediate emotional support and promote systemic change by advocating for policy improvements. The availability of such networks is, however, shaped by socioeconomic and cultural contexts—families in rural or under-resourced regions may face reduced access to these supports (Hartley et al., 2012). Thus, fostering social support is both an individual and structural responsibility. When families are embedded in strong relational networks, they are less vulnerable to stress and more capable of sustaining adaptive functioning.

Optimism and Hope

Optimism and hope serve as essential cognitive-emotional resources that promote resilience by shaping how parents interpret and respond to challenges. Optimism involves a general expectation that positive outcomes are possible, while hope represents a future-oriented belief that one's actions can influence desired results (Snyder, 2002).

Parents who maintain an optimistic mindset tend to use adaptive coping strategies, focus on achievable goals, and demonstrate greater emotional regulation under pressure. Research has shown that optimism predicts lower stress levels and higher life satisfaction among parents of children with developmental disabilities (Bayat, 2007). Hope, as a motivational construct, sustains parents through uncertainty and setbacks. It provides psychological energy to persist in the face of barriers—whether navigating bureaucratic systems or supporting a child's slow developmental progress. Hope also enhances meaning-making, allowing parents to perceive caregiving not merely as hardship but as a meaningful, purpose-driven endeavor. Practitioners can nurture optimism and hope by highlighting progress (however small), facilitating goal-setting, and reinforcing the parent's role as an active agent in the child's growth. Optimism and hope thus serve as emotional anchors that sustain motivation and protect against despair in the long trajectory of caregiving.

Family Cohesion and Adaptability

At the family level, cohesion (emotional bonding among members) and adaptability (the ability to adjust roles and routines in response to changing demands) are vital protective factors. Families characterized by open communication, emotional warmth, and cooperative problem-solving are more resilient to stress (Walsh, 2016).

Partner support plays a particularly critical role. Studies have shown that couples who share caregiving responsibilities equitably and maintain emotional intimacy experience lower levels of stress and marital conflict (Lickenbrock et al., 2011). Conversely, when caregiving burdens are unequally distributed or communication breaks down, both partners are at risk of emotional fatigue and relationship strain. Adaptive families often demonstrate flexibility in redefining expectations and roles—for example, adjusting work schedules or modifying family activities to accommodate the child's needs. This adaptability prevents role overload and maintains family harmony. Moreover, sibling involvement can foster empathy and collective identity, further strengthening the family's resilience.

Interventions that target family cohesion—such as family systems therapy or psychoeducation—help enhance communication and joint problem-solving. When family members operate as a coordinated, supportive unit, they create a stable emotional environment that supports both the child's development and the parents' mental health.

Cultural and Spiritual Beliefs

Cultural and spiritual frameworks profoundly influence how parents interpret disability and construct resilience. In many cultures, spirituality offers a source of comfort, meaning, and acceptance. Religious faith can help parents contextualize their experiences within a broader moral or existential narrative, transforming suffering into purpose (Skinner et al., 2001).

Spiritual practices such as prayer, meditation, or communal worship provide not only emotional solace but also opportunities for social connection and ritualized expression of hope. For instance, in some communities, religious institutions serve as informal support networks, offering both guidance and practical assistance. Cultural context also determines societal attitudes toward disability. In collectivist societies, caregiving is often distributed across extended families and community members, reducing the burden on individual parents. Communal child-rearing practices, characteristic of many non-Western cultures, act as natural resilience enhancers by embedding families in networks of reciprocal care (McCabe, 2007).

However, cultural beliefs can also present barriers if disability is stigmatized or attributed to supernatural causes. In such cases, parental resilience depends on reconciling personal beliefs with external judgment and finding empowerment through advocacy and community education. Recognizing and respecting cultural and spiritual diversity is therefore essential for practitioners aiming to support parental resilience. Incorporating culturally sensitive practices strengthens trust and ensures interventions are meaningful within the family's worldview.

An Ecological View of Resilience

Ultimately, resilience emerges through the interplay of protective factors across multiple ecological levels. Individual traits such as self-efficacy and optimism interact with relational factors like family cohesion and social support, all within broader societal and cultural frameworks. This aligns with Bronfenbrenner's ecological systems theory (1979), which conceptualizes resilience as a multi-layered process influenced by micro- (family), meso- (community), and macro- (cultural and policy) systems. When these protective systems align harmoniously—when families are embedded in supportive networks, guided by hopeful belief systems, and empowered through inclusive policies—parents are most likely to adapt positively and sustain well-being across the lifespan of caregiving.

THEORETICAL MODELS OF FAMILY RESILIENCE

A range of theoretical frameworks has been developed to explain how families adapt to adversity. These models underscore the relational and systemic dimensions of resilience.

Bronfenbrenner's ecological systems theory (1979) provides a foundational framework for understanding how resilience operates within interrelated environmental systems. According to this model, parental resilience is shaped not only by personal coping capacities but also by interactions across the child's immediate environment (microsystem), the relationships between these settings (mesosystem), the broader social and institutional context (exosystem), and overarching cultural norms and policies (macrosystem). For example, inclusive educational environments and disability-supportive policies can strengthen resilience by reducing external stressors and promoting empowerment.

Building upon ecological principles, Walsh's Family Resilience Framework (2016) identifies three core domains that enable families to adapt to crisis and prolonged stress: belief systems, organizational patterns, and communication processes. Belief systems influence how families make meaning of adversity, whether through faith, shared values, or collective optimism. Organizational patterns refer to family flexibility, connectedness, and access to social and economic resources. Communication processes involve clarity, emotional sharing, and collaborative problem-solving. When these domains function cohesively, families are better able to recover and even grow through adversity.

The positive psychology perspective complements these systemic models by focusing on the strengths and virtues that allow individuals to thrive. It shifts the narrative from "coping with deficits" to "building strengths." Concepts such as optimism, gratitude, and meaning-making are not viewed as denial mechanisms but as active processes that enhance well-being and foster psychological endurance (Seligman, 2011). Lastly, resilience-as-process models (Masten, 2018) emphasize that adaptation unfolds over time. Rather than a single recovery event, resilience represents an ongoing negotiation between risk and protective influences. This temporal understanding aligns with the lived experiences of parents who describe their journey as one of continual adjustment, learning, and redefinition.

Cultural and Contextual Considerations

Resilience among parents of children with intellectual disabilities cannot be fully understood without considering cultural and contextual influences. Culture shapes beliefs about disability, caregiving roles, and acceptable coping practices. In many Western societies, the emphasis on individualism and autonomy can place additional pressure on parents to act as primary advocates and self-sufficient caregivers. Conversely, in collectivist cultures, caregiving responsibilities are often shared among extended family members, which can mitigate stress and promote resilience through communal support (McCabe, 2007).

Cultural frameworks also influence how disability is interpreted—either as a source of stigma or as a variation of human diversity. In societies where disability is heavily stigmatized, parents may experience social exclusion, which erodes social support and increases psychological burden (Shin et al., 2006). However, in communities where disability is viewed through a spiritual or moral lens—such as "a test of faith" or "a gift from God"—parents often report higher levels of acceptance and hope (Gona et al., 2016). These interpretations can serve as meaning-making mechanisms that support resilience, even amid structural disadvantage.

Socioeconomic context further moderates resilience outcomes. Families in low-resource environments often face compounded stressors such as limited access to healthcare, educational support, and respite services. Yet, research shows that even in the absence of extensive formal resources, informal community networks, mutual aid groups, and faith-based organizations can play a crucial role in sustaining parental resilience (Hartley et al., 2012).

Policy and societal attitudes also matter. Countries that invest in inclusive education, disability rights legislation, and family support services create environments that foster resilience not only at the individual level but also at the systemic level. These supportive ecosystems illustrate that resilience is not merely a personal characteristic—it is an outcome of social justice, equitable access, and inclusive policy frameworks.

PRACTICAL IMPLICATIONS FOR SUPPORTING PARENTAL RESILIENCE

The insights from resilience research have significant implications for practitioners, policymakers, and service providers working with families of children with intellectual disabilities.

Promoting Family-Centered Services

Professionals who work with families of children with intellectual disabilities must embrace a family-centered philosophy of care—one that recognizes parents not merely as recipients of professional expertise but as collaborative partners in the therapeutic and educational process. Family-centered services are grounded in principles of respect, empowerment, and individualized care. They acknowledge that parents possess unique, experiential knowledge of their child's needs, strengths, and preferences (Dunst, Trivette, & Deal, 2007).

A holistic approach entails tailoring interventions to the family's values, culture, and circumstances rather than imposing standardized models. This may involve joint goal-setting, regular feedback, and shared decision-making between professionals and families. Family-centered approaches also prioritize strengths-based assessment, focusing on family resources and competencies rather than deficits.

Empirical evidence shows that when parents feel respected and actively involved in intervention planning, they exhibit greater satisfaction, lower stress, and improved adherence to therapeutic recommendations. Professionals, in turn, benefit from enhanced trust and more accurate insights into the child's day-to-day functioning. Ultimately, the family-centered model redefines professional practice—from "doing for" families to "working with" them.

Facilitating Social Support Networks

Social support represents a cornerstone of parental resilience. Many parents of children with intellectual disabilities report experiencing isolation due to societal stigma, caregiving demands, or limited access to understanding peers. Structured support networks—whether community-based, virtual, or peer-led—offer vital emotional and practical resources.

Programs that foster peer-to-peer connection allow parents to share experiences, exchange coping strategies, and validate one another's emotional struggles. Research has demonstrated that these networks reduce perceived isolation, enhance problem-solving confidence, and contribute to positive mental health outcomes (Smith et al., 2013). In addition to informal peer groups, professional and community organizations play an important role in facilitating connections between families and relevant services. Schools, early intervention centers, and disability advocacy groups can serve as bridging institutions, linking parents to mental health resources, respite services, and financial assistance programs. Beyond practical benefits, social support networks foster a collective sense of identity among parents. They transform individual struggles into shared resilience, allowing families to feel seen, supported, and valued within their communities.

Strengthening Parental Self-Efficacy

Parental self-efficacy—the belief in one's capacity to effectively manage caregiving challenges—is a powerful predictor of adaptive coping and psychological well-being. Parents who perceive themselves as competent are more likely to engage in proactive problem-solving, seek information, and maintain hope during stressful periods (Hastings & Brown, 2002).

Interventions aimed at enhancing self-efficacy should focus on skill-building, mastery experiences, and cognitive restructuring. Structured training programs that teach parents behavior management, communication strategies, and advocacy skills can empower them to navigate complex systems confidently. Psychoeducational workshops also provide parents with evidence-based information about their child's condition, reducing uncertainty and enhancing their sense of control.

Cognitive-behavioral approaches (Hastings & Beck, 2004) have proven particularly effective in helping parents identify and modify negative self-beliefs (e.g., "I'm not doing enough") and replace them with more realistic, affirming perspectives. As parents experience success in managing daily challenges, their self-efficacy strengthens, creating a positive feedback loop that sustains resilience. Ultimately, fostering self-efficacy requires consistent reinforcement from professionals, peers, and social systems that recognize and celebrate parental competence.

Integrating Mental Health and Respite Services

Caring for a child with intellectual disabilities can be emotionally and physically exhausting, often resulting in caregiver burnout if adequate supports are not in place. To prevent long-term strain, comprehensive service systems must integrate mental health care and respite options as essential—not supplementary—components of family support.

Accessible counseling, stress management programs, and therapeutic interventions can help parents process complex emotions such as guilt, frustration, or grief. Mental health support also mitigates risks of depression and anxiety, which are disproportionately high among parents of children with disabilities (Emerson et al., 2010). Respite care, whether formal (e.g., short-term residential programs) or informal (e.g., extended family assistance), provides temporary relief from caregiving duties, allowing parents to rest, attend to personal needs, or spend quality time with other family members. Research indicates that regular respite use is associated with lower stress levels, improved marital satisfaction, and greater long-term caregiving sustainability (Chan & Sigafoos, 2001).

Integrating these services into existing community frameworks requires policy commitment and collaboration across health, education, and social sectors. Prioritizing parental well-being through mental health and respite services is not only compassionate—it is a prerequisite for the sustained resilience of the entire family unit.

Encouraging Positive Meaning-Making

A crucial dimension of resilience lies in the ability to derive meaning and growth from adversity. Parents who engage in meaning-making processes often describe a redefined sense of purpose, identity, and relational depth as outcomes of their caregiving journey. Practitioners can facilitate this transformative process through structured interventions such as narrative therapy, reflective journaling, and strengths-based counseling.

These approaches encourage parents to articulate their experiences, identify moments of pride or progress, and reframe hardship within a broader story of endurance and love. Meaning-making does not eliminate pain but integrates it into a coherent narrative that affirms personal growth. Positive psychology offers additional tools for meaning reconstruction, including gratitude practices, mindfulness, and values clarification (Tedeschi & Calhoun, 2004; Seligman, 2011). Encouraging parents to recognize their achievements and the positive impact of their care on their children's lives promotes a sense of agency and emotional balance. Ultimately, facilitating meaning-making allows parents to move beyond survival toward post-traumatic growth—an enduring transformation characterized by increased empathy, strengthened relationships, and a deeper appreciation of life.

Advocating for Inclusive Policy

Resilience is not solely an individual or family attribute—it is deeply shaped by structural and policy environments. Policymakers play a critical role in creating conditions that support families raising children with intellectual disabilities.

Inclusive policies must ensure that family support is embedded across education, health, and social service systems. This includes accessible early intervention programs, inclusive schooling practices, financial assistance, and flexible workplace policies that accommodate caregiving responsibilities. Evidence shows that families in societies with strong welfare systems and inclusive legislation report lower stress and higher life satisfaction (Tøssebro, 2016).

Advocacy also extends to addressing social attitudes. Public awareness campaigns, community education, and media representation can challenge stigma and promote disability acceptance. When parents feel supported and their children valued, the broader culture itself becomes a protective environment that reinforces resilience. In essence, building parental resilience requires systemic commitment. Investment in inclusive infrastructure—educational, psychological, and economic—ensures that no parent's strength depends solely on personal endurance but is sustained by a compassionate and equitable society.

CONCLUSION

Raising a child with an intellectual disability is one of the most demanding yet potentially transformative experiences a parent can face. While the journey is characterized by chronic stressors, emotional complexity, and systemic barriers, it is equally marked by profound acts of endurance, adaptability, and growth. Parental resilience, as explored throughout this chapter, is not a static trait but a dynamic, multifaceted process shaped by personal, familial, cultural, and structural factors.

Resilience manifests through coping mechanisms, protective factors, and supportive environments that collectively allow parents to navigate adversity while maintaining emotional well-being. Theoretical frameworks—from Bronfenbrenner's ecological model to Walsh's family resilience paradigm—underscore that resilience is relational and systemic. It flourishes when individual capacities are supported by family cohesion, community solidarity, and equitable social policies.

Ultimately, understanding parental resilience in the context of intellectual disabilities demands that researchers and practitioners look beyond pathology toward strength-based models of adaptation. By recognizing and fostering the conditions that enable parents to thrive, we not only improve their quality of life but also contribute to more inclusive, compassionate societies that honor the diversity of human experience.

REFERENCES

Bandura, A. (1997). *Self-efficacy: The exercise of control*. W. H. Freeman.

Bayat, M. (2007). Evidence of resilience in families of children with autism. *Journal of Intellectual Disability Research*, *51*(9), 702–714. DOI: 10.1111/j.1365-2788.2007.00960.x PMID: 17845239

Bonanno, G. A. (2004). Loss, trauma, and human resilience: Have we underestimated the human capacity to thrive after extremely aversive events? *The American Psychologist*, *59*(1), 20–28. DOI: 10.1037/0003-066X.59.1.20 PMID: 14736317

Bronfenbrenner, U. (1979). *The ecology of human development: Experiments by nature and design*. Harvard University Press. DOI: 10.4159/9780674028845

Chan, J. B., & Sigafoos, J. (2001). Does respite care reduce parental stress in families with developmentally disabled children? *Child and Youth Care Forum*, *30*(5), 253–263. DOI: 10.1023/A:1014467226528

Dunst, C. J., Trivette, C. M., & Deal, A. G. (2007). *Enabling and empowering families: Principles and guidelines for practice*. Brookline Books.

Emerson, E., Hatton, C., Llewellyn, G., Blacher, J., & Graham, H. (2010). Socio-economic position, household composition, health status and indicators of child well-being in families of children with and without intellectual disabilities. *Journal of Intellectual Disability Research*, *54*(12), 1086–1098.

Folkman, S., & Moskowitz, J. T. (2000). Positive affect and the other side of coping. *The American Psychologist*, *55*(6), 647–654. DOI: 10.1037/0003-066X.55.6.647 PMID: 10892207

Gona, J. K., Newton, C. R., Hartley, S., & Bunning, K. (2016). Developing and validating the 'parenting a child with disabilities' scale in a rural context in Kenya. *Disability and Rehabilitation*, *38*(20), 2019–2030.

Gupta, A., & Singhal, N. (2005). Psychosocial support for families of children with intellectual disabilities. *British Journal of Special Education*, *31*(4), 214–221.

Hartley, S. L., Barker, E. T., Seltzer, M. M., Floyd, F. J., Greenberg, J. S., Orsmond, G. I., & Bolt, D. (2012). The relative risk and timing of divorce in families of children with an autism spectrum disorder. *Journal of Family Psychology*, *24*(4), 449–457. DOI: 10.1037/a0019847 PMID: 20731491

Hastings, R. P., & Beck, A. (2004). Practitioner review: Stress intervention for parents of children with intellectual disabilities. *Journal of Child Psychology and Psychiatry, and Allied Disciplines*, *45*(8), 1338–1349. DOI: 10.1111/j.1469-7610.2004.00357.x PMID: 15482495

Hastings, R. P., & Brown, T. (2002). Behavior problems of children with autism, parental self-efficacy, and mental health. *American Journal of Mental Retardation*, *107*(3), 222–232. DOI: 10.1352/0895-8017(2002)107<0222:BPOCWA>2.0.CO;2 PMID: 11966335

Hastings, R. P., Kovshoff, H., Brown, T., Ward, N. J., Espinosa, F. D., & Remington, B. (2005). Coping strategies in mothers and fathers of preschool and school-age children with autism. *Autism*, *9*(4), 377–391. DOI: 10.1177/1362361305056078 PMID: 16155055

Hastings, R. P., & Taunt, H. M. (2002). Positive perceptions in families of children with developmental disabilities. *American Journal of Mental Retardation*, *107*(2), 116–127. DOI: 10.1352/0895-8017(2002)107<0116:PPIFOC>2.0.CO;2 PMID: 11853529

Jones, J., & Passey, J. (2004). Family adaptation, coping and resources: Parents of children with developmental disabilities and behavior problems. *Journal on Developmental Disabilities*, *11*(1), 31–46.

Katsarou, D., Efthymiou, E., Kougioumtzis, G., Sofologi, M., & Theodoratou, M. (2024). Identifying Language Development in Children with ADHD: Differential Challenges, Interventions, and Collaborative Strategies. *Children (Basel, Switzerland)*, *11*(7), 841–850. DOI: 10.3390/children11070841 PMID: 39062289

Katsarou, D., Kougioumtzis, G., Efthymiou, E., Sofologi, M., & Mantsos, E. (2025). School-based mental health interventions for adolescents: supporting typically developing students and students with neurodevelopmental disorders. *Review of Clinical Pharmacology and Pharmacokinetics, International Edition*, 39(1), 11-22.

Katsarou, D., Mantsos, E., Papadopoulou, S., Sofologi, M., Efthymiou, E., Vasileiou, I., Megari, K., Theodoratou, M., & Kougioumtzis, G. (2025). Exploring AI technology in grammar performance testing for children with learning disabilities. *Education Sciences*, *15*(3), 351–365. DOI: 10.3390/educsci15030351

Lazarus, R. S., & Folkman, S. (1984). *Stress, appraisal, and coping*. Springer.

Lickenbrock, D. M., Ekas, N. V., & Whitman, T. L. (2011). Feeling good, feeling bad: Influences of maternal perceptions of the child and child behavior problems on maternal affect in families of children with autism spectrum disorders. *Journal of Autism and Developmental Disorders, 41*(7), 848–858. DOI: 10.1007/s10803-010-1105-9 PMID: 20839039

Lloyd, T., & Hastings, R. P. (2008). Psychological variables as correlates of adjustment in mothers of children with intellectual disabilities: Cross-sectional and longitudinal relationships. *Journal of Intellectual Disability Research, 52*(1), 37–48. DOI: 10.1111/j.1365-2788.2007.00974.x PMID: 18173571

Masten, A. S. (2014). *Ordinary magic: Resilience in development.* Guilford Press.

Masten, A. S. (2018). Resilience theory and research on children and families: Past, present, and promise. *Journal of Family Theory & Review, 10*(1), 12–31. DOI: 10.1111/jftr.12255

McCabe, H. (2007). Parent advocacy in the face of adversity: Autism and families in the People's Republic of China. *Focus on Autism and Other Developmental Disabilities, 22*(1), 39–50. DOI: 10.1177/10883576070220010501

McConnell, D., & Savage, A. (2015). Stress and resilience among families caring for children with intellectual disability: Expanding the research agenda. *Current Developmental Disorders Reports, 2*(2), 100–109. DOI: 10.1007/s40474-015-0040-z

Olshansky, S. (1962). Chronic sorrow: A response to having a mentally defective child. *Social Casework, 43*(4), 190–193. DOI: 10.1177/104438946204300404

Rutter, M. (2012). Resilience as a dynamic concept. *Development and Psychopathology, 24*(2), 335–344. DOI: 10.1017/S0954579412000028 PMID: 22559117

Seligman, M. E. P. (2011). *Flourish: A visionary new understanding of happiness and well-being.* Free Press.

Shin, J. Y., Nhan, N. V., Crittenden, K. S., Hong, H. T., Flory, M., & Ladinsky, J. (2006). Parenting stress of mothers and fathers of young children with cognitive delays in Vietnam. *Journal of Intellectual Disability Research, 50*(10), 748–760. DOI: 10.1111/j.1365-2788.2006.00840.x PMID: 16961704

Skinner, D., Correa, V., Skinner, M., & Bailey, D. (2001). Role of religion in the lives of Latino families of young children with developmental delays. *American Journal of Mental Retardation, 106*(4), 297–313. DOI: 10.1352/0895-8017(2001)106<0297:RORITL>2.0.CO;2 PMID: 11414871

Smith, L. E., Seltzer, M. M., Tager-Flusberg, H., Greenberg, J. S., & Carter, A. S. (2013). A comparative analysis of well-being and coping among mothers of children with autism spectrum disorder, Down syndrome, and fragile X syndrome. *American Journal on Intellectual and Developmental Disabilities*, *118*(4), 273–292.

Snyder, C. R. (2002). Hope theory: Rainbows in the mind. *Psychological Inquiry*, *13*(4), 249–275. DOI: 10.1207/S15327965PLI1304_01

Solomon, M., Pistrang, N., & Barker, C. (2001). The benefits of mutual support groups for parents of children with disabilities. *American Journal of Community Psychology*, *29*(1), 113–132. DOI: 10.1023/A:1005253514140 PMID: 11439824

Tedeschi, R. G., & Calhoun, L. G. (2004). Posttraumatic growth: Conceptual foundations and empirical evidence. *Psychological Inquiry*, *15*(1), 1–18. DOI: 10.1207/s15327965pli1501_01

Thoits, P. A. (2011). Mechanisms linking social ties and support to physical and mental health. *Journal of Health and Social Behavior*, *52*(2), 145–161. DOI: 10.1177/0022146510395592 PMID: 21673143

Tøssebro, J. (2016). Scandinavian disability policy: From deinstitutionalisation to non-discrimination and beyond. *Alter (Paris)*, *10*(2), 111–123. DOI: 10.1016/j.alter.2016.03.003

Totsika, V., Hastings, R. P., Emerson, E., Lancaster, G. A., & Berridge, D. M. (2011). A population-based investigation of behavioral and emotional problems and maternal mental health: Associations with autism spectrum disorder and intellectual disability. *Journal of Child Psychology and Psychiatry, and Allied Disciplines*, *52*(1), 91–99. DOI: 10.1111/j.1469-7610.2010.02295.x PMID: 20649912

Walsh, F. (2016). *Strengthening family resilience* (3rd ed.). Guilford Press.

White, M., & Epston, D. (1990). *Narrative means to therapeutic ends*. Norton.

Chapter 5
Psychological Resilience and Meaning-Making After Prenatal Detection of Genetic Syndromes

Dimitra V. Katsarou
http://orcid.org/0000-0001-8690-0314
University of the Aegean, Greece

Evangelos Mantsos
http://orcid.org/0009-0002-8490-2660
University of Western Macedonia, Greece

Kalliopi Megari
http://orcid.org/0000-0002-5861-7199
Aristotle University of Thessaloniki, Greece

Maria Sofologi
http://orcid.org/0000-0003-0380-2220
University of Ioannina, Greece

Georgios A. Kougioumtzis
http://orcid.org/0000-0002-2362-2094
National and Kapodistrian University of Athens, Greece

Effie Efthymiou
Zayed University, UAE

Miltiadis Karvounis
Hellenic Open University, Greece

Ilias Vasileiou
http://orcid.org/0009-0001-0530-4463
ICPS College, Greece

ABSTRACT

Receiving a prenatal diagnosis of a genetic syndrome creates a profound psychological and existential crisis for expectant mothers, prompting a deep need for meaning-making and identity reconstruction, a process this study explored qualitatively through interviews with 10 mothers diagnosed with Trisomy 21, 13, or 18. The findings established four major themes: the initial Disruption and Diagnosis,

DOI: 10.4018/979-8-3373-6294-6.ch005

marked by shock, grief, and guilt; Meaning-Making through spiritual reframing and symbolic rituals; the Reconfiguring Maternal Identity around advocacy, resilience, and unconditional love, which reflects post-traumatic growth; and the role of Social Support and Silences, where compassionate care offered resilience, while judgment and directive pressure exacerbated isolation. Ultimately, a prenatal diagnosis acts as a developmental inflection point whose outcomes are heavily shaped by risk and protective factors in psychological, cultural, and relational systems, underscoring the necessity of providing narrative-informed, trauma-sensitive, and culturally competent care.

INTRODUCTION

The prenatal period is marked by profound emotional and psychological transformation, and these dynamics become even more complex following the diagnosis of a genetic syndrome such as Trisomy 21, Trisomy 13, or Trisomy 18. Such diagnoses often disrupt the anticipated joy of pregnancy, instead evoking grief, fear, and uncertainty. Parents who choose to continue pregnancies after diagnoses like Trisomy 13 or 18 frequently describe their children as "not a diagnosis," emphasizing the tension between medical prognoses and parental identity formation (Guon et al., 2013).

Research consistently shows that a prenatal diagnosis of chromosomal abnormalities introduces high levels of psychological distress, with mothers reporting shock, sadness, and feelings of helplessness (Walker et al., 2008). The diagnosis often forces parents to grapple with prognostic uncertainty and existential questions about caregiving, disability, and the value of life (Statham, 2002). These experiences are compounded by the challenging medical realities, as survival outcomes for Trisomy 13 and Trisomy 18 are poor, leaving families in a prolonged state of anticipatory grief (Lakovschek et al., 2011).

Parental decision-making in these contexts is shaped not only by medical information but also by moral and cultural frameworks. Some families report that continuing the pregnancy contributes positively to their long-term emotional health and sense of parental identity, despite the anticipated loss (Winn et al., 2018). Others, who choose termination, describe complex grief reactions that can persist for years (Statham, 2002). Importantly, the quality of counseling and the structure of healthcare support significantly influence maternal coping. Patient-centered, multidisciplinary care helps families navigate decisions and mitigate psychological harm (Haug et al., 2017; Kim et al., 2024).

Ultimately, prenatal diagnoses of Trisomy 21, Trisomy 13, and Trisomy 18 illustrate how medical information reshapes maternal identity, emotional trajectories, and moral reasoning during pregnancy. The journey is one of profound emotional complexity, demanding compassionate healthcare responses that acknowledge both the medical and existential dimensions of parenting in the context of genetic syndromes (Merritt et al., 2012).

Maternal psychological responses often include shock, sadness, and existential questioning, as women face prognostic uncertainty and must reconcile their expectations of motherhood with the realities of parenting a child with significant medical needs. Families report that these diagnoses raise deep moral and existential dilemmas around the meaning of caregiving, disability, and social belonging (Ritchie et al., 2024). For some, the decision to terminate following diagnosis carries lasting psychological consequences, with themes of guilt, stigma, and disrupted identity shaping the experience (Atienza-Carrasco et al., 2019; Statham, 2002).

Termination of pregnancy after a prenatal diagnosis is frequently associated with intense grief, guilt, and even anger. Studies reveal that many women experience shame and stigma after termination, which can complicate their mourning process and impact long-term psychological well-being (McCoyd, 2007; Maguire et al., 2015). Some mothers describe being "branded" by the social perception of abortion, particularly when the pregnancy was initially desired, leading to ongoing identity struggles and feelings of isolation (McCoyd, 2007).

Comparative research further indicates that women who terminate after a fetal anomaly report higher levels of psychological distress—including guilt, depression, and intrusive memories—than women experiencing other pregnancy losses (Coleman, 2015). Feelings of self-blame are common, with some women questioning their decision or perceiving it as a moral failure (Atienza-Carrasco et al., 2019). Conversely, supportive and respectful healthcare interactions, including patient-centered counseling, can mitigate some of these negative outcomes, reinforcing the importance of compassionate clinical practice (Hodgson et al., 2016).

Ultimately, the psychological aftermath of prenatal diagnosis and subsequent decision-making reflects the intersection of individual grief, cultural stigma, and the broader social narratives surrounding disability and reproductive choice. Whether mothers continue or terminate a pregnancy, the experiences often leave a profound emotional imprint, shaped by moral dilemmas and the perceived meaning of their decision (Statham, 2002; Ngan et al., 2020).

Other studies emphasize that the way healthcare systems and professionals deliver the diagnosis plays a significant role in shaping maternal adjustment. Patient-centered communication and compassionate counseling can help parents navigate the emotional turbulence of prenatal genetic diagnoses (Haug et al., 2017). Such approaches respect maternal autonomy, reduce feelings of isolation, and promote coping even in the context of life-limiting conditions such as Trisomy 13 and 18 (Cleary et al., 2021).

By contrast, directive or overly medicalized counseling has been linked to higher rates of termination, as it can subtly pressure families toward certain choices while undermining their sense of agency (Jacobs et al., 2016). In contrast, when women feel heard and supported through shared decision-making processes, they report greater satisfaction with their care and lower levels of decisional regret (Farrell et al., 2013). Multidisciplinary and individualized counseling frameworks further ensure that families receive consistent information across specialties and are empowered to align decisions with their values (Lugli et al., 2024).

Communication style also matters at the interpersonal level. Research has shown that midwives' and genetic counselors' use of empathetic, non-directive verbal and nonverbal communication fosters trust and facilitates informed choices (Martin et al., 2016; Scott & Watermeyer, 2024). Conversely, when families perceive a lack of compassion or feel that information is delivered in a rushed or directive manner, it can exacerbate psychological distress and hinder adjustment (van der Steen et al., 2019). Thus, healthcare communication after a prenatal diagnosis is not merely informational but deeply relational, influencing both immediate emotional outcomes and long-term parental adaptation.

Ultimately, the prenatal diagnosis of chromosomal conditions such as Trisomy 21 or 13 not only transforms the psychological landscape of pregnancy but also demands that mothers navigate new moral terrains, reframe identity, and engage with shifting social narratives around disability and parenthood (Thompson et al., 2024; Walker et al., 2008).

THEORETICAL AND CONCEPTUAL FRAMEWORK

This study is grounded in a multidimensional psychological framework that integrates four complementary perspectives to understand maternal responses to prenatal diagnosis of genetic syndromes.

First, developmental psychology provides a foundation through Erikson's (1982) model of psychosocial development, which situates pregnancy as a critical period of identity transformation. Motherhood represents a turning point in the life cycle, where women negotiate shifts in self-concept and social roles, often accompanied by heightened vulnerability and opportunities for growth (Thomson et al., 2017).

Second, the transactional model of stress and coping (Lazarus & Folkman, 1984) emphasizes the dynamic appraisal processes mothers undergo following a stressful diagnosis. Coping strategies—ranging from problem-focused approaches to emotion regulation—are central in mediating psychological outcomes. This model has been widely applied to perinatal contexts, showing how maternal adaptation depends on cognitive appraisals of both the stressor and available resources (Hollander-Goldfein et al., 2012).

Third, meaning-making theory highlights how individuals strive to reconstruct coherence and significance when confronted with adversity (Park, 2010). In the context of prenatal diagnosis, expectant mothers often engage in narrative meaning-making to reconcile medical prognoses with deeply held values surrounding motherhood, caregiving, and disability. Research shows that meaning-making can buffer distress, facilitating resilience and adaptive identity reconstruction (Taubman-Ben-Ari, 2014; Davis, 2001).

Finally, the concept of post-traumatic growth (Tedeschi & Calhoun, 2004) captures how psychological adversity may catalyze profound personal transformation. Mothers navigating the challenges of prenatal diagnoses often report new perspectives on life, strengthened relationships, and greater appreciation for personal resilience (Athan, 2011; Berger, 2015). These outcomes demonstrate how adversity, while disruptive, may also serve as a catalyst for flourishing and self-development in the perinatal period.

Taken together, these frameworks offer a rich and integrative lens, illuminating how mothers draw upon cognitive, spiritual, social, and behavioral resources to cope with and sometimes transcend the disruptions of prenatal diagnosis. This multidimensional approach allows for nuanced exploration of both the vulnerabilities and the transformative potentials embedded in the maternal experience.

STUDY DESIGN AND METHODOLOGY

Research Design

This qualitative study employed a phenomenological approach to explore the lived experiences of mothers following a prenatal diagnosis of a genetic syndrome. This design was chosen to capture the depth and complexity of maternal responses, emphasizing subjective meaning-making and identity reconstruction.

Participants

Ten mothers between the ages of 24 and 42 participated in the study. All had received a prenatal diagnosis of a genetic syndrome—including Trisomy 21, Trisomy 13, or Trisomy 18—during the second trimester of pregnancy. Purposive sampling was used to ensure diversity across maternal background variables such as marital status, educational attainment, religious affiliation, and prior pregnancy experience.

Recruitment was conducted through prenatal care centers, genetic counseling clinics, and maternal support networks in urban and semi-urban regions.

Table 1. Demographics

Participant	Age	Marital Status	Education	Genetic Diagnosis	Previous Pregnancies
P1	24	Married	High school	Trisomy 21	0
P2	27	Single	College	Trisomy 13	1
P3	29	Married	College	Trisomy 18	2
P4	31	Cohabiting	Postgraduate	Trisomy 21	1
P5	33	Married	College	Trisomy 18	3
P6	35	Single	High school	Trisomy 21	0
P7	37	Married	Postgraduate	Trisomy 13	2
P8	39	Married	College	Trisomy 21	1
P9	40	Cohabiting	Postgraduate	Trisomy 18	4
P10	42	Married	College	Trisomy 21	2

Data Collection

Semi-structured interviews were conducted either in private consultation rooms at clinics or via secure video conferencing platforms, depending on participant preference and accessibility. Each interview lasted between 60 and 90 minutes, providing sufficient time for in-depth narrative exploration. The interview guide included open-ended questions on themes such as:

- Emotional reactions to the diagnosis (e.g., shock, grief, hope).
- Changes in maternal identity.
- Spiritual or religious coping strategies.
- Perceptions of healthcare communication.
- Expectations of caregiving and disability.

Probing questions were used to encourage participants to elaborate on turning points, metaphors, and personal narratives that shaped their adjustment. All interviews were audio-recorded with informed consent and transcribed verbatim. Pseudonyms were assigned to preserve anonymity.

Data Analysis

Thematic analysis was carried out using Braun and Clarke's (2006) six-phase framework: familiarization, coding, generating initial themes, reviewing themes, defining and naming themes, and producing the report. Two coders independently analyzed the transcripts and compared coding decisions during regular meetings to ensure reliability. NVivo 12 software was used to manage data and support the organization of codes and themes. Reflexive journaling and memo-writing were incorporated to document the researchers' assumptions, insights, and evolving interpretations throughout the process.

The analysis emphasized processes of adaptation, identity reconstruction, and meaning-making across individual narratives. Three overarching themes were identified: "navigating uncertainty," "redefining motherhood," and "finding strength in community." These themes capture both the shared and unique ways mothers made sense of the diagnosis and its implications for their lives.

Trustworthiness

To enhance the rigor of the study, Lincoln and Guba's (1985) criteria for trustworthiness were applied:

- Credibility was ensured through prolonged engagement with participants, member-checking of summaries, and peer debriefing within the research team. Participants were invited to review transcripts and preliminary findings to validate accuracy.
- Transferability was supported through thick descriptions of participants' demographic backgrounds, healthcare contexts, and experiences, enabling readers to judge the applicability of findings in other settings.
- Dependability was achieved by maintaining an audit trail of methodological decisions, coding frameworks, and reflexive memos that documented the research process.
- Confirmability was strengthened through reflexive journaling, where researchers critically examined their assumptions and emotional responses to reduce bias and maintain grounding in participants' narratives.

Together, these strategies ensured that the findings present a trustworthy and authentic account of maternal experiences following prenatal diagnosis of genetic syndromes.

FINDINGS

Disruption and Diagnosis: "Everything Changed in That Moment"

All participants described the moment of diagnosis as a profound rupture, a point in time that radically altered the imagined trajectory of their pregnancies and future motherhood. The diagnosis was consistently narrated as an intrusion—an external force that derailed expectations of a healthy baby and reshaped the meaning of their maternal journey. Words like *"hijacked," "detoured,"* and *"stolen"* were repeatedly invoked, underscoring a deep sense of disorientation and loss of agency.

Themes of shock and disbelief were often intertwined with waves of grief, as mothers spoke of mourning not only for the child they had envisioned but also for their own anticipated role as a "typical" mother. Some described this grief as silent and invisible, hidden beneath the surface because their pregnancies were ongoing, yet emotionally altered. Feelings of guilt emerged in different forms—some mothers blamed themselves for perceived genetic or lifestyle contributions, while others internalized broader societal messages about maternal responsibility and control over pregnancy outcomes.

Fear of judgment surfaced frequently, particularly in relation to family members, healthcare providers, and broader social circles. Several mothers worried that their decisions—whether to continue or consider termination—would be scrutinized, leaving them feeling isolated or misunderstood. This fear was not only about judgment from others but also self-judgment, as many wrestled with doubts about their adequacy as mothers and their ability to care for a child with complex needs.

Existential confusion added another layer of complexity. Mothers spoke of questioning notions of fairness, fate, and purpose. For some, the diagnosis destabilized spiritual or religious beliefs, while for others it deepened their search for meaning in the midst of crisis. These reflections often marked the beginning of a longer process of reconstructing identity and values in the face of uncertainty.

In the immediate aftermath of diagnosis, mothers struggled to integrate the medical reality with their prenatal expectations. Several reported difficulty bonding with the pregnancy, describing feelings of detachment or ambivalence toward their unborn child. This detachment was not necessarily a rejection but rather a protective strategy, an attempt to shield themselves from potential loss or disappointment. The tension between wanting to connect and fearing emotional vulnerability created an emotional limbo that many found exhausting.

Overall, this stage of disruption revealed the extent to which diagnosis reshaped not only maternal expectations but also the very foundation of identity, belonging, and agency in pregnancy. It was less a single moment of shock and more an unfolding process of disorientation that set the stage for subsequent coping, adaptation, and meaning-making.

Meaning-Making: *"She Is Still My Baby"*

Eight mothers described engaging in deliberate meaning-making processes as a way to navigate the emotional weight of diagnosis. For many, this involved reframing the experience through spiritual or religious beliefs. Some spoke of seeing the diagnosis as part of a divine plan, a calling to nurture a child who carried unique significance, or a test of faith that would strengthen their resilience. Prayer, scripture, and conversations with faith leaders provided both comfort and a lens through which to interpret the uncertainty of their circumstances.

Others turned to narrative restructuring, using storytelling, journaling, or private reflection to reclaim their voice and reimagine their role as mothers. Several participants described writing letters to their unborn child, not only as an act of love but also as a way to affirm connection and resist the clinical detachment that medical prognoses seemed to demand. Symbolic rituals—such as creating memory boxes, attending blessing ceremonies, or incorporating the pregnancy into family traditions—offered tangible ways to integrate the child into their lives and honor their place within the family.

A powerful recurring theme was the tension between medical language and maternal intuition. Mothers recalled being overwhelmed by diagnostic terminology that reduced their child to probabilities, deficits, and limitations. Many resisted what they perceived as dehumanizing labels and instead reasserted the child's identity as a baby, not a diagnosis. The simple act of naming the child, speaking to them, or using affectionate terms during pregnancy was described as an act of defiance against a system that spoke in terms of pathology rather than personhood.

This reclamation of the child's humanity was central to maternal resilience. Mothers often drew strength from affirming statements such as, *"She is still my baby,"* which allowed them to hold onto a sense of continuity between their prenatal hopes and their present reality. In doing so, they created a bridge between loss and love, diagnosis and identity.

These processes of reframing, ritualizing, and resisting medical reductionism revealed how mothers actively worked to reconstruct meaning and coherence. Rather than passively absorbing the shock of diagnosis, they engaged in practices that restored agency, reconnected them emotionally to their pregnancies, and offered a framework for resilience. Meaning-making, in this sense, was not a single act but an ongoing negotiation between external medical realities and deeply personal maternal values.

Reconfiguring Maternal Identity: *"I Became a Different Mother"*

Participants consistently reported that the prenatal diagnosis marked not only a disruption but also a redefinition of their maternal identity. Prior to diagnosis, many envisioned motherhood in terms of developmental milestones—first words, first steps, school readiness—or social benchmarks such as comparison with peers. After diagnosis, these expectations gave way to a more values-centered orientation. Parenting goals were reframed around advocacy, unconditional love, and moral strength. Rather than measuring success by milestones, mothers spoke of celebrating presence, resilience, and small, everyday victories.

This transformation was often described as a profound personal shift. Several mothers explained that they became more emotionally attuned—listening closely to their own feelings as well as to the subtle cues of their unborn child. Others shared that they grew spiritually grounded, drawing on faith practices not only for comfort but also as a guide for parenting with purpose. Advocacy emerged as a central feature of maternal identity, with mothers describing a newfound confidence in challenging healthcare professionals, seeking second opinions, or educating family members about the realities of their child's condition.

A recurring theme was the discovery of inner strength. Mothers expressed that the diagnosis, while initially devastating, had awakened capacities they had not previously recognized. Some framed this as resilience: the ability to withstand uncertainty and remain present in the face of fear. Others spoke of it as courage: the willingness to advocate fiercely for their child's dignity in contexts where medical or social systems tended to marginalize or reduce them to their condition.

This identity reconstruction was not always smooth or immediate; participants acknowledged moments of doubt, fatigue, and grief. Yet many reflected that they had "become different mothers" through the process—more assertive, more compassionate, and more deeply connected to values of justice, care, and unconditional love. For some, this transformation extended beyond their immediate family, inspiring involvement in advocacy groups, support networks, or faith-based initiatives aimed at creating broader awareness and inclusion.

In these ways, maternal identity was not dismantled by diagnosis but reshaped into a more expansive and resilient form. What began as an experience of loss and disruption evolved, for many, into a source of personal growth and strength that redefined how they saw themselves not only as mothers, but as individuals navigating life's uncertainties with courage and conviction.

Social Support and Silences

Mothers identified both formal and informal sources of support as vital to their ability to cope with the emotional upheaval of diagnosis. Formal support often came in the form of compassionate, non-directive genetic counseling. Participants described these interactions as "lifelines," moments when they felt listened to and empowered rather than overwhelmed by medical jargon or pressured into particular decisions. Counselors who emphasized autonomy and affirmed maternal capacity were especially valued, as their approach helped mothers regain a sense of agency during a time of vulnerability.

Equally important were informal networks of support. Peer connections with other mothers who had faced similar diagnoses were repeatedly described as transformative. Sharing stories, practical advice, and emotional solidarity created a sense of belonging that counteracted feelings of isolation. Some mothers sought out online forums, while others engaged with local support groups or faith-based communities. In these spaces, they found validation of their grief, their hopes, and their struggles—experiences often minimized or misunderstood in their broader social environments.

At the same time, mothers highlighted the profound impact of silences. Several described encounters with medical professionals who delivered the diagnosis in a detached or overly clinical manner, leaving them feeling dehumanized and unsupported. Others recounted family members who avoided discussing the diagnosis altogether, either out of discomfort or denial. These silences could be just as painful as overt judgment, intensifying mothers' sense of being alone in their experience.

Some participants also reported feeling pressured by professionals or relatives toward particular decisions, such as termination or continuation of pregnancy, without adequate space to explore their own values. Such pressure compounded guilt and uncertainty, reinforcing the emotional burden of an already difficult situation. Conversely, when family members offered open listening and unconditional support—"I'm here for you, whatever you decide"—mothers described feeling anchored and more confident in their choices.

Overall, the presence or absence of supportive voices shaped not only how mothers processed the diagnosis but also how they saw themselves as capable and resilient. Support was not merely a practical resource but a form of recognition—an affirmation that their experiences and emotions were valid. By contrast, silences, dismissals, or coercion eroded trust, deepened isolation, and made the already heavy emotional weight of diagnosis even harder to carry.

DISCUSSION

The findings of this study highlight the profound psychological and existential disruption that accompanies a prenatal diagnosis of genetic syndromes. Consistent with earlier research, the moment of diagnosis was experienced as a rupture in the imagined trajectory of motherhood, triggering grief-like responses and destabilization of maternal identity (Lafarge et al., 2013; McCoyd, 2007). Participants' descriptions of shock, guilt, and existential questioning echo Souka et al.'s (2010) observation that prenatal diagnosis often initiates a cycle of anticipatory grief, in which women mourn both the "idealized child" and the anticipated experience of typical motherhood.

A central contribution of this study lies in illuminating the active processes of meaning-making employed by mothers. Mothers resisted purely medicalized interpretations of diagnosis, instead reframing their experience through spiritual belief, narrative practices, and symbolic rituals. This mirrors Park's (2010) framework on global and situational meaning-making, suggesting that constructing significance is a protective factor in maternal resilience. Similar patterns have been documented by Taubman-Ben-Ari (2014), who found that mothers often draw upon spiritual and existential resources to preserve a sense of coherence when faced with perinatal adversity.

The reconfiguration of maternal identity observed in this study further aligns with Tedeschi and Calhoun's (2004) model of post-traumatic growth. Mothers described becoming more assertive, spiritually grounded, and resilient in advocating for their child, reflecting findings from Athan (2011) that motherhood in contexts of adversity can serve as a catalyst for personal transformation. Rather than undermining maternal identity, diagnosis prompted many participants to redefine their motherhood in terms of advocacy, unconditional love, and moral strength.

Social support—or the lack thereof—was also a decisive factor shaping maternal adjustment. Empathic, autonomy-supportive counseling was described as protective, enabling mothers to regain agency and reduce isolation. These findings reinforce prior studies emphasizing the importance of non-directive, compassionate communication in prenatal genetic counseling (Skirton & Barr, 2007; Hodgson et al., 2016). Conversely, participants' accounts of silence, pressure, and invalidation align with evidence that social minimization exacerbates distress and compounds feelings of stigma (Maguire et al., 2015). The contrast between supportive and dismissive responses underscores the relational nature of resilience: psychological outcomes were influenced not only by individual coping but also by the quality of interpersonal and systemic interactions.

Taken together, these findings contribute to the growing body of literature emphasizing the multidimensional impact of prenatal diagnosis. They suggest that maternal adaptation is best understood not simply as an individual psychological process but as a dynamic negotiation of meaning, identity, and support embedded within social, cultural, and medical contexts.

IMPLICATIONS FOR HEALTH PSYCHOLOGY PRACTICE

This study underscores the importance of approaching prenatal diagnosis not only as a biomedical event but as a developmental and psychological turning point. A **developmental psychopathology lens** emphasizes how individual adaptation emerges from dynamic interactions between risk and protective factors across time. From this perspective, the maternal response to diagnosis can be understood as a critical developmental juncture, where identity, coping strategies, and support systems shape both immediate psychological outcomes and longer-term trajectories for maternal and child well-being.

1. **Narrative-informed approaches.** Narrative interventions, such as guided storytelling, journaling, or symbolic rituals, offer mothers opportunities to integrate the diagnosis into a coherent life narrative. From a developmental psychopathology standpoint, these practices reduce fragmentation in maternal identity and foster adaptive meaning-making, which can buffer against maladaptive trajectories such as prolonged grief or depressive symptomatology.
2. **Trauma-informed care.** The diagnostic moment often functions as a potential traumatic stressor, disrupting normative developmental processes of pregnancy. Training clinicians to use trauma-informed approaches—marked by attunement, continuity, and sensitivity—acknowledges the event's developmental significance. By responding with empathy and continuity of care, clinicians can interrupt the risk pathway toward chronic distress and promote resilience.
3. **Cultural and spiritual competence.** Cultural and spiritual frameworks are integral developmental contexts in which mothers construct meaning. Recognizing and validating these interpretations supports not only coping in the short term but also strengthens maternal identity over time. Developmental psychopathology highlights that resilience emerges through multiple pathways; religious and cultural practices can serve as protective factors that help mothers reestablish coherence and stability.
4. **Peer support integration.** Peer networks create protective relational contexts that counterbalance risks of stigma, isolation, and identity disruption. Structured programs that connect mothers with others facing similar diagnoses can provide corrective experiences, normalizing grief and fostering a sense of belonging. Viewed through developmental psychopathology, these relational supports

act as buffers that reduce vulnerability to maladaptive outcomes and reinforce positive adaptation across time.

5. **Identity-based care planning.** Because prenatal diagnosis reshapes maternal identity, care planning should explicitly support the reconstruction of this identity. Clinicians can help mothers articulate new parenting goals—centered on advocacy, unconditional love, and moral strength—while reinforcing competencies that bolster self-efficacy. This approach reduces vulnerability to psychopathology, while supporting healthier mother–infant relationships and long-term developmental outcomes for both mother and child.

In sum, applying a developmental psychopathology framework to health psychology practice highlights that maternal adjustment to prenatal diagnosis is not a singular event but a process unfolding across time, shaped by multiple interacting systems—biological, psychological, social, and cultural. By recognizing diagnosis as a developmental inflection point, clinicians can design interventions that address immediate distress while also fostering trajectories of resilience, growth, and relational health.

FUTURE RESEARCH DIRECTIONS

The findings of this study point to several important areas for future research. One priority is the need for longitudinal studies that follow mothers across time, from the moment of diagnosis through pregnancy, postpartum, and early childhood. Such research would provide valuable insights into how processes such as meaning-making, identity reconstruction, and social support evolve and interact across developmental stages. A longitudinal, developmental psychopathology approach could also clarify which early risk and protective factors predict resilient trajectories and which contribute to vulnerability, offering evidence for targeted interventions.

Another important direction lies in expanding the scope beyond maternal voices to include fathers, partners, siblings, and extended family members. Prenatal diagnosis is rarely an isolated maternal experience; rather, it reverberates through family systems. Understanding how families collectively negotiate caregiving roles, decision-making, and meaning-making will provide a fuller picture of the psychological and relational consequences of diagnosis.

Cross-cultural perspectives also warrant greater attention. Maternal responses to diagnosis are embedded within broader cultural, religious, and healthcare contexts, which shape the narratives of disability, motherhood, and caregiving available to women. Comparative studies across diverse populations would help to illuminate how cultural frameworks both constrain and enable resilience, while also highlighting disparities in access to supportive counseling and peer networks.

In addition, there is a need for intervention studies that design, implement, and evaluate evidence-based practices informed by narrative, trauma-informed, and identity-based approaches. Such interventions could be tested for their ability to enhance resilience, reduce distress, and strengthen maternal–infant bonding. Evaluating these programs through rigorous mixed-methods or randomized controlled trials would provide critical data to guide best practices in prenatal and maternal care.

Finally, future research should explicitly integrate developmental psychopathology models to refine our theoretical understanding of maternal adjustment to prenatal diagnosis. By examining how risk factors such as stigma, guilt, and isolation interact with protective resources like peer support, spiritual frameworks, and narrative meaning-making, researchers can better conceptualize diagnosis as a developmental inflection point. Such work would contribute to theory-building while also shaping clinical practices aimed at supporting families over the long term.

This study has illuminated the profound psychological, emotional, and existential challenges faced by mothers following a prenatal diagnosis of a genetic syndrome. Across narratives, the moment of diagnosis emerged as a disruptive turning point—one that radically altered expectations of pregnancy and motherhood. Mothers described feelings of shock, grief, guilt, and isolation, experiences that echoed grief-like processes of loss while also destabilizing maternal identity. These findings resonate with research documenting the grief and anticipatory mourning that often accompany prenatal diagnoses (Lafarge et al., 2013; Maguire et al., 2015). Yet within this disruption, mothers engaged in deliberate strategies of meaning-making, narrative reconstruction, and spiritual or symbolic reframing that allowed them to reclaim a sense of agency and reassert the humanity of their child, echoing Park's (2010) framework on meaning-making.

The findings also demonstrate that prenatal diagnosis can catalyze significant transformations in maternal identity. Many mothers described becoming more assertive, spiritually grounded, and resilient, reframing motherhood in terms of advocacy, unconditional love, and moral strength. These shifts align with Tedeschi and Calhoun's (2004) model of post-traumatic growth, showing that adversity can open pathways for deep personal change and reorientation. At the same time, the presence—or absence—of supportive relationships shaped the trajectory of adjustment. Empathic counseling, peer support, and open family dialogue served as powerful protective factors, while silences, judgment, and directive pressures compounded distress and deepened feelings of isolation, consistent with prior work on the relational dynamics of prenatal decision-making (Hodgson et al., 2016; Skirton & Barr, 2007).

Taken together, these results suggest that maternal adjustment to prenatal diagnosis is best understood as a multidimensional process. It is simultaneously psychological, social, cultural, and developmental. From a developmental psychopathology perspective, diagnosis can be seen as an inflection point where risk and protective factors converge to shape long-term trajectories for both mothers and their children. Whether outcomes follow maladaptive or resilient pathways depends on the interplay between personal resources, relational supports, cultural frameworks, and healthcare practices (Souka et al., 2010; McCoyd, 2007).

The study carries important implications for health psychology practice. Narrative-informed, trauma-sensitive, and culturally competent approaches can empower mothers to integrate diagnosis into their evolving identities. Structured peer support and identity-based care planning can strengthen resilience, enhance bonding, and improve long-term well-being. These findings also highlight a need for systemic change within healthcare, where diagnostic communication should be approached as a relational and potentially traumatic event rather than a purely medical disclosure.

Future research should extend these insights through longitudinal designs, cross-cultural comparisons, and family-centered approaches, while testing interventions that draw upon meaning-making, identity reconstruction, and developmental psychopathology frameworks. By deepening our understanding of how mothers navigate the disruptive yet transformative terrain of prenatal diagnosis, future scholarship and practice can better support families not only in surviving disruption, but in discovering new forms of resilience, meaning, and growth.

REFERENCES

Athan, A. M. (2011). *Postpartum flourishing: Motherhood as opportunity for positive growth and self-development.* ProQuest Dissertations Publishing. https://search.proquest.com/openview/e31d26d93e356c201d593c371d69578c/1

Atienza-Carrasco, J., Linares-Abad, M., Padilla Ruiz, M., & Morales Gil, I. M. (2019). Experiences and outcomes following diagnosis of congenital foetal anomaly and medical termination of pregnancy: A phenomenological study. *Journal of Clinical Nursing*, *29*(1-2), 93–104. DOI: 10.1111/jocn.15162 PMID: 31887230

Berger, R. (2015). *Stress, trauma, and posttraumatic growth: Social context, environment, and identities*. Routledge., DOI: 10.4324/9780203118795

Cleary, J. P., Janvier, A., Farlow, B., Weaver, M., Hammel, J., & Lantos, J. (2021). Cardiac interventions for patients with trisomy 13 and trisomy 18: Experience, ethical issues, communication, and the case for individualized family-centered care. *Journal of Patient Experience*, *9*, 1–8. DOI: 10.1177/21501351211044132 PMID: 34919485

Coleman, P. K. (2015). Diagnosis of fetal anomaly and the increased maternal psychological toll associated with pregnancy termination. *Issues in Law & Medicine*, *30*(1), 3–23. https://www.researchgate.net/publication/279308414 PMID: 26103706

Davis, C. G. (2001). The tormented and the transformed: Understanding responses to loss and trauma. In Neimeyer, R. A. (Ed.), *Meaning reconstruction & the experience of loss* (pp. 137–155). American Psychological Association., DOI: 10.1037/10397-007

Erikson, E. H. (1982). *The life cycle completed.* W. W. Norton & Company.

Farrell, R. M., Nutter, B., & Agatisa, P. K. (2013). Patient-centered prenatal counseling: Aligning obstetric healthcare professionals with needs of pregnant women. *Women & Health*, *55*(3), 302–316. DOI: 10.1080/03630242.2014.996724 PMID: 25794055

Guon, J., Wilfond, B. S., Farlow, B., Brazg, T., & Janvier, A. (2013). Our children are not a diagnosis: The experience of parents who continue their pregnancy after a prenatal diagnosis of trisomy 13 or 18. *American Journal of Medical Genetics. Part A*, *164A*(2), 308–318. DOI: 10.1002/ajmg.a.36298 PMID: 24311520

Haug, S., Goldstein, M., Cummins, D., Fayard, E., & Merritt, A. (2017). Using patient-centered care after a prenatal diagnosis of trisomy 18 or trisomy 13: A review. *JAMA Pediatrics*, *171*(4), 382–387. https://jamanetwork.com/journals/jamapediatrics/article-abstract/2601244. DOI: 10.1001/jamapediatrics.2016.4798 PMID: 28192554

Hodgson, J., Pitt, P., Metcalfe, S., Halliday, J., Menezes, M., Fisher, J., Hickerton, C., Petersen, K., & McClaren, B. (2016). Experiences of prenatal diagnosis and decision-making about termination of pregnancy: A qualitative study. *Australian and New Zealand Journal of Obstetrics and Gynaecology*, *56*(6), 605–613. DOI: 10.1111/ajo.12501 PMID: 27402530

Hollander-Goldfein, B., Isserman, N., & Goldenberg, J. E. (2012). *Transcending trauma: Survival, resilience and clinical implications in survivor families*. Routledge.

Jacobs, M., Cooper, S. A., McGowan, R., Nelson, S. M., & Pell, J. (2016). Pregnancy outcome following prenatal diagnosis of chromosomal anomaly: A record linkage study of 26,261 pregnancies. *PLoS One*, *11*(1), e0166909. DOI: 10.1371/journal.pone.0166909 PMID: 27907018

Lafarge, C., Mitchell, K., & Fox, P. (2013). Women's experiences of coping with pregnancy termination for fetal abnormality. *Qualitative Health Research*, *23*(7), 924–936. DOI: 10.1177/1049732313484198 PMID: 23558712

Lakovschek, I. C., Streubel, B., & Ulm, B. (2011). Natural outcome of trisomy 13, trisomy 18, and triploidy after prenatal diagnosis. *American Journal of Medical Genetics. Part A*, *155*(11), 2616–2626. DOI: 10.1002/ajmg.a.34284 PMID: 21990236

Lazarus, R. S., & Folkman, S. (1984). *Stress, appraisal, and coping*. Springer.

Lugli, L., Rossi, C., Berardi, A., Pugliese, M., Ceccarelli, P., Sileo, G., Chiossi, G., Contu, G., Calabrese, O., Marca, A., & Bertucci, E. (2024). Prenatal multidisciplinary counseling for fetal congenital anomalies: A narrative review. *International Journal of Gynaecology and Obstetrics: the Official Organ of the International Federation of Gynaecology and Obstetrics*, *160*(1), 45–55. DOI: 10.1002/ijgo.16068 PMID: 39660910

Maguire, M., Light, A., Kuppermann, M., Dalton, V. K., Steinauer, J. E., & Kerns, J. L. (2015). Grief after second-trimester termination for fetal anomaly: A qualitative study. *Contraception*, *91*(3), 234–239. DOI: 10.1016/j.contraception.2014.11.015 PMID: 25499590

Martin, L., Gitsels-van der Wal, J. T., Pereboom, M. T., Spelten, E. R., Hutton, E. K., & van Dulmen, S. (2016). Clients' psychosocial communication and midwives' verbal and nonverbal communication during prenatal counseling for anomaly screening. *Patient Education and Counseling*, *99*(1), 85–91. DOI: 10.1016/j.pec.2015.07.020 PMID: 26298217

McCoyd, J. L. M. (2007). Pregnancy interrupted: Loss of a desired pregnancy after diagnosis of fetal anomaly. *Health Care for Women International, 28*(1), 3–18. DOI: 10.1080/07399330601003473 PMID: 17148106

Merritt, T. A., Catlin, A., Wool, C., Peverini, R., Goldstein, M., & Oshiro, B. (2012). Trisomy 18 and trisomy 13: Treatment and management decisions. *NeoReviews, 13*(1), e40–e48. DOI: 10.1542/neo.13-1-e40

Ngan, O. M. Y., Yi, H., Bryant, L., Sahota, D. S., Chan, O. Y. M., & Ahmed, S. (2020). Parental expectations of raising a child with disability in decision-making for prenatal testing and termination of pregnancy: A mixed methods study. *Patient Education and Counseling, 103*(11), 2373–2383. DOI: 10.1016/j.pec.2020.05.010 PMID: 32507714

Park, C. L. (2010). Making sense of the meaning literature: An integrative review of meaning making and its effects on adjustment to stressful life events. *Psychological Bulletin, 136*(2), 257–301. DOI: 10.1037/a0018301 PMID: 20192563

Ritchie, Z., Teachman, G., Shaul, R. Z., & Smith, M. J. (2024). "She was finally mine": The moral experience of families in the context of trisomy 13 and 18–a scoping review with thematic analysis. *BMC Medical Ethics, 25*(1), 94. DOI: 10.1186/s12910-023-00994-x PMID: 38431625

Scott, M., Watermeyer, J., & Wessels, T.-M. (2024). A balancing act: Non-directive communication, risk perceptions, and meeting patient needs in genetic counseling: A South African case study. *Journal of Genetic Counseling, 33*(2), 1741–1752. DOI: 10.1002/jgc4.1741 PMID: 37323090

Skirton, H., & Barr, O. (2007). Influences on uptake of antenatal screening for down syndrome: A review of the literature. *Evidence-Based Midwifery, 5*(1), 4–10.

Souka, A. P., Michalitsi, V. D., Skentou, H., Euripioti, H., Papadopoulos, G. K., Kassanos, D., Messinis, I. E., & Salamalekis, E. E. (2010). Attitudes of pregnant women regarding termination of pregnancy for fetal abnormality. *Prenatal Diagnosis, 30*(10), 977–980. DOI: 10.1002/pd.2600 PMID: 20730784

Statham, H. (2002). Prenatal diagnosis of fetal abnormality: The decision to terminate the pregnancy and the psychological consequences. *Fetal and Maternal Medicine Review, 13*(4), 213–247. DOI: 10.1017/S0965539502000414

Taubman-Ben-Ari, O. (2014). Well-being and personal growth in emerging motherhood: and what about meaning? In Batthyany, A., & Russo-Netzer, P. (Eds.), *Meaning in positive and existential psychology* (pp. 417–438). Springer. DOI: 10.1007/978-1-4939-0308-5_21

Tedeschi, R. G., & Calhoun, L. G. (2004). Posttraumatic growth: Conceptual foundations and empirical evidence. *Psychological Inquiry*, *15*(1), 1–18. DOI: 10.1207/s15327965pli1501_01

Thompson, T., Tisher, J., Davis, S., Miller, C., Kirk, J., Tartaglia, N., & Howell, S. (2024). The emotional journey of adapting to prenatally identified trisomy X. *Journal of Genetic Counseling*, *33*(1), 177–190. DOI: 10.1002/jgc4.1778 PMID: 37691399

Thomson, G., & Schmied, V. (2017). *Psychosocial resilience and risk in the perinatal period*. Routledge., DOI: 10.4324/9781315656854

van der Steen, S. L., Houtman, D., Bakkeren, I. M., Galjaard, R.-J., Polak, M., Busschbach, J., Tibben, A., & Riedjik, S. (2019). Offering a choice between NIPT and invasive PND in prenatal genetic counseling: The impact of clinician characteristics on patients' test uptake. *European Journal of Human Genetics : EJHG*, *27*(1), 103–111. DOI: 10.1038/s41431-018-0287-z PMID: 30297905

Walker, L. V., Miller, V. J., & Dalton, V. K. (2008). The health-care experiences of families given the prenatal diagnosis of trisomy 18. *Journal of Perinatology*, *28*(1), 12–19. DOI: 10.1038/sj.jp.7211860 PMID: 18165828

Winn, P., Acharya, K., Peterson, E., & Leuthner, S. (2018). Prenatal counseling and parental decision-making following a fetal diagnosis of trisomy 13 or 18. *Journal of Perinatology*, *38*(5), 588–595. DOI: 10.1038/s41372-018-0107-x PMID: 29740195

Chapter 6
Health Psychology in Practice:
Coping, Meaning, and Resilience in Therapists Supporting CSA Survivors

Blessy Lenin
http://orcid.org/0009-0007-0282-116X
Martin Luther Christian University, Canada

ABSTRACT

Child sexual abuse (CSA) profoundly affects both survivors and the therapists who support them. Drawing on Blessy Lenin's qualitative study of fourteen Indian counsellors, this chapter examines how coping, resilience, and meaning-making sustain therapists exposed to trauma narratives. Participants reported secondary trauma, burnout, and psychosomatic distress, yet employed mindfulness, supervision, spirituality, and cultural practices to maintain well-being. Framed within the biopsychosocial model and resilience theory, the chapter highlights how meaning-making transforms suffering into growth and strengthens professional identity. It advocates trauma-informed, culturally sensitive frameworks within health psychology to promote therapist self-care, resilience, and holistic well-being while enhancing outcomes for CSA survivors.

INTRODUCTION

Child sexual abuse (CSA) has long been recognized as one of the most pervasive forms of human rights violations and a global public health concern. The World

DOI: 10.4018/979-8-3373-6294-6.ch006

Health Organization (WHO, 1999) defines CSA as the involvement of a child in sexual activity that he or she does not fully comprehend, is unable to give informed consent to, or that violates laws or social taboos of society. In India, surveys reveal that nearly one in two children report experiences of sexual abuse before adulthood (Hindustan Times, 2017; BBC, 2017). Despite legislative frameworks such as the Protection of Children from Sexual Offences (POCSO) Act, cultural silence and stigmatization continue to obscure both survivor recovery and professional intervention.

The trauma of CSA manifests not only in survivors' physical and psychological domains but also resonates deeply within the therapists who engage empathetically in this work. Mental health professionals working with CSA survivors are repeatedly exposed to narratives of violence, helplessness, and betrayal, leading to what Figley (1995) conceptualized as *secondary traumatic stress disorder*. Such exposure often results in symptoms akin to post-traumatic stress disorder (PTSD), including intrusive thoughts, avoidance behaviors, emotional numbing, and physiological arousal (Follette, Polusny, & Milbeck, 1994).

Within health psychology, therapist well-being is increasingly recognized as a vital aspect of healthcare systems. The biopsychosocial framework emphasizes that health is determined by the complex interaction between biological, psychological, and social processes (Engel, 1977). For therapists, this translates into understanding how emotional labor, professional exposure, and sociocultural context jointly influence mental health. Lenin's doctoral ongoing study in India expands this framework to include spiritual and cultural determinants of resilience factors that have historically been underexplored in Western psychology.

Therapists often report paradoxical experiences: deep exhaustion coexists with profound fulfillment; emotional vulnerability accompanies a strengthened sense of purpose. This dialectic aligns with the concept of *post-traumatic growth* (Tedeschi & Calhoun, 2004), wherein professionals derive meaning and transformation from their exposure to trauma work. Within the Indian context, spirituality, religious faith, and collective cultural identity play a significant role in this transformation. Many counselors frame their therapeutic practice as *seva* a form of service imbued with ethical and spiritual meaning.

Furthermore, gender and social norms shape therapists' coping trajectories. The majority of CSA counselors in India are women, a demographic reality that compounds the emotional labor associated with trauma work (Baum, 2016). These women not only face the internal demands of professional empathy but also external societal expectations of caregiving, modesty, and resilience. Lenin's notes that for many female therapists, the work triggers a reevaluation of self, morality, and boundaries what one participant described as "a dismantling and rebuilding of who I am, both as a woman and as a professional."

Despite the psychological toll, the counselors interviewed by Lenin frequently described their engagement with CSA survivors as transformative. They experienced heightened self-awareness, compassion, and professional maturity. This phenomenon aligns with health psychology's interest in understanding not merely pathology but adaptive recovery and growth in the face of stress (Richardson, 2002).

In this chapter, therapist experiences are analyzed through the lens of health psychology. The discipline's holistic view of health encompassing physical, psychological, social, and spiritual domains provides an apt theoretical scaffolding for understanding how counselors maintain equilibrium amid trauma exposure. By exploring coping strategies, resilience mechanisms, and meaning-making processes among therapists, this chapter contributes to expanding the scope of health psychology from patient-focused to practitioner-centered well-being.

2. BACKGROUND OF THE STUDY

Child sexual abuse (CSA) constitutes one of the most severe forms of interpersonal trauma, with profound repercussions extending far beyond the survivor (Putnam, 2009). According to UNICEF (2017), nearly 15 million adolescent girls aged 15–19 globally have experienced forced sex, with 9 in 10 of these incidents perpetrated by someone known to the child. The psychological toll on survivors includes depression, post-traumatic stress disorder (PTSD), dissociation, and personality changes (Hailes et al., 2019).

However, the impact of CSA extends secondarily to those who witness or therapeutically engage with survivors' narratives. Mental health practitioners particularly trauma therapists are repeatedly exposed to distressing accounts, forming what Figley (1995) terms *secondary traumatic stress*. These professionals often internalize their clients' suffering, resulting in symptoms mirroring primary trauma such as intrusive imagery, avoidance, somatic tension, and changes in worldview (Pearlman & Saakvitne, 1995).

While secondary traumatization is a recognized occupational hazard in clinical psychology, the magnitude of its impact depends on contextual factors such as social support, cultural beliefs, and access to supervision (Cunningham, 2003). Studies in Western contexts have established that therapists working with survivors of sexual abuse report significantly higher emotional exhaustion and disrupted cognitive schemas compared to those working with other trauma populations such as cancer patients or refugees (Cunningham, 2003; Brady et al., 1999).

In the Indian setting, however, this professional suffering occurs within distinctive sociocultural structures marked by patriarchal attitudes, social silence, and moral ambivalence toward sexual violence (Choudhry et al., 2018). The lack of systemic acknowledgment of therapists' emotional labor contributes to a hidden layer of distress within the caregiving profession. Blessy Lenin's study addresses this gap by foregrounding the voices of Indian counselors and framing their lived experiences within health psychology and cultural resilience theory.

India presents a paradoxical landscape in addressing CSA. Despite progressive laws such as the Protection of Children from Sexual Offences (POCSO) Act of 2012, sociocultural taboos surrounding sexuality, purity, and family honor often inhibit disclosure and intervention (Hemanth Kumar et al., 2024). For therapists, this creates a dual challenge: working with survivors who struggle against societal denial, and confronting their own internalized cultural conditioning regarding gender and morality.

Lenin's ongoing research highlights that many counselors encounter personal and professional dissonance in such environments. Female therapists who form the overwhelming majority in this field face unique vulnerabilities. They are not only more likely to empathically identify with young female survivors but also to internalize anger and helplessness toward patriarchal structures that perpetuate abuse (Baum, 2016).

Therapists often report psychosomatic symptoms including headaches, digestive issues, and fatigue resulting from accumulated emotional strain. One participant described the physical manifestation of trauma as "tightness in my chest and stomach when I hear a child narrate her abuse" (Lenin, in progress). These experiences align with Engel's (1977) biopsychosocial model, which posits that health is the outcome of intertwined biological, psychological, and social influences.

The scarcity of institutional support further compounds therapists' vulnerability. Most Indian NGOs and child welfare agencies lack structured supervision systems, and counsellors are expected to manage high caseloads, documentation, and legal coordination independently (Lenin, in progress). Over time, the absence of psychological containment mechanisms such as peer consultation, case debriefing, and reflective supervision erodes resilience and increases burnout risk.

Yet within this adversity, Lenin's identifies a remarkable counter current: the creative and culturally embedded strategies that therapists employ to sustain themselves. These include prayer, meditation, community gatherings, family engagement, music, and journaling forms of *indigenous coping* deeply intertwined with India's spiritual heritage. This reliance on culturally congruent practices resonates with cross-cultural health psychology findings that spirituality and social relatedness can buffer against occupational stress (Comas-Díaz & Jacobsen, 1991; Ungar, 2011).

The relationship between therapist and client in CSA work is characterized by deep emotional reciprocity. Exposure to intense trauma narratives often provokes *countertransference* the therapist's unconscious emotional response to the client's experiences (Prasko et al., 2022). In Lenin's study, many participants reported oscillating between empathy, anger, and helplessness. These reactions, if unacknowledged, risk impairing therapeutic judgment and personal well-being.

The emotional ecology of trauma therapy involves complex processes of attunement, projection, and internalization. Therapists serve as both witnesses and containers for their clients' pain. When this containment fails, secondary traumatization manifests not merely as emotional exhaustion but as existential disorientation. One therapist noted, *"There were days when I felt I could no longer distinguish between my pain and the client's"* (Lenin, in progress)

Such emotional blurring is intensified in collectivist societies where personal and professional boundaries are often fluid. Indian therapists frequently navigate overlapping identities as caregivers, community members, and advocates. These intersecting roles contribute to both empathy and vulnerability. As Comas-Díaz and Jacobsen (1991) observe, in cultures where communal values dominate, therapists' sense of self becomes inherently relational making them more susceptible to vicarious emotional resonance.

This relational orientation, however, also also enables resilience. Many of Lenin's participants described moments of renewal through *shared emotional release* crying during supervision, praying collectively, or expressing gratitude with peers. Such practices represent not weakness but adaptive emotional regulation, aligning with contemporary understandings of resilience as a dynamic, socially situated process rather than an individual trait (Richardson, 2002; Ungar, 2011).

Coping has long been conceptualized as the cognitive and behavioral effort to manage internal or external demands that exceed personal resources (Lazarus & Folkman, 1984). Health psychology extends this framework by considering how coping behaviors influence physiological and psychological health outcomes. Lenin's study identifies a spectrum of coping mechanisms employed by CSA therapists, including both adaptive (e.g., mindfulness, physical exercise, supervision) and maladaptive strategies (e.g., emotional suppression, avoidance).

Mindfulness practices deep breathing, grounding techniques, and body awareness emerged as crucial tools for emotional regulation. Several participants attributed their sustained engagement in trauma work to regular mindfulness routines: "Breathing helped me return to the present moment when I felt overwhelmed" (Lenin, in progress)Empirical research supports these findings, showing that mindfulness reduces physiological stress responses and fosters cognitive flexibility (Shapiro, Brown, & Biegel, 2007).

Another critical dimension of resilience identified in the study is spiritual coping. Therapists reported using prayer, reading sacred texts, and engaging in rituals as mechanisms of self-soothing and meaning reconstruction. Spirituality served as both a psychological anchor and a moral compass enabling therapists to view their work as part of a larger existential purpose. This resonates with Linley et al.

(2005), who found that individuals with a strong sense of coherence comprising comprehensibility, manageability, and meaningfulness demonstrate higher levels of post-traumatic growth.

Social connectedness also emerged as a protective factor. Counselors described finding solace in peer discussions, professional supervision, and informal debriefing sessions. These relational processes exemplify the *social ecology of resilience* (Ungar, 2011), which emphasizes that the availability of supportive environments significantly influences the capacity to recover from stress.

Meaning-making represents a central process in transforming trauma exposure into personal growth. Park (2010) defines meaning-making as the process through which individuals reconcile discrepancies between global beliefs and situational meaning following stressful events. In Lenin's study, therapists often reframed their distress as an opportunity for self-discovery and professional evolution.

One participant stated: *"Working with these children has changed how I see pain it's no longer something to fear but something that can teach."* Such narratives reflect post-traumatic growth (PTG) a construct referring to positive psychological change resulting from struggle with highly challenging circumstances (Tedeschi & Calhoun, 2004).

Therapists in the study reported three domains of growth:

1. **Personal Strength:** Gaining confidence and emotional maturity.
2. **Relational Depth:** Developing heightened empathy and authenticity in relationships.
3. **Existential Awareness:** Experiencing a renewed sense of purpose and connection with the divine or community.

Health psychology's integration of PTG provides a holistic lens to interpret these outcomes. It recognizes that stress-related growth does not negate suffering but reconfigures its meaning within a broader narrative of resilience. Lenin's participants often viewed their professional endurance not as resistance to pain but as transformation through it.

This reorientation aligns with the meaning-centered approach to health (Steger, 2012), which posits that individuals who derive meaning from adversity exhibit greater well-being and lower burnout. Therapists' ability to make sense of their emotional suffering becomes a mechanism of resilience, allowing them to sustain therapeutic engagement despite repeated exposure to trauma.

While research on vicarious trauma and burnout among Western therapists is substantial, studies addressing these phenomena within the Indian or broader South Asian context remain sparse. Existing literature predominantly focuses on survivor outcomes rather than caregiver well-being. Furthermore, cross-cultural variables such as spirituality, collectivism, and gendered caregiving roles are are often underrepresented in mainstream trauma literature.

Lenin's study contributes a rare, contextually grounded perspective by integrating cultural, spiritual, and emotional dimensions of therapist experience. However, translating thesc insights into broader frameworks of health psychology can deepen their applicability. Specifically, this chapter aims to:

- Bridge micro-level (individual coping) and macro-level (organizational, cultural) determinants of therapist health.
- Expand resilience theory by incorporating indigenous spiritual practices as valid psychological resources.
- Highlight the need for trauma-informed supervision and systemic self-care models in Indian mental health settings.

In doing so, the chapter aligns with global movements within health psychology to humanize healthcare providers as whole beings embedded within cultural and relational networks (Engel, 1977; Ungar, 2011). By focusing on the therapists who carry the emotional weight of others' suffering, this work advocates a paradigm shift from viewing mental health professionals as neutral agents to acknowledging them as participants in a shared process of healing and growth.

In summary, the background of this study underscores the multidimensional nature of therapist well-being in CSA counseling. Grounded in Blessy Lenin's qualitative exploration, the review reveals that therapists experience significant psychological and physical strain, but also possess remarkable capacities for adaptation and transformation. Their coping strategies rooted in mindfulness, spirituality, and community exemplify health psychology principles of resilience and meaning-making.

Culturally, the Indian context adds complexity: gendered expectations, social silence, and spiritual collectivism shape both the experience of stress and the pathways to recovery. The biopsychosocial model provides an integrative scaffold to understand these interactions, while resilience and meaning-making theories elucidate how therapists derive growth from adversity.

This foundation sets the stage for the next sections of the chapter, which elaborate the theoretical and methodological frameworks, present the empirical findings, and discuss their implications for health psychology, counseling training, and trauma-informed practice.

3. THEORETICAL AND CONCEPTUAL FRAMEWORK

3.1 The Biopsychosocial Model of Therapist Health

George Engel's (1977) biopsychosocial model revolutionized the understanding of health by proposing that illness and well-being arise from the complex interplay of biological, psychological, and social factors. Within the context of trauma work, this model serves as a holistic framework for understanding how counselors' physical symptoms, cognitive reactions, and social realities interconnect.

In Lenin's study, therapists described a range of biological symptoms fatigue, headaches, nausea, sleep disturbances, and somatic tension manifesting during or after counseling sessions with CSA survivors. One participant recalled, "After listening to the details of abuse, I would physically ache. It felt as though the pain had entered my body" (Lenin, in progress).

The psychological dimension of the model captures secondary trauma, emotional exhaustion, and cognitive schema disruptions. Counselors often experienced intrusive imagery and pervasive sadness, reflecting Figley's (1995) model of secondary traumatic stress disorder. Lenin's reported that therapists struggled to separate their professional identity from their emotional self, indicating blurred boundaries and internalized trauma.

The social dimension encompasses societal attitudes, organizational systems, and cultural values that shape how therapists perceive and manage their distress. In the Indian context, stigma surrounding mental illness and the idealization of self-sacrifice limit professionals' willingness to seek help. This cultural suppression amplifies burnout and feelings of isolation.

Thus, Engel's (1977) model underscores that addressing therapist well-being demands multi-level interventions self-care at the individual level, supportive supervision at the institutional level, and cultural reframing at the societal level. The model's strength lies in its compatibility with health psychology's emphasis on mind-body unity and contextual determinants of behavior.

3.2 Resilience Theory

Resilience theory, as articulated by Richardson (2002), conceptualizes resilience as a dynamic process involving disruption, reintegration, and growth following adversity. Rather than viewing resilience as a static trait, the theory portrays it as a continual cycle where individuals adapt through coping and meaning-making.

In Lenin's study, participants demonstrated resilience through adaptive reintegration using personal, social, and spiritual resources to re-establish psychological equilibrium after distressing sessions. Several reported findings renewed motivation and empathy after confronting their emotional breakdowns. One therapist reflected: "I used to question why I was doing this work. But every time I saw a child heal, it reminded me why I began" (Lenin, in progress).

Richardson's framework identifies four resilience outcomes: (a) dysfunctional reintegration (maladaptive coping), (b) recovery (return to baseline), (c) resilient reintegration (growth), and (d) loss. The therapists in Lenin's study predominantly reflected resilient reintegration, characterized by emotional maturity and deepened professional identity.

Health psychology integrates resilience theory to understand behavioral and cognitive mechanisms that facilitate adaptation. Practices such as mindfulness, supervision, and boundary setting foster emotional regulation and cognitive restructuring core mechanisms of resilience. In collectivist cultures, relational and spiritual dimensions play additional roles. As Ungar (2011) observes, resilience is embedded in social ecologies that provide meaning and belonging. The Indian therapists' reliance on faith communities and familial networks illustrates this cultural contextualization of resilience.

3.3 Meaning-Making Models

Meaning-making theory (Park, 2010) posits that individuals maintain global meaning systems beliefs, goals, and worldviews that help interpret experiences. When traumatic events disrupt these systems, individuals engage in cognitive processing to reconcile discrepancies between their beliefs and new realities.

For therapists working with CSA survivors, meaning-making becomes both a coping strategy and a professional transformation. Lenin's participants frequently redefined their work as spiritual vocation or moral duty. As one counselor expressed, *"I stopped asking why these things happen and started asking how I can be part of the healing"* (p. 172).

This reframing mirrors the meaning-centered approach to health (Steger, 2012), which emphasizes that purpose and coherence enhance psychological well-being. By finding meaning in suffering, therapists transform vicarious trauma into post-traumatic growth (PTG). Linley, Joseph, and Loumidis (2005) identified PTG as comprising enhanced relationships, appreciation of life, and existential growth all of which were echoed in Lenin's findings.

Meaning-making thus serves as both an explanatory and therapeutic construct: it illuminates how health professionals reconstruct identity in response to the emotional burdens of caregiving, positioning growth as an outcome rather than the absence of distress.

3.4 Cultural Psychology and Contextual Resilience

Cultural psychology recognizes that coping, emotion, and resilience are socially embedded and culturally mediated (Comas-Díaz & Jacobsen, 1991). Indian therapists operate within a context where spirituality, collectivism, and family are central to identity. Lenin's study shows that counselors drew on faith, ritual, and cultural idioms to sustain emotional energy.

For example, several participants employed prayer or meditation before sessions to "invoke strength." Others used collective rituals such as lighting candles or expressing gratitude as closure. These practices functioned as psychological boundaries and emotional grounding mechanisms. From a health-psychology standpoint, they exemplify culturally congruent coping behaviors that align with personal belief systems and community values, enhancing their efficacy (Kuo, 2013).

Cultural perspectives also contextualize gender. Female therapists navigated dual expectations: professional competence and emotional nurturing. While these expectations heightened vulnerability to compassion fatigue, they also facilitated deeper empathy and relational attunement. Such duality reflects the cultural embodiment of resilience as relational harmony rather than individual toughness (Ungar, 2011).

Hence, the theoretical integration of biopsychosocial, resilience, and meaning-making models anchored in cultural context offers a comprehensive lens for understanding therapist well-being within health psychology.

4. METHODOLOGY

4.1 Research Design

Blessy Lenin's study employed a qualitative, grounded-theory design within the discipline of psychology, focusing on the lived experiences of therapists who counsel CSA survivors. This approach allowed for an inductive exploration of subjective meaning, emotional complexity, and cultural nuance.

The study was conducted across four Indian metropolitan regions Bengaluru, Chennai, Delhi, and Mumbai chosen for their diverse cultural contexts and established child protection infrastructures. Data collection occurred over one year (2022–2023), combining in-depth semi-structured interviews and reflexive journaling.

4.2 Participants

Fourteen professional counselors (12 female, 2 male) participated. All held postgraduate degrees in counseling or clinical psychology and had a minimum of three years' experience working with CSA survivors. Participants represented NGOs, hospitals, and child protection organizations. Ages ranged from 28 to 45, with an average of 8.5 years in practice.

4.3 Data Collection

Each interview lasted 60–90 minutes, conducted either in person or via secure online platforms. Open-ended questions explored emotional, physical, spiritual, and professional impacts of trauma work. Example prompts included:

- "What are some of the emotional experiences you undergo after sessions with CSA survivors?"
- "How do you cope with feelings of distress or helplessness?"
- "In what ways do your cultural or spiritual beliefs influence your work?"

Interviews were audio-recorded, transcribed verbatim, and coded using Taguette, an open-source qualitative analysis software. Reflexivity journals captured the researcher's personal responses, ensuring awareness of bias.

4.4 Data Analysis

Data were analyzed using Braun and Clarke's (2006) six-step thematic analysis framework: familiarization, coding, theme generation, review, definition, and write-up. Two independent coders cross-validated themes for reliability. The iterative process produced 26 core themes, grouped into five domains:

1. Physical and emotional effects of trauma work.
2. Self-care and supervision.
3. Spirituality and cultural influence.
4. Professional boundaries and identity.
5. Meaning-making and growth.

4.5 Ethical Considerations

Ethical clearance was obtained from the institutional review board. Participants provided informed consent, ensuring confidentiality and withdrawal rights. Given the sensitive nature of the topic, counselors were provided access to peer support if interviews triggered emotional discomfort. The researcher's reflexive stance ensured empathy and ethical mindfulness throughout data collection (Lenin, in progress).

5. FINDINGS AND DISCUSSION

Lenin's thematic findings, interpreted through health psychology theories, reveal a dynamic balance between distress and growth. The discussion below integrates empirical evidence with conceptual frameworks.

5.1 Physical and Psychological Effects

Therapists reported substantial psychosomatic manifestations, including headaches, stomach pain, appetite loss, and fatigue. The bodily dimension of trauma underscores the embodiment of empathy: the physical translation of emotional pain (van der Kolk, 2014). These findings corroborate Engel's (1977) biopsychosocial principle that psychological stress manifests physiologically.

Emotionally, participants described anger, guilt, helplessness, and sadness. These experiences align with countertransference phenomena described by Prasko et al. (2022). Therapists often oscillated between compassion and avoidance, revealing an ongoing struggle to maintain emotional boundaries.

Yet, awareness of these reactions prompted self-regulation. Many counselors adopted grounding techniques to prevent emotional flooding. This adaptive self-awareness illustrates the stress and coping model of Lazarus and Folkman (1984) where cognitive appraisal and behavioral strategies determine stress outcomes.

5.2 Self-Care and Coping Strategies

Self-care emerged as both necessity and challenge. Lenin notes that many therapists initially undervalued self-care, perceiving it as indulgent rather than essential. Over time, they recognized its critical role in sustaining empathy and efficacy.

Adaptive coping mechanisms included:

- **Mindfulness and breathing exercises:** Used to restore focus during distressing sessions.
- **Physical activity:** Walking, yoga, and dance to release tension.
- **Journaling:** To externalize emotions and reflect on professional boundaries.
- **Supervision and peer consultation:** Providing normalization and shared understanding.

These strategies demonstrate a health-psychology application of behavioral self-regulation. Shapiro, Brown, and Biegel (2007) emphasize that mindfulness enhances interoceptive awareness and reduces emotional exhaustion, findings echoed in Lenin's sample.

Spiritual practices such as prayer and gratitude constituted another form of coping. For many Indian therapists, faith-based reflection provided a sense of coherence and moral renewal. This *spiritual resilience* aligns with Linley et al. (2005), who linked sense of coherence with positive post-traumatic change.

5.3 Supervision, Boundaries, and Ethical Containment

Effective supervision mitigates burnout and vicarious trauma (Pearlman & Saakvitne, 1995). However, Lenin's reports that structured supervision remains limited in India. Counselors often rely on informal peer support rather than institutionalized systems. The absence of professional containment contributes to over-identification and boundary erosion.

Participants described difficulty "switching off" after sessions and carrying emotional residue home. This phenomenon, labeled emotional spillover, exemplifies the breakdown of professional boundaries (Rose et al., 2025). However, through reflective practice and self-awareness, many therapists gradually learned to compartmentalize demonstrating adaptive boundary formation as a resilience mechanism.

5.4 Spirituality and Cultural Influences

Spirituality permeated nearly all narratives. Counselors interpreted their vocation as divinely guided, framing their work as service (*seva*). Spiritual coping involved prayer, meditation, gratitude, and surrender to higher purpose. Such orientation reduced moral distress and cultivated meaning a protective factor against compassion fatigue (Linley et al., 2005).

Cultural influences shaped both coping and vulnerability. In collectivist contexts, emotional expression through shared rituals or storytelling enabled catharsis. Religion offered a moral framework for understanding suffering. However, cultural stigma around sexuality also intensified isolation; counselors hesitated to discuss CSA-related distress with family or clergy for fear of judgment.

Health psychology's acknowledgment of cultural determinants (Engel, 1977; Comas-Díaz & Jacobsen, 1991) is essential here: resilience emerges not merely from individual willpower but from the congruence between personal coping styles and cultural meaning systems.

5.5 Meaning-Making and Professional Growth

Perhaps the most transformative finding was the evolution of meaning-making. Many therapists described initial despair evolving into deeper purpose and existential insight. Through continuous engagement with trauma, they reconstructed their worldview:

- **Enhanced empathy:** "I no longer see pain as something to fix but something to sit with."
- **Strengthened identity:** "I have become more authentic, both as a therapist and as a person."
- **Moral reorientation:** "I found faith not as dogma, but as the strength to keep showing up."

These statements exemplify post-traumatic growth (Tedeschi & Calhoun, 2004). Rather than succumbing to burnout, counselors experienced self-expansion illustrating Richardson's (2002) model of resilient reintegration.

Meaning-making served a restorative function: by aligning their professional suffering with higher purpose, therapists converted vulnerability into strength. From a health-psychology standpoint, this process reflects psychological immunity the cognitive reframing of stress that preserves mental equilibrium (Steger, 2012).

5.6 Integrating Findings with Health Psychology

The synthesis of Lenin's empirical data with theoretical constructs yields several overarching insights:

1. **Health as Integration:** The biopsychosocial model encapsulates how emotional exposure (psychological), somatic distress (biological), and sociocultural context (social) intersect in therapist experiences.
2. **Resilience as Process:** Consistent with Richardson's (2002) framework, resilience among therapists is cyclical alternating between breakdown, reflection, and reintegration.
3. **Meaning as Medicine:** Spiritual and existential meaning-making transforms distress into growth, functioning as an intrinsic coping mechanism (Park, 2010).
4. **Culture as Context:** Coping behaviors derive potency from cultural alignment; spiritual collectivism and relational support enhance resilience (Ungar, 2011).

These insights demonstrate that therapist well-being is not peripheral but central to the health-psychology enterprise. The profession's emphasis on patient care must expand to include caregiver health as a determinant of therapeutic efficacy.

6. RECOMMENDATIONS AND SOLUTIONS

6.1 Institutional and Organizational Support

Therapists who work with CSA survivors operate in emotionally demanding environments where sustained exposure to trauma narratives can lead to burnout and secondary traumatization. Lenin's study clearly demonstrates that many Indian organizations lack the structural frameworks to support therapists' mental health. Addressing this gap requires systemic reform across three tiers **supervision, workload management, and organizational culture.**

1. **Supervision and Reflective Practice**
    - o Establish formal, structured supervision frameworks within child welfare and counseling organizations.
    - o Supervisors should be trained in trauma-informed supervision (Pearlman & Saakvitne, 1995), focusing on empathic containment and reflective processing rather than mere performance evaluation.
    - o Incorporate group supervision and peer debriefing sessions that enable normalization and mutual validation, reducing feelings of isolation.
2. **Workload Regulation and Burnout Prevention**
    - o Institutional policies must cap the number of trauma cases per therapist to ensure emotional sustainability.
    - o Rotational case assignments or "cool-down" periods after intense cases can prevent emotional exhaustion.
    - o Regular wellness audits and mental health check-ins should be mandatory for all trauma counselors.
3. **Organizational Culture**
    - o Promote a culture of compassion and open dialogue where self-care is encouraged rather than stigmatized.
    - o Integrate employee assistance programs that provide access to confidential counseling for staff members.
    - o Recognize emotional labor as a legitimate component of professional output during performance reviews.

Health psychology emphasizes that environmental conditions significantly shape health outcomes (Engel, 1977). Institutional reforms, therefore, represent a vital component of the biopsychosocial approach to therapist well-being.

6.2 Training and Curriculum Enhancement

Counseling and psychology curricula in India and similar contexts often emphasize clinical skills while neglecting practitioner self-awareness and emotional resilience (Lenin, in progress). The following recommendations address this gap:

- **Integrate Self-Care and Mindfulness Modules:**

Incorporate training on mindfulness-based stress reduction (MBSR) and compassion-focused therapy (CFT) techniques (Shapiro et al., 2007).

- **Trauma-Informed Education:**

Include courses on trauma physiology, vicarious trauma, and secondary stress management within counseling programs.

- **Supervision Pedagogy:**

Train emerging supervisors in reflective supervision, which emphasizes empathy, process analysis, and boundary management (Rose et al., 2025).

- **Cultural Competence Training:**

Expose students to indigenous models of healing, community-based care, and spiritual integration. This decolonizes psychological education and ensures that coping practices remain culturally congruent (Kuo, 2013).

Such curricular reforms align with health psychology's commitment to bridging scientific knowledge with lived human experience, fostering a generation of counselors who can sustain their health while supporting others.

6.3 Enhancing Coping and Resilience in Practice

From Lenin's findings, resilience is not innate it is cultivated through intentional coping mechanisms. Health psychology frameworks suggest that adaptive coping promotes both psychological and physiological well-being. Thus, practical strategies include:

1. **Mindfulness and Embodied Awareness**

Daily mindfulness practices—such as breath awareness, yogic movement, and contemplative exercises—facilitate the reconnection of mind and body, contributing to reduced cortisol levels and enhanced emotional regulation (Shapiro et al., 2007). As Mindfulness-Based Interventions (MBIs) gain increasing prominence across educational, clinical, and organizational settings, their application within both Western and Indian psychological traditions necessitates a culturally sensitive, evidence-informed, and ethically grounded approach to practice and research. Drawing on the comparative insights of Singha and Singha (2024), mindfulness practices must be adapted to respect indigenous belief systems, linguistic diversity, and socio-spiritual values. In the Indian context, this involves anchoring mindfulness in traditional contemplative systems such as yoga, Vedantic psychology, and Buddhist Vipassana, thereby ensuring conceptual continuity with native philosophical traditions. Western adaptations, by contrast, may continue to emphasize secular and cognitive frameworks (e.g., MBSR, MBCT), while incorporating multicultural competence training to mitigate the risks of cultural appropriation.

Beyond therapeutic and educational domains, mindfulness assumes critical relevance within contemporary socio-political contexts characterized by polarization and the rise of populist movements. As examined by Singha and Singha (2024b), mindfulness functions as a psychological resource that enables young individuals to resist the affective appeal of populist rhetoric by strengthening emotional regulation, critical awareness, and resilience. In emotionally dysregulated environments, fear-based narratives and divisive ideologies are often amplified. When combined with emotional intelligence, mindfulness equips young people with the capacity to engage reflectively with contentious ideas rather than responding reactively. The authors further emphasize the importance of culturally responsive strategies and awareness-building initiatives to ensure that mindfulness-based approaches remain contextually relevant and ethically grounded. Integrating mindfulness into everyday practices thus emerges as a practical and preventive strategy for fostering psychologically resilient, socially aware, and critically engaged youth capable of navigating complex ideological landscapes.

At a deeper theoretical level, mindfulness operates in a reciprocal relationship with social cognitive processing. As articulated by Singha (2024), present-moment awareness both shapes and is shaped by social interactions, norms, and relational contexts. This bidirectional dynamic enhances social cognition by fostering empathy, compassion, and prosocial behaviour, while simultaneously cultivating a more integrated and harmonious sense of self. The multifunctionality of mindfulness becomes evident across interpersonal, organizational, and educational domains, where it contributes to reduced psychological tension, improved team dynamics, and more adaptive social engagement. Longitudinal evidence further underscores the durability of these effects, demonstrating sustained improvements in well-being and social functioning over time. Consequently, mindfulness emerges as a powerful catalyst for positive social change, with the potential to nurture communities that are more interconnected, empathetic, and responsive to collective challenges.

Mindfulness must also be situated within the broader socio-economic realities shaping contemporary educational and professional environments. Addressing precarity within neoliberal education systems requires comprehensive interventions that integrate mindfulness with addiction prevention and resilience-building strategies. As Singha (2026) argues, addiction, resilience, and mindfulness constitute interlinked dimensions in responding to the psychological strain experienced by learners and educators under conditions of instability. Substance use frequently emerges as a maladaptive coping response to stress and uncertainty, underscoring the importance of robust mental health support systems and structured mentoring initiatives. Within this framework, mindfulness serves as a protective mechanism by enhancing emotional regulation, tolerance of uncertainty, and adaptive resilience. Accordingly, a holistic strategy that integrates mindfulness practices, addiction-responsive interventions, and resilience-oriented support systems is essential for advancing educational equity, well-being, and sustainable engagement in precarious learning environments.

Extending these insights into pedagogical practice, mindfulness and meditation offer transformative benefits that extend beyond academic achievement. As highlighted by Singha (2025), the systematic incorporation of mindfulness within educational settings enhances cognitive functioning, emotional regulation, and attentional capacity, thereby strengthening resilience and fostering a positive, future-oriented outlook among learners. Over time, such practices contribute to the development of emotionally resilient, socially competent, and intrinsically motivated individuals, while also promoting overall well-being and sustained inspiration. Importantly, the cultivation of mindfulness is not limited to students alone; educators play a pivotal role by embodying mindfulness principles in their pedagogical approaches and serving as role models within the learning ecosystem. This integrative educational methodology encourages the continuous adaptation of instructional strategies, ensuring that learners are equipped with the psychological resources necessary to navigate uncertainty and envision more resilient and meaningful futures.

Building upon this foundation, the integration of mindfulness with compassion and service learning in higher education offers a comprehensive pedagogical framework for transformative learning. As proposed by Singha (2024b), drawing on service-learning frameworks, compassion education models, contemplative pedagogy, transformative learning theory, and holistic education paradigms enables educators to design learning experiences that foreground civic responsibility, self-awareness, and critical reflection. Through engagement with this integrated conceptual terrain, learners are nurtured as conscientious, empathetic, and socially accountable individuals—qualities essential for engaging with the complexities of contemporary life and fostering meaningful and sustainable social change.

These frameworks must further be extended to address the needs of neurodiverse individuals, who often experience distinct cognitive, emotional, and social challenges that may heighten vulnerability to addictive behaviours. Conventional addiction models frequently overlook the lived realities of neurodiverse populations, underscoring the need for more inclusive and responsive approaches. Building on this recognition, the chapter advocates for the systematic incorporation of mindfulness practices into professional preparation programmes as an inclusive strategy for addiction prevention and recovery. Mindfulness approaches grounded in present-moment awareness and non-judgmental observation of thoughts and emotions can be adapted to accommodate diverse cognitive and sensory profiles. Such practices function not only as therapeutic tools for addiction recovery, but also as mechanisms for enhancing emotional regulation, self-awareness, and adaptive coping. Embedding mindfulness-based approaches within professional preparation programmes thus fosters more equitable, supportive, and effective pathways for recovery and inclusive professional development (Singha & Singha, 2024c).

Finally, the discourse on mindfulness, addiction, and social well-being must also account for the pivotal role of women-led collective action in community transformation. In the Indian context, women's empowerment initiatives and self-help groups have proven to be largely effective at the grassroots level. However, their impact can be further strengthened through the incorporation of standardized quality parameters within training programmes. While locally organized skill-training initiatives facilitated by empowerment cells operate efficiently, there remains a need for structured training frameworks that enable self-help groups to meet international standards in production, management, and sustainability.

A significant challenge lies in the decentralized and remote nature of many training programmes, which often limits sustained engagement by facilitators. Establishing clear criteria for trainer selection and implementing context-sensitive, well-planned curricula are therefore essential. Beyond structural constraints, social impediments—most notably drug and alcohol addiction reinforced by certain cultural and societal norms—continue to undermine empowerment efforts. Women's collectives have demonstrated considerable capacity to confront these challenges. Notably, the Naga Mothers' Association has played a transformative role in reducing substance abuse through community mobilization, moral authority, and sustained advocacy, although stronger legislative and institutional support remains necessary.

Similarly, the women's wing of the Koch Rajbongshi Students' Union has effectively mobilized communities and disseminated awareness regarding the harmful effects of addiction, illustrating the broader potential of women-led grassroots movements in addressing entrenched social evils. These initiatives underscore the importance of integrating mindfulness—rooted in Buddhist contemplative traditions—as a foundational mechanism for social change. As argued by Singha and Kanna (2022), mindfulness and compassion are central to addressing addiction and social degradation, while reflective awareness enables informed, ethical, and contextually grounded decision-making. When mindfulness, compassion, and reflective practice are embedded within empowerment and training programmes, women emerge not only as economic agents but also as moral leaders capable of catalyzing sustainable and transformative social change in Indian society (Singha & Kanna, 2022

2. **Cognitive Reframing and Meaning-Making**

Cognitive reframing and meaning-making are essential processes for helping therapists navigate professional distress, particularly when working in emotionally demanding contexts. Rather than viewing distress solely as a sign of burnout or impairment, therapists can be guided to reinterpret challenging experiences as opportunities for personal and professional growth. Cognitive reframing enables individuals to shift maladaptive interpretations of stress toward more constructive perspectives, thereby enhancing psychological resilience and sustaining professional commitment.

Meaning-making practices play a central role in this process. Reflective writing allows therapists to process complex emotional experiences, identify recurring themes, and gain insight into how their work aligns with personal values and professional purpose. Gratitude journaling further supports this process by redirecting attention toward positive experiences, accomplishments, and relational strengths, counterbalancing the emotional weight of therapeutic work. Such practices foster emotional balance and reinforce a sense of efficacy and appreciation.

Existential inquiry offers an additional layer of depth by encouraging therapists to explore questions related to meaning, purpose, suffering, and growth. Through this reflective engagement, distressing experiences can be integrated into a coherent personal narrative rather than remaining fragmented or overwhelming. As Park (2010) emphasizes, meaning-making is a dynamic process that supports psychological adjustment to stressful life events. When embedded within professional support and training contexts, cognitive reframing and meaning-making not only reduce distress but also promote long-term well-being, professional identity development, and post-adversarial growth among therapists.

3. **Boundary Setting**

Boundary setting is a critical self-care and ethical practice for therapists, particularly those working with trauma, vulnerability, and high emotional demand. Establishing clear physical, emotional, and temporal boundaries helps prevent role overload, emotional exhaustion, and secondary traumatization. As Baum (2016) highlights, blurred boundaries and excessive case overlap can intensify exposure to clients' distress, increasing the risk of compassion fatigue and reduced professional effectiveness.

Clear temporal boundaries are especially important. Defining therapy hours, limiting after-hours communication, and scheduling regular breaks allow therapists to maintain psychological distance from work-related stressors. Avoiding excessive case overlap—particularly when working with clients experiencing similar forms of trauma—reduces cumulative emotional strain and supports sustained attentional focus. Physical boundaries, such as maintaining dedicated workspaces and minimizing work-related intrusions into personal environments, further reinforce this separation.

4. Equally important is the intentional preservation of personal life. Maintaining boundaries between professional and personal roles enables therapists to engage in restorative activities, relationships, and identities beyond their clinical work. This separation not only supports emotional recovery but also enhances therapeutic presence and ethical practice. Boundary setting should be understood not as disengagement, but as a proactive strategy for sustaining empathy, competence, and long-term professional well-being. When integrated into training and supervision, boundary awareness empowers therapists to protect their mental health while delivering effective and compassionate care (Baum, 2016).**Social Support Networks**

Cultivate supportive communities through professional networks, workshops, and retreats. Social connectedness serves as a buffer against occupational stress (Ungar, 2011).

5. **Spiritual Engagement**

Spiritual engagement can serve as a vital source of comfort, coherence, and resilience for therapists working in emotionally demanding and trauma-exposed contexts. Encouraging therapists to draw upon their personal or culturally rooted spiritual practices allows them to reconnect with deeper sources of meaning, hope, and inner stability. Spirituality, in this sense, need not be confined to formal religious traditions; it may also encompass personal belief systems, contemplative practices, values-based reflection, or culturally embedded rituals that foster a sense of purpose and transcendence.

Findings from Lenin's study highlight the protective role of spiritual practices such as prayer, gratitude, and ritual in sustaining professionals' emotional endurance. These practices helped therapists maintain hope, process moral and emotional strain, and regain a sense of coherence amid repeated exposure to client suffering. Prayer and reflective rituals offered moments of pause and surrender, while gratitude practices enabled therapists to acknowledge positive experiences and affirm the meaningful impact of their work.

Spiritual engagement also supports ethical grounding and compassion, allowing therapists to remain connected to their core values while navigating professional challenges. When respected as a personal resource rather than imposed as a clinical requirement, spirituality can complement psychological self-care strategies and enhance overall well-being. Integrating space for spiritual reflection within supervision and self-care planning can therefore strengthen therapists' resilience, support long-term engagement in practice, and promote a balanced integration of professional competence and inner life.These strategies align with the meaning-centered approach to health (Steger, 2012), which asserts that the capacity to find coherence amid adversity is fundamental to psychological resilience.

6.4 Policy-Level Recommendations

To institutionalize therapist well-being at the systemic level, policymakers and professional associations must implement structural changes:

- **National Guidelines for Therapist Well-Being:**

The development of national guidelines for therapist well-being is essential to ensure ethical, sustainable, and effective mental health practice. Regulatory bodies such as the Rehabilitation Council of India (RCI) and other professional governing institutions play a critical role in shaping standards of care, professional conduct, and practitioner accountability. Recognizing therapist self-care as an ethical responsibility—not merely a personal choice—marks a crucial shift toward safeguarding both practitioner well-being and client outcomes.

Therapists working in high-demand clinical, educational, and community settings are routinely exposed to emotional distress, trauma narratives, and systemic pressures that place them at increased risk of burnout, compassion fatigue, and secondary traumatization. National ethical guidelines that explicitly address therapist well-being can provide a formal framework for preventive care, emphasizing manageable caseloads, adequate supervision, regular breaks, and access to mental health support services. Such guidelines would also legitimize self-care practices as integral to professional competence and ethical responsibility.

Embedding therapist well-being within ethical codes encourages institutions and employers to share accountability for practitioner health rather than placing the burden solely on individuals. It further promotes a culture of openness, reducing stigma around help-seeking among mental health professionals. By institutionalizing self-care as an ethical mandate, national regulatory bodies can strengthen professional sustainability, enhance quality of care, and foster a healthier, more resilient mental health workforce across the country.

- **Funding for Counselor Support Programs:**

Allocating dedicated government and Corporate Social Responsibility (CSR) funding for counselor support programs is a critical step toward strengthening the mental health workforce, particularly within trauma-focused non-governmental organizations (NGOs). Counselors and therapists working in trauma-related settings are frequently exposed to high levels of emotional distress, secondary trauma, and resource constraints, which significantly increase the risk of burnout and reduced service quality. Establishing well-funded resilience centers and professional supervision services can provide essential structural support to address these challenges.

Resilience centers can function as safe spaces where counselors access psychological support, peer consultation, mindfulness-based stress reduction, and skills for emotional regulation and coping. Such centers may also offer workshops on boundary setting, self-care, and trauma-informed practice, fostering sustained professional well-being. Equally important are structured supervision services, which allow counselors to reflect on complex cases, manage emotional overload, and maintain ethical and professional standards. Regular supervision has been shown to reduce isolation, enhance clinical competence, and support long-term engagement in trauma care.

Government funding and CSR initiatives can play a complementary role in sustaining these programs, particularly in under-resourced NGOs. By investing in counselor well-being, funding bodies indirectly improve the quality, continuity, and ethical integrity of trauma services. Institutionalizing such support systems signals a commitment to workforce sustainability, ensuring that those who care for others are themselves adequately supported, resilient, and empowered to continue their vital work.

- **Mandatory Debriefing in High-Trauma Settings:**

Mandatory debriefing in high-trauma settings is a crucial organizational practice for protecting the psychological well-being of mental health professionals. Counselors, therapists, and frontline workers who are repeatedly exposed to critical incidents—such as abuse cases, disaster response, or severe violence—face heightened risks of secondary traumatic stress, emotional exhaustion, and burnout. Requiring structured debriefing sessions after exposure to such cases helps mitigate these risks by providing a formal space for emotional processing, reflection, and support.

Structured debriefing, modeled on crisis intervention approaches used in disaster management, allows professionals to articulate emotional responses, normalize stress reactions, and integrate challenging experiences in a supportive environment. These sessions are not intended to evaluate performance, but rather to promote psychological safety and collective coping. Facilitated by trained supervisors or mental health professionals, debriefings can include guided reflection, stress regulation techniques, and peer support, helping individuals regain emotional equilibrium before returning to routine responsibilities.

Institutionalizing mandatory debriefing also signals organizational responsibility for staff well-being, reducing stigma around emotional vulnerability in professional settings. When embedded within trauma-informed organizational policies, debriefing practices enhance resilience, prevent cumulative stress, and support ethical and effective service delivery. Ultimately, mandatory debriefing ensures that professionals exposed to high-impact trauma are not left to process distress in isolation, fostering sustainable practice and long-term workforce health.

- **Research Incentives:**

Providing targeted research incentives is essential for advancing a culturally grounded and evidence-based understanding of therapist resilience. Encouraging systematic studies on indigenous coping strategies and cross-cultural models of well-being allows mental health practice to move beyond Western-centric frameworks and better reflect the diverse socio-cultural contexts in which therapists operate. Such research is particularly important in countries with rich indigenous traditions, where community-based healing practices, spiritual resources, and collective coping mechanisms have long supported psychological resilience but remain underrepresented in mainstream literature.

Research incentives such as dedicated grants, fellowships, and institutional recognition can motivate scholars and practitioners to document, validate, and critically examine these indigenous approaches. Studies focusing on culturally embedded practices, including mindfulness traditions, ritual, storytelling, community support, and spiritual engagement, can offer valuable insights into sustainable coping mechanisms for therapists working in high-stress environments. Cross-cultural comparative research further enables the identification of universal and context-specific resilience factors, supporting the development of adaptable intervention models.

Integrating findings from such research into training curricula, supervision frameworks, and organizational policies strengthens evidence-based practice while respecting cultural diversity. Moreover, incentivizing practitioner-led research encourages reflective practice and bridges the gap between theory and lived professional experience. By prioritizing research on indigenous and cross-cultural resilience strategies, institutions can foster more inclusive, ethical, and effective approaches to therapist well-being, ultimately enhancing the quality and sustainability of mental health care delivery. Such policies align with the World Health Organization's (2013) call to protect caregiver health as an integral component of sustainable healthcare systems.

7. FUTURE DIRECTIONS

While Lenin's study provides a rich foundation for understanding therapists' lived experiences, several areas warrant further exploration to expand the scope of health psychology and trauma care.

7.1 Longitudinal Studies on Therapist Adaptation

Longitudinal research designs are essential for developing a nuanced understanding of how therapists' coping strategies, resilience, and professional well-being evolve over time. Unlike cross-sectional studies, longitudinal approaches allow researchers to track changes in psychological, emotional, and physiological functioning across different stages of a therapist's career. Such designs are particularly valuable for examining whether early-career counselors differ from more experienced professionals in their responses to stress, exposure to trauma, and capacity for emotional regulation.

Future longitudinal studies could explore how repeated exposure to high-intensity clinical work influences therapists' adaptation processes, including shifts in coping styles, meaning-making, and professional identity. Tracking cohorts from training through advanced practice may reveal critical periods of vulnerability or growth, informing targeted interventions. Importantly, long-term data can help determine whether structured supports—such as mindfulness-based training, supervision, and reflective practices—produce sustained benefits rather than short-term relief.

Incorporating physiological indicators (e.g., cortisol levels, heart rate variability) alongside psychological measures (e.g., burnout, compassion satisfaction, resilience) would strengthen the evidence base by linking subjective experience with objective outcomes. Such integrative research can clarify causal pathways and identify protective factors that buffer against cumulative stress. Ultimately, longitudinal studies on therapist adaptation can inform evidence-based training models, organizational policies, and ethical guidelines, contributing to the development of a resilient, sustainable, and well-supported mental health workforce.

7.2 Gendered Dimensions of Trauma Work

A gendered analysis of trauma work is essential, particularly in the context of child sexual abuse (CSA) counseling, where women constitute the majority of the professional workforce. The predominance of women in this field means that emotional labor—such as sustained empathy, nurturing, and relational engagement—is often implicitly expected and unevenly distributed. These expectations are frequently shaped by gender norms that position women as natural caregivers, which can intensify emotional demands and increase vulnerability to burnout, compassion fatigue, and secondary traumatic stress.

Gender norms also influence boundary setting and help-seeking behaviors within professional contexts. Women therapists may experience greater pressure to maintain availability, flexibility, and emotional responsiveness, making it more challenging to establish clear professional boundaries or refuse excessive workloads. Access to supervision and institutional support may further be shaped by gendered power dynamics, organizational hierarchies, and cultural expectations, affecting how women navigate professional vulnerability and self-care. Additionally, professional identity formation among women counselors is often intertwined with societal narratives of self-sacrifice and moral responsibility, which may discourage the prioritization of personal well-being.

Exploring these gendered dimensions through systematic research can inform the development of gender-sensitive training and support systems. Such approaches may include supervision models attentive to emotional labor, training on assertive boundary setting, and organizational policies that recognize and redistribute care work. Addressing gendered patterns in trauma work is therefore crucial for fostering equitable, sustainable, and psychologically safe professional environments.

7.3 Technological Interventions and Digital Resilience

The rapid expansion of teletherapy and digital mental health platforms has transformed the delivery of psychological services, creating new opportunities for access, continuity of care, and professional support. At the same time, this digital shift introduces distinct stressors for therapists, including prolonged screen exposure, blurred work–life boundaries, digital fatigue, and a heightened risk of compassion fatigue. The absence of physical co-presence with clients can intensify cognitive load and emotional strain, requiring therapists to adapt new modes of attentional and emotional regulation.

Within this evolving landscape, technological interventions offer promising avenues for strengthening digital resilience among mental health professionals. AI-assisted supervision tools, for instance, can support reflective practice by identifying patterns in case documentation, flagging potential risk indicators, and offering structured feedback to complement human supervision. Virtual mindfulness programs and guided digital interventions can provide flexible, on-demand resources for stress reduction, emotional regulation, and self-care, particularly for practitioners in remote or under-resourced settings. Mobile applications tailored to counselor well-being may further facilitate daily mindfulness practices, mood tracking, and boundary management.

However, the integration of technology must remain ethically grounded, trauma-informed, and supportive rather than intrusive. Research is needed to evaluate the effectiveness, acceptability, and long-term impact of digital tools on therapist well-being. By thoughtfully leveraging technological innovations, mental health systems can enhance accessibility, scalability, and sustainability of support while fostering adaptive digital resilience in an increasingly virtual therapeutic environment.

7.4 Cross-Cultural Comparisons

Cross-cultural comparative research offers valuable insights into how cultural contexts shape therapists' resilience, coping strategies, and professional well-being. Comparing practitioners working in collectivist societies such as India and Sri Lanka with those in more individualist contexts like the United States and the United Kingdom can illuminate culturally specific pathways through which resilience is cultivated and sustained. In collectivist cultures, resilience is often embedded within relational networks, community support, shared responsibility, and spiritual or cultural practices, whereas individualist societies may emphasize personal autonomy, self-efficacy, and individualized coping mechanisms.

Such comparisons can reveal how cultural values influence therapists' perceptions of stress, boundary setting, help-seeking behavior, and meaning-making in professional roles. For example, collectivist frameworks may normalize shared emotional labor and communal coping, while individualist models may prioritize personal self-care and professional independence. Understanding these differences can help identify both protective and risk factors unique to each cultural context.

Importantly, cross-cultural studies can contribute to the development of more inclusive global health psychology frameworks by integrating indigenous and non-Western models of resilience that are often marginalized in mainstream research. By valuing culturally rooted practices—such as mindfulness traditions, ritual, community engagement, and collective reflection—researchers can enrich theoretical models and inform culturally responsive training, supervision, and policy interventions. Ultimately, cross-cultural comparisons foster a more nuanced, equitable, and globally relevant understanding of therapist resilience and well-being.

7.5 Neuroscientific Integration

Integrating neuroscientific perspectives into the study of therapist well-being offers a powerful avenue for advancing understanding of compassion fatigue, empathy fatigue, and resilience. Emerging research employing neuroimaging techniques—such as functional magnetic resonance imaging (fMRI), electroencephalography (EEG), and neuroendocrine assessments—has begun to illuminate how repeated exposure to trauma narratives and emotional distress alters brain functioning. Prolonged empathic engagement with clients may affect neural networks involved in emotion regulation, threat detection, and stress responsivity, including the amygdala, prefrontal cortex, and insular regions.

Understanding these neural mechanisms can clarify why therapists may experience emotional exhaustion, reduced empathic capacity, or heightened reactivity over time. Importantly, neuroscientific findings can be meaningfully integrated with psychological theories of stress, coping, and meaning-making to create a more comprehensive model of therapist adaptation. For instance, mindfulness and compassion-based practices have been shown to modulate neural activity associated with emotional regulation and attentional control, suggesting their potential to counteract the neurobiological effects of chronic stress and secondary trauma.

By bridging neuroscience and psychology, future resilience training programs can be grounded in both subjective experience and objective biological evidence. Such integration may lead to the development of targeted interventions that enhance neural plasticity, support emotional balance, and sustain empathic engagement. Ultimately, neuroscientific integration holds promise for revolutionizing therapist training, supervision, and self-care by aligning clinical practice with emerging insights into brain–behavior relationships.

7.6 Policy-Oriented Action Research

Policy-oriented action research offers a pragmatic and collaborative pathway for translating theoretical insights on therapist well-being into sustainable practice. By fostering partnerships among universities, non-governmental organizations (NGOs), and government bodies, such research can bridge the longstanding gap between academic knowledge and policy implementation. These collaborations enable the co-creation, testing, and refinement of contextually relevant interventions that respond directly to the lived challenges faced by therapists working in high-trauma and resource-constrained environments.

One promising avenue involves the development and evaluation of pilot initiatives such as "therapist resilience clinics," which can provide integrated services including psychological support, peer consultation, supervision, and mindfulness-based self-care. Similarly, trauma-informed training modules designed through collaborative action research can be embedded within professional education and in-service training programs, ensuring alignment with regulatory standards and institutional realities. Action research methodologies allow for iterative feedback, continuous improvement, and stakeholder engagement, enhancing both effectiveness and acceptability.

Importantly, policy-oriented action research positions therapists not merely as recipients of interventions but as active contributors to knowledge generation and policy design. Findings from such projects can inform evidence-based guidelines, funding priorities, and regulatory reforms at institutional and national levels. By grounding policy in empirical practice-based evidence, this approach supports scalable, culturally responsive, and sustainable solutions that strengthen therapist resilience while advancing ethical and effective mental health systems.

8. CONCLUSION

Therapists who work with survivors of child sexual abuse occupy a paradoxical position: they are both healers and witnesses to suffering. Blessy Lenin's study unveils the hidden emotional costs of caregiving in the Indian context while highlighting the transformative potential of coping, resilience, and meaning-making.

From a health psychology perspective, this work redefines therapist well-being as a multidimensional construct influenced by biological stress responses, psychological regulation, social support, and cultural meaning systems (Engel, 1977). The findings demonstrate that resilience is not the absence of distress but the ability to adaptively reintegrate after disruption (Richardson, 2002).

Meaning-making emerges as the cornerstone of this reintegration allowing therapists to derive purpose and identity from their encounters with trauma (Park, 2010; Steger, 2012). In a society where silence and stigma persist, Indian therapists model courage through service, spiritual grounding, and cultural creativity. Their stories expand the boundaries of global health psychology, reminding us that healing is reciprocal and that caregivers, too, need care.

To sustain trauma professionals, systemic support must complement individual coping: organizations must institutionalize supervision, education must emphasize reflective self-care, and policy must recognize counselor well-being as essential public health.

Ultimately, this chapter advances a holistic vision of health psychology one that integrates behavior, resilience, and meaning into a unified model of human flourishing. By nurturing the healers, we safeguard the healing process itself.

REFERENCES

Baum, N. (2016). Secondary traumatization in mental health professionals: A systematic review of gender findings. *Traumatology, 22*(2), 144–151. DOI: 10.1177/1524838015584357 PMID: 25964278

Brady, J. L., Guy, J. D., Poelstra, P. L., & Brokaw, B. F. (1999). Vicarious traumatization, spirituality, and the treatment of sexual abuse survivors: A national survey of women psychotherapists. *Professional Psychology, Research and Practice, 30*(4), 386–393. https://psycnet.apa.org/doi/10.1037/0735-7028.30.4.386. DOI: 10.1037/0735-7028.30.4.386

Braun, V., & Clarke, V. (2006). Using thematic analysis in psychology. *Qualitative Research in Psychology, 3*(2), 77–101. DOI: 10.1191/1478088706qp063oa

Choudhry, V., Dayal, R., Pillai, D., Kalokhe, A., Beier, K., & Patel, V. (2018). Child sexual abuse in India: A systematic review. *PLoS One, 13*(10), e0205086. DOI: 10.1371/journal.pone.0205086 PMID: 30300379

Comas-Díaz, L., & Jacobsen, F. M. (1991). Ethnocultural transference and countertransference in the therapeutic dyad. *The American Journal of Orthopsychiatry, 61*(3), 392–402. https://psycnet.apa.org/doi/10.1037/h0079267. DOI: 10.1037/h0079267 PMID: 1951646

Cunningham, M. (2003). Impact of trauma work on social work clinicians: Empirical findings. *Social Work, 48*(4), 451–459. DOI: 10.1093/sw/48.4.451 PMID: 14620102

Engel, G. L. (1977). The need for a new medical model: A challenge for biomedicine. *Science, 196*(4286), 129–136. DOI: 10.1126/science.847460 PMID: 847460

Figley, C. R. (1995). *Compassion fatigue: Coping with secondary traumatic stress disorder in those who treat the traumatized.* DOI: 10.4324/9780203777381

Follette, V. M., Polusny, M. M., & Milbeck, K. (1994). Mental health and law enforcement professionals: Trauma history, psychological symptoms, and impact of providing services to child sexual abuse survivors. *Professional Psychology, Research and Practice, 25*(3), 275–282. DOI: 10.1037/0735-7028.25.3.275

Hailes, H. P., Yu, R., Danese, A., & Fazel, S. (2019). Long-term outcomes of childhood sexual abuse: An umbrella review. *The Lancet. Psychiatry, 6*(10), 830–839. DOI: 10.1016/S2215-0366(19)30286-X PMID: 31519507

Hemanth Kumar, T., Naga Kumari, Y. V., & Narasimha Rao, A. (2024). Child sexual abuse in India: Understanding the problem, responding to the challenges, and charting a way forward. In Shaik, A., Thota, S. L., & Atmakuri, L. R. (Eds.), *Child sexual abuse* (pp. xx–xx). Springer., DOI: 10.1007/978-981-99-8745-0_5

Kuo, B. C. H. (2013). Collectivism and coping: Current theories, evidence, and measurements of collective coping. *International Journal of Psychology, 48*(3), 374–388. DOI: 10.1080/00207594.2011.640681 PMID: 22335198

Lazarus, R. S., & Folkman, S. (1984). *Stress, appraisal, and coping.* Springer. https://link.springer.com/rwe/10.1007/978-1-4419-1005-9_215

Lenin, B. P. (in progress). *Therapist experiences in counselling sexually abused children* (Unpublished doctoral thesis). Martin Luther Christian University.

Linley, P. A., Joseph, S., & Loumidis, K. (2005). Positive and negative changes following vicarious trauma: Associations with sense of coherence. *Journal of Traumatic Stress, 18*(6), 751–758. DOI: 10.1002/jts.20083 PMID: 16382431

Park, C. L. (2010). Making sense of the meaning literature: An integrative review of meaning-making and its effects on adjustment to stressful life events. *Psychological Bulletin, 136*(2), 257–301. https://psycnet.apa.org/doi/10.1037/a0018301. DOI: 10.1037/a0018301 PMID: 20192563

Pearlman, L. A., & Saakvitne, K. W. (1995). *Trauma and the therapist: Countertransference and vicarious traumatization in psychotherapy with incest survivors.* W. W. Norton. https://wwnorton.com/books/Trauma-and-the-Therapist/

Prasko, J., Ociskova, M., Vanek, J., Burkauskas, J., Slepecky, M., Bite, I., Krone, I., Sollar, T., & Juskiene, A. (2022). Managing transference and countertransference in cognitive behavioral supervision: Theoretical framework and clinical application. *Psychology Research and Behavior Management, 15*, 2129–2155. DOI: 10.2147/PRBM.S369294 PMID: 35990755

Richardson, G. E. (2002). The metatheory of resilience and resiliency. *Journal of Clinical Psychology, 58*(3), 307–321. DOI: 10.1002/jclp.10020 PMID: 11836712

Rose, S., McCusker, P., Mitchell, M., Roesch-Marsh, A., Jian, M., & Petrova, L. (2025). Self-care in social work: An imperative or beyond reach? *British Journal of Social Work, 55*(3), 1455–1473. DOI: 10.1093/bjsw/bcae204

Shapiro, S. L., Brown, K. W., & Biegel, G. M. (2007). Teaching self-care to caregivers: Effects of mindfulness-based stress reduction on mental health of therapists in training. *Training and Education in Professional Psychology, 1*(2), 105–115. https://psycnet.apa.org/doi/10.1037/1931-3918.1.2.105. DOI: 10.1037/1931-3918.1.2.105

Singha, R. (2024). Mindfulness and social cognitive processing. In Reddy, K. (Ed.), *Principles and clinical interventions in social cognition* (pp. 104–124). IGI Global Scientific Publishing., DOI: 10.4018/979-8-3693-1265-0.ch007

Singha, R. (2024b). Fostering mindfulness and compassion: Strategies, benefits, and challenges. In S. Watson (Ed.), *Applications of service learning in higher education* (pp. 45–64). IGI Global Scientific Publishing. https://doi.org/DOI: 10.4018/979-8-3693-2133-1.ch00

Singha, R. (2025). Empowering students through mindfulness and meditation practices. In Gonçalves, S. (Ed.), *Nurturing student well-being in the modern world* (pp. 141–170). IGI Global Scientific Publishing., DOI: 10.4018/979-8-3693-1455-5.ch006

Singha, R. (2026). Resilience in education: Addressing addiction and cultivating mindfulness for well-being. In Collister, R. (Ed.), *Facing precarity in adult, community, and vocational education: Role of meaningful work* (pp. 253–278). IGI Global Scientific Publishing., DOI: 10.4018/979-8-3693-1099-1.ch011

Singha, R., & Kanna, Y. S. (2022). Women's empowerment, mindfulness, and role of women in eradicating alcohol and drug addiction from Indian society. *Journal of International Women's Studies*, *24*(7), 7. https://vc.bridgew.edu/jiws/vol24/iss7/7

Singha, R., & Singha, S. (2024). Mindfulness-Based Interventions: Applications in Western and Indian Psychology. In Sathiyaseelan, A., & Balasundaram, S. (Eds.), *Global Applications of Indian Psychology: Therapeutic and Strategic Models* (pp. 192–212). IGI Global Scientific Publishing., DOI: 10.4018/978-1-6684-9778-4.ch011

Singha, R., & Singha, S. (2024b). Mindfulness in the Age of Populism. In Chennattuserry, J. C., Deshpande, M., & Hong, P. (Eds.), *Encyclopedia of New Populism and Responses in the 21st Century*. Springer., DOI: 10.1007/978-981-99-7802-1_437

Singha, R., & Singha, S. (2024c). Understanding neurodiversity and mindfulness: A holistic approach to addiction in professional preparation programs. In Jamanis, S., & Vogler-Elias, D. (Eds.), *Autism, neurodiversity, and equity in professional preparation programs* (pp. 255–275). IGI Global Scientific Publishing., DOI: 10.4018/979-8-3693-0163-0.ch012

Steger, M. F. (2012). Making meaning in life. *Psychological Inquiry*, *23*(4), 381–385. DOI: 10.1080/1047840X.2012.720832

Tedeschi, R. G., & Calhoun, L. G. (2004). Posttraumatic growth: Conceptual foundations and empirical evidence. *Psychological Inquiry*, *15*(1), 1–18. DOI: 10.1207/s15327965pli1501_01

Ungar, M. (2011). The social ecology of resilience: Addressing contextual and cultural ambiguity of a nascent construct. *The American Journal of Orthopsychiatry*, *81*(1), 1–17. https://psycnet.apa.org/doi/10.1111/j.1939-0025.2010.01067.x. DOI: 10.1111/j.1939-0025.2010.01067.x PMID: 21219271

UNICEF. (2017). *A familiar face: Violence in the lives of children and adolescents.* United Nations Children's Fund. https://www.unicef.org/media/48671/file/Violence_in_the_lives_of_children_and_adolescents.pdf

van der Kolk, B. A. (2014). *The body keeps the score: Brain, mind, and body in the healing of trauma.* Penguin Books. https://www.penguinrandomhouse.com/books/313183/the-body-keeps-the-score-by-bessel-van-der-kolk-md/

World Health Organization. (2013). *Mental health action plan 2013–2020.* WHO Press. https://www.who.int/publications/i/item/9789241506021

KEY TERMS AND DEFINITIONS

Child Sexual Abuse (CSA): Any sexual activity involving a child that is exploitative, coercive, or developmentally inappropriate, violating legal, ethical, and psychological boundaries, often resulting in long-term psychological and social consequences.

Coping: Cognitive, emotional, and behavioral strategies used to manage stressors and demands, influencing psychological adjustment, well-being, and professional sustainability in challenging contexts.

Cultural Context: The shared beliefs, values, norms, traditions, and social structures that shape individual behavior, meaning-making, coping strategies, and mental health experiences.

Health Psychology: A field of psychology examining how biological, psychological, social, and cultural factors influence health, illness, coping, and health-related behaviors.

India: A culturally diverse South Asian nation where historical, spiritual, social, and community-oriented contexts significantly shape mental health experiences, coping practices, and therapeutic approaches.

Meaning-Making: The process of interpreting and integrating stressful or traumatic experiences into a coherent personal framework that restores purpose, understanding, and psychological equilibrium.

Resilience: The dynamic capacity to adapt, recover, and grow in the face of stress, adversity, or trauma, supported by personal, relational, cultural, and systemic protective factors.

Secondary Trauma: Psychological distress experienced by professionals through indirect exposure to clients' traumatic experiences, leading to emotional exhaustion, intrusive symptoms, and altered cognitive or emotional responses.

Self-Care: Intentional practices that promote physical, emotional, and psychological well-being, including rest, reflection, boundaries, and support, essential for sustaining professional effectiveness.

Spirituality: A personal or cultural orientation involving meaning, purpose, values, or connection to something transcendent, often supporting hope, ethical grounding, and resilience during adversity.

Supervision: A structured professional relationship providing guidance, reflection, ethical oversight, and emotional support to practitioners, enhancing competence, accountability, and well-being.

Therapist Well-Being: The psychological, emotional, and physical health of therapists, sustained through self-care, supervision, supportive work environments, and adaptive coping to ensure ethical and effective professional functioning.

Trauma-Informed Care: An approach to practice that recognizes trauma's impact, prioritizes safety, empowerment, and collaboration, and avoids re-traumatization while promoting healing and resilience.

Chapter 7

A Theoretical Perspective on Determinants and Implications of Mental Health With Reference to South Asian Countries

Chitralekha Thapliyal
http://orcid.org/0009-0006-8792-8830
Department of Humanities and Social Sciences, Graphic Era (Deemed to be) University, Dehradun

Ajay Kumar Singh
http://orcid.org/0000-0003-0429-0925
Department of Humanities and Social Sciences, Graphic Era (Deemed to be) University, Dehradun

ABSTRACT

Appropriate mental health is necessary to maintain social, economic, psychological, technical and skill wellbeing of people. Mental health is also helpful to increase the intellect of people. While mental health depends on above-mentioned activities, and other indicators that are associated with livelihood security of people. This chapter, therefore, explores the determinants, measurement and implications of mental health as per existing literature. Thereupon, it provides the overall mental health status of India with comparison to South Asian countries as per the availability of secondary data. It used 10 different indicators which measure the mental health of people. This chapter found multiple indicators in the area of psychology, economic, social

DOI: 10.4018/979-8-3373-6294-6.ch007

and environmental sectors that are highly supportive to increase mental health. It provides a list of indicators that are leading to mental disorders. This chapter makes a significant contribution in the theoretical literature in medical psychology.

1. INTRODUCTION

Mental health is significant to maintain the overall health of the people (Manwell et al., 2015). It ensures the efficiency of an individual to cope with stressors, contribute to society and realise their potential towards different responsibilities (WHO, 2024a). It means that human body does not have illness and mental health helps to increase the performance of people in different perspectives. Further, it maintains the equilibrium with physical and social surroundings of people (Galderisi, 2015). Appropriate mental health of people depends on food, accommodation, survival, safety, society, social support and freedom from suffering (Maslow, 1958). An individual is mentally healthy if he/she has an ability to maintain relationships with others, recognise, acknowledge and manage emotions of self and others, and function according to the social norms. Mental health involves positive emotions like love, emotions, and empathy towards self and others (Bhugra et al., 2013). A person's beliefs and feelings about themselves and their situations determine their mental health (MHF, 2008). Human health manages stress and other diseases which cause to increase mental problems. It means that "*There is no health without mental health*" (WHO, 2024b).

Mental health measures the capability of an individual to comprehend a difficult situation, and manage it (Huber et al., 2011). The sense of coherence enhances the connection between body and mind and quality of life. Coherence fosters coping skills, supports the recovery from severe psychological stress, and prevents mental disorders. The capacity for self-management and adaptation, enhanced by the "sense of coherence," enhances subjective well-being of people (Huber et al., 2011). Moreover, mental health helps to attain basic cognitive and social skills, self-awareness, and positive emotion regulation. It is, therefore, a core constituent of overall health. Mental health improves the quality of life and lessens medical costs (Manwell et al., 2015). The components of mental health include cognitive ability (to understand and process information), emotions (emotional knowledge, intelligence and regulation), mental health literacy (being aware of the symptoms and warning signs to recognise both new and old disorders) (Degan et al., 2018; Singh et al., 2025). Attitude towards mental health disorder (i.e., understanding, showing compassion, and having empathy) (Fusar-Poli, 2019), social skills (Soto-Icaza et al., 2015), relationships (the capacity to build deep connections with family members and other significant individuals) are also a key component of mental health. Positive communication and engagement are made possible by having healthy relationships and the concept of self (acknowledging and valuing individual psychological traits, self-worth, and positive self-esteem) (Fusar-Poli, 2019).

Bad mental health leads to increased mental disorders that impact behaviour, emotion, and thought processes and significantly impair the ability to function in daily life of an individual. Mental disorder tends to run in the family. The prevalence, onset, and infirmity of mental disorders may influence the overall burden of disease. Mental disorders are compilations of syndromes that impair a person's ability to think, control their emotions, or behave. A mental illness is a condition marked by a clinically substantial disruption in one's behaviour, regulation of emotions, or thought processes that indicates a dysfunction in the biological, psychological, or evolving mechanisms that underlie mental operational (APA, 2022). Mental health of people can be detected from following psychological aspects:

Depression: It measures mood disorders and feelings of sadness in human life. It is also associated with fatiguability and diminished activity, loss of interest and enjoyment, low self-esteem and confidence, unworthiness, negative thoughts, sleep disturbance, low appetite and suicidal thoughts among the people (WHO, 1992). It is divided into mild, moderate and severe depression as per the severity of the symptoms (Singh et al., 2025).

Schizophrenia: It is defined by the fundamental and characteristic distortion of cognitive and motor function. It changes the function of thinking, feelings and behaviour in a person. Further, it is characterised by hallucinations, delusions, cognitive and motor impairment, disorganised behaviour, speech and thoughts, and reduction of expression of emotions. It can be divided in following categories: paranoid hebephrenic, catatonic, undifferentiated, residual, simple, other schizophrenia and schizophrenia, and unspecified (WHO, 1992).

Bipolar Disorder: It is a tool for examine the mood disorder characterised by episodes of significant fluctuation of mood and energy either increases (mania or hypomania) or decreases (depression) (WHO, 1992). Bipolar is further divided into two parts i.e., Bipolar I (involving episodes of mania) and Bipolar II (hypermania and MDD) (APA, 2022).

Anxiety Disorders: It comes under (F40-F48) neurotic, stress-related and somatoform disorders in ICD-10 characterised by feelings of fear and anxiety. Anxiety disorders include phobias, panic disorder and general anxiety disorder (WHO, 1992).

Alcohol Use Disorder (AUD): It is a psychological disorder described as addiction to consuming alcohol that leads to increased chronic illness and distress in humanity (APA, 2022). Alcohol use disorder is also reflecting the mental ability and attitude of its consumers.

Drug Use Disorder: It also known as substance use disorder or drug addiction. It is described as a negative pattern of drug use that is leading to increased impairment and/or distress in humanity (APA, 2022).

Eating Disorder: It is a behaviour disorder characterised by critical and relentless disturbance in eating patterns. It is associated with negative thoughts, emotions and body image. Anorexia Nervosa (self-famishment) and Bulimia Nervosa (purging) are two types of eating disorders (WHO, 1992).

Autism and Asperger Syndrome: The prevalence of autism and Asperger syndrome are considered as a child-development disorder. These are defined as abnormal development and functioning in social relations, interaction and constrained recurring behaviour. Autism is more severe than Asperger syndrome among children (WHO, 1992). Furthermore, childhood behavioural disorders can be segregated in following forms: a) Attention-deficit/Hyperactivity Disorder (ADHD) – It is a childhood behavioural disorder that is described as inattention, less co-ordinate, hyperactive, prone to injuries and accidents and impulsive (APA, 2022), and b) Conduct disorder – A childhood behavioural disorder characterised as antisocial, aggressive, violent behaviour towards others and social norms (WHO, 1992).

Intellectual disability: It is a developmental disorder formerly known as mental retardation and it is characterised by deficit cognitive functioning (abstract and critical) and motor functioning that hampers one's social interaction, communication, and self-care (APA, 2022).

1.1. Psychological Assessment Tools for Measuring Mental Health

1.1.1. Depression

The Beck Depression Inventory and the Patient Health Questionnaire can be used as the best assessment tools for measuring the level of depressive disorder in adults.

Beck Depression Inventory (BDI): Beck et al. (1961) developed the BDI self-report tool for measuring the level of depression. This tool includes 21 items (questionnaires) as an assessment of BDI-II. While it has a high internal consistency between 0.86 to 0.81 for people over 13 years (APA, 2011).

Hamilton Depression Rating Scale (HDRS): This tool was developed by Hamilton (1960). It includes 17 items for measuring the rating scale of depression among the youth. The techniques measure levels of depression pre, during, and post-treatment with a high internal consistency. Self-assessment tools and the Geriatric Depression Scale (GDS) can be applied to measure the stage of depression.

1.1.2. Schizophrenia

Positive and Negative Syndrome Scale (PANSS): This scale is introduced by Kay et al. (1987). It consists of 30 items for measuring the syndrome scale of schizophrenia. Further, it measures positive symptoms including hallucinations (false sensory perception that is not present), delusions (unreal belief), paranoia (distorted belief), and repetitive movements and negative symptoms for instance blunted affect (lack of emotional expression), alogia (narrow speech range), avolition (lack of energy), asociality (low desire to be social), Anhedonia (lack of ability to experience pleasure) and distress along with general psychopathology (Kumari et al., 2018).

Brief Negative Symptom Scale (BNSS): Clinicians also use 5 subscales (with 13-items) to assess the negative effects of schizophrenia. BNSS has high reliability with strong internal consistency, test-retest and interrator (Kumari et al., 2018).

1.1.3. Bipolar Disorder

Mood Disorder Questionnaire (MDQ): MDQ is developed by Hirschfeld et al. (2000) and it is based on 15-items. It is a self-report inventory used in a diagnosis of bipolar disorder with 0.73 sensitivity (Baldassano, 2005).

Bipolar Spectrum Diagnostic Scale (BSDS): It is a narrative-based 19-items scale developed by Pies to determine the probability of bipolar spectrum disorder. Clinicians narrate the items and individuals score the narration on how well they describe their situation. High scores indicate a high chance of the presence of bipolar disorder (Baldassano, 2005). Moreover, Structural clinical interviews and the hypomanic Personality scale are also used to assess bipolar disorders among the patients.

1.1.4. Anxiety Disorder

Generalized Anxiety Disorder–7 (GAD7): A 7-item scale developed by Spitzer et al. (2006) to measure GAD with strong internal consistency (0.89) and sensitivity (0.80). GAD-7 is a self-report inventory used for the patient in the presence of a clinician or practitioner (Rose & Devine, 2014).

Hospital Anxiety and Depression Scale (HADS): HADS is used to assess anxiety, and depression is a 14-item scale (7 each). The scale developed by Zigmond and Snaith (1983) with strong internal consistency (0.76) and sensitivity (0.85) (Rose & Devine, 2014). Anxiety Screening Questions and Anxiety Disorder Diagnostic Questions. (ADDQ) are also used to measure anxiety disorders by the clinical psychologists.

1.1.5. Alcohol Use Disorder (AUD)

The Alcohol Use Disorders Identification Test (AUDIT): It includes test–retest reliability of 0.84 consists of 10 questions. It assesses the extent of alcohol consumption, and its detrimental effects, and proof that others have observed the respondent's drinking issue.

1.1.6. Drug Use Disorder

Drug Abuse Screening Test (DAST): This test comprises a 10-item screening tool condensed from 28 items to assess illicit drug use problems with strong validity and reliability. The tool is proposed by Skinner (1982).

1.1.7. Eating Disorder

Eating Disorders Inventory (EDI): It is developed by Garner et al. (980) to measure anorexia nervosa and bulimia nervosa behavioural, and psychological traits. The scale has 8 subdivisions that assess beliefs about body shape, weight, and other psychological traits. The latest version of this tool is EDI-3 with 91-item and it shows strong test-retest reliability (0.79 to 0.95) (Túry et al., 2009).

Eating Disorder Examination Questionnaire (EDE-Q): EDE-Q, a 33- item questionnaire with excellent internal consistency and test-retest reliability ranging from 0.78 to 0.93 and 0.81 to 0.94 developed by Fairburn and Beglin (1994) to assess eating disorders. EDE-Q uses a semi-structured interview format to determine the severity of eating attitudes and behaviour of individuals (Túry et al., 2009).

1.1.8. Autism and Asperger Syndrome

Autism Spectrum Screening Questionnaire (ASSQ): ASSQ was developed by Ehlers et al. (1999). This technique has a 27-item questionnaire with 0.62-0.82 sensitivity and 0.90 to 0.91 specificity for children and adolescents, respectively. ASSQ has 3 subscales for measuring mental health of a person (Sappok, 2015).

Asperger Syndrome Diagnostic Scale (ASDS): A 50-item developed by Myles et al. (2001) for children and adolescents based on yes and no answers provided by parents, caregivers, guardians, and teachers conducted by clinicians. It consists of 5 subscales that are learning, social, maladaptive, cognitive, and sensorimotor (Sappok, 2015).

1.1.9. Attention Deficit/Hyperactivity Disorder

ADHD Symptom Inventory (ADHD-SI): This 18-item scale with strong test-retest reliability (0.87) was developed by Cox et al. (1999). It has two subscales (inattention and hyperactivity/impulsivity) for measuring mental health of the people (Penberthy et al., 2005).

ADHD Rating Scale-IV: This rating scale has good reliability developed by DuPaul et al. (1998). It consists of two subscales ADHD-SI inattention and hyperactivity-impulsivity with 9 items. ADHD rating scale-IV is a home version of this test (Penberthy et al., 2005).

1.1.10. Conduct Disorder

Child Behaviour Checklist (CBCL): Total 113 items are scored under CBCL from teacher's reports and self-report to measure social problems, rule-breaking and aggression. CBCL is widely utilised, and it is a highly valid and reliable psychometric tool (Raine et al., 2022).

Conduct and Oppositional Defiant Disorder Scales (CODDS): A 23-item report by parents or caregivers as well as a self-report instrument used to measure conduct disorder (CD) along with oppositional defiant disorder (ODD) was developed by Raine et al. (2022). The internal reliability for both caregivers and self-reports for CD is high (0.86) (Raine et al., 2022).

1.1.11. Intellectual Disability

The Child and Adolescent Intellectual Disability Screening Questionnaire (CAIDS-Q): It is a 7-item instrument that is used to screen prevalence of intellectual disability among children and adolescents. Lower scores indicate the presence of intellectual disability in the subject (McKenzie et al., 2018).

The Wechsler Intelligence Scale (WISC-IV): WISC-IV contains 10 subtests to measure the intellectual ability of a child. It is a widely used test with high reliability and validity with high sensitivity and specificity (McKenzie et al., 2018). Table 1 listed the crucial assessment tools for measuring the mental disorder among the people.

Table 1. Indicators for measuring mental disorders

Types of Mental Disorders	Indicators (Assessment Tools)	Measurement	Assessment conduction
Depressive disorder	HDRS	HDRS is used for assessing depression among adults	Self-report
	BDI	A 13-item tool for depression in adolescents and adults	Self-report
Schizophrenia	PANSS	It measures positive and negative symptoms of schizophrenia along with general psychopathology	Clinicians
	BNSS	BNSS measures the negative symptoms of schizophrenia	Clinicians
Bipolar disorder	MDQ	It measures bipolar disorder	Self-report
	BSDS	It determines the bipolar spectrum disorder	Clinician
Anxiety disorder	GAD-7	It assesses general anxiety disorder	Self-report
	HADS	It measures anxiety disorders	Self-report
Alcohol use disorder	AUDIT	It is a screening test to identify alcohol use problems	Self-report
Drug use disorder	DAST	It assesses drug use problems in patients	Self-report
Eating disorder	EDI-3	It measures eating disorders	Self-report
	EDE-Q	It measures eating disorders	Clinicians
Autism and Asperger syndrome	ASSQ	It assesses autism spectrum disorders	Clinicians
	ASDS	It determines Asperger syndrome	Clinicians
Attention Deficit/ Hyperactivity Disorder	ADHD-SI	It assesses inattention and hyperactivity-impulsivity in children	Clinician
	ADHD Rating Scale-IV	It assesses inattention and hyperactivity-impulsivity in children	Clinician
Conduct Disorder	CBCL	It assesses behavioural problems in a child	Clinicians and answered by parents, caregivers and teachers
	CODDS	It examines Conduct and Oppositional Defiant Disorder	Clinicians and answered by parents, caregivers and teachers as well as self-report

continued on following page

Table 1. Continued

Types of Mental Disorders	Indicators (Assessment Tools)	Measurement	Assessment conduction
Idiopathic intellectual disability	CAIDS-Q	It assesses the presence or absence of intellectual disability	Clinicians
	WISC-IV	It assesses the intellectual ability of the child	Clinicians

Source: Author's compilation as per the past literature.

The preceding sections provide definitions of different forms of mental health. However, existing literature could not explain the determinants and implications of mental health. This chapter, therefore, highlighted different definitions, determinants and implications of mental health. Further, this study explores the position of India in the prevalence of mental disorders as compared to the South Asian countries (SAC) and the world. Although there are ample numbers of studies on mental health and mental disorders that have been investigated by the researchers. There are only a few studies that target the Indian population. While few studies could estimate India's mental strength at the global level. As India, the most populous country in the world with different religions, cultures, and geographical settings. Thus, it is necessary to analyse the causes and treatment gaps of increasing mental disorders of people in India. Hence, this paper explains the factors affecting mental health and its implications, and measurement of mental health with reference to India and SAC. The comprehensive review of this chapter provides the amalgamation of many topics related to mental health. This chapter is written to assess the answers to the following research questions:

- What are the determinants of mental health as per existing literature?
- What are the main implications of mental health?
- How is it possible to measure mental health?
- What is India's strength in mental health as compared to the world's average?
- What is the impact of these factors on mental health?

This chapter has following objectives:

- To explore the determinants, measurement and implications of mental health as per existing literature.
- To provide the overall mental health status of India with comparison to SAC.
- To provide policy suggestions to increase mental health.

2. LITERATURE REVIEW

There are numerous factors affecting mental health and the development of mental disorders. These factors can be divided into the following categories: lifestyle, nutritional and food quality, biological, gender, social and economic, technological addiction, and environment.

2.1. Lifestyle

Lifestyle-related activities have impact on mental health of people. Lifestyle and health behaviour of an individual have a great effect on their mental health. For instance, smoking, drinking alcohol, and drug abuse reduce the mental health of people (Kim & Kim, 2017). Addiction to smoking is also a cause for mental disorders. Further, individuals with smoking and alcohol addiction are less likely to cope with stress and other mental difficulties (Buser & Scinicariello, 2017). However, initially people start alcohol consumption to avoid their personal stress and mental depression. Adequate sleeping, nutrition intake, physical activity, and meditation are beneficial for improving mental health (Kim & Kim, 2017). Therefore, it is advisable to get sufficient sleep to function cognitively well. Sufficient sleep significantly improves mental health and decreases stress and depression, and vice versa.

Learning and memory processing are facilitated by getting enough good-quality sleep for an appropriate amount of time. It supports memory acquisition, sensorimotor processing and coordination, regulatory cognitive functioning, and concentration of an individual (Laishram et al., 2025). For the best health benefits, this measurement should preferably be 85% or higher (Laishram et al., 2025). Song et al. (2015) noticed that sleep deprivation increases the production of cortisol (a stress hormone) and has a lasting impact on one's mental health. The findings of Song et al. (2015)'s study is based on a survey of military servicemen. Further, physical activity or exercise promotes sleep quality, energy, and stamina, helps to lower stress, and anxiety and prevents dementia and other psychotic disorders (Song et al., 2015). An individual who works out 45 minutes to one hour, three to five times in a week is negatively related to depression. Depression exercise helps to reduce the possibility of dementia, cognitive deterioration and cognitive impairment (Tikka et al., 2020).

2.2. Nutritional and Food Quality

Obesity is indeed a significant social problem. Data suggest that approximately 30% of the world population is obese, consuming high-energy foods with mal-nutritional value, processed food (Grajek et al., 2022). Nutrition has a direct and indirect effect on mental health. For instance, inflammation mostly derived from low nutrition intake can develop many mental disorders (Dal & Bilici, 2024). Appropriate nutritional content in the food has a significant impact on mental health. Macronutrients like Fatty Acids, phosphoglyceride, vitamin B6, B12 and D are beneficial for improving mental health. These macronutrients improve cognitive and memory abilities and reduce mental disorders (Lakhan & Vieira, 2008). There is a significant deficiency in dietary intake patterns of people in Asian and American countries (Rao, 2008). Also, most people's dietary patterns do not have proper nutrients (Rao, 2008). Consumption of less fibre and malnourished food when combined with smoking, lack of physical activity, and hazardous alcohol use has a negative impact on health. Further, lack of food and nutritional deficiency is caused to increase mental disorders (Grajek et al., 2022).

Food availability and quality influence the gut microbial profile and its activity. Research has indicated that increased consumption of fibre, probiotics, and prebiotics alters the gut microbes that have a direct impact on the gut-brain connection (Dal & Bilici, 2024). In the early stages of brain development, nutrients play a crucial role. Macronutrients like saturated fatty acids and cholesterol are associated with cognitive impairment that leads to increased neurological disorders (dementia and Alzheimer's) (Beilharz et al., 2015). It also causes to increase in the risk for metabolic disorders (diabetes) and cardiovascular diseases (Lim et al., 2016). Additionally, the presence of nutrients in meals is necessary for the antioxidant system to work properly. Foods affect the amount of brain-derived neurotrophic factor, which influences the neurodegenerative and developmental processes. A nutritional supplement or treatment is emerging as a key therapeutic intervention for improving mental health. Increased microbiome diversity has been linked to a plant-based diet and healthful eating patterns. These can be used to control and, to some extent, prevent mental problems like anxiety disorders, eating disorders, depressive disorders, ADHD, and abuse disorders among the population (Rao, 2008).

2.3. Biological (Gender and Genetics)

Gender-specific patterns and mental health are significantly connected with each other. Males and females face different mental problems due to their biological property (GBD, 2021). For instance, males are more likely to suffer from ADHD, autism, and substance use disorders, (Hyman, 2000). Further, research also supports the above finding females are more susceptible to experience greater levels of stress and depressive symptoms than counterparts (Barua et al., 2010; Lee et al., 2015). The prevalence of common health disorders is much higher in females than males in India (Jayasankar et al., 2022). The prevalence of mental illness is greater in females than males in the US (NIMH, 2022).

Nature also plays a crucial role in an individual life course (positive and negative). These two factors may cause several mental disorders in humanity (Stoewen, 2022). Certain genes and their variation are associated with certain mental disorders like anxiety, depressive disorders (MDD and bipolar), schizophrenia and addictive disorders (Rauf & Freese, 2024). Further, numerous studies based on twin studies support the substantial correlation between genetic factors and mental health (Kendler et al., 2011). The twin studies reported that genetic makeup is responsible for variation in depression and anxiety (Rauf & Freese, 2024).

Furthermore, nature also plays an important role in changing a person's genetics. The concept of de novo genetic mutation occurs in recent generations based on how they interact with their environment (Stoewen, 2022). The genome-wide association studies reported that a phenotypic variation in genes can occur through the integration of gene and environmental interaction (Rauf & Freese, 2024). A polygenic score of sensitivity (a person's risk of developing a disease based on their genetic makeup) can act as a moderator to develop mental health problems (Assary et al., 2024). For instance, a parent's poor health or risky conduct may have genetic effects that cause depression in their child through the exposure to a negative family environment and manifest in the child's genetic composition (Rauf & Freese, 2024). Furthermore, finding the genes that transmit risk for mental disorders is a major global endeavour. By improving diagnoses and treatments, linking the gene or genes that cause or increase exposure to a problem can help to recognise the biological cause of the development of mental illness (Hyman, 2000).

Neurotransmitters are also linked with mental health. Depression is frequently linked to irregularities in neurotransmitters including the secretion of serotonin, dopamine, noradrenaline, and other happy hormones. Many studies have demonstrated that the amino acids methionine, phenylalanine, tyrosine, and tryptophan help treat depression and other mood disorders. Tryptophan, a precursor to serotonin, promotes calmness and better sleep. This implies that depression caused by serotonin shortage is lessened when serotonin levels are increased (Rao, 2008).

2.4. Social and Economic, and Cultural Diversity

Social ties of an individual with his/her close ones and society are linked with his/her psychological and mental well-being. Few close relationships, low social support, poverty, and bad relationships have all been linked with depression. Socioeconomic status and poverty are firmly associated with mental disorders and poor mental health. Low income leads to increased illiteracy and low level of education also increase high risk of mental disorders like anxiety, panic, phobia and substance use disorders (Reddy, 2019). Cohen et al. (2000) proposed two effective models of social ties and mental health (direct and stress-buffered). The direct model explains different ways through which high social networking can affect one's mental health. Social networks are linked with a sense of purpose, belongingness and security. According to the Maslow hierarchy of needs safety and security, love and belonging are crucial for individual self-esteem, self-growth and self-actualization (Maslow, 1958). A positive social network is beneficial for mental health as well as in neuroendocrine response to difficult situations or stressors. The stress-buffered model explains that social support acts as a buffer in a stressful situation and helps a person to cope with the stressors and thus help maintain positive mental health (Kawachi & Berkman, 2001).

Moreover, an individual's cultural background also impacts mental health. Culture is identified as the set of values and belief systems carried out from generation (Hwang et al., 2007). Culture is an important part of the system; it provides us with the meaning, values, language, knowledge, customs and traditions that make us a social living being. Culture also can affect psychological distress and mental illness, thus affecting the mental health of an individual (Hwang et al., 2007). Culture breaks into many parts and hence makes them vulnerable minorities that are prone to violence, war, political persecution and other traumatic experiences (Sundquist et al., 2005).

Social networks and support are positive to increase mental health. It is proposed that social support signifies how one perceives and copes with stress. When an individual feels supported and accepted, stress tends to be reduced (Acoba, 2024). High social support (from parents, spouses, other relationships, and friends) is positively related with good mental health (Mohd et al., 2019). While low support is significantly related to depressive symptoms and self-harm (Bedaso et al., 2021; Singh et al., 2025). Low support also hinders the treatment and recovery from depression or other mental health disorders. Social support and women are negatively associated with each other. Gender discrimination, social exclusion, and gender disadvantages can lead to increased early marriage, worry about the husband's substance abuse, and domestic violence all increase the likelihood that women may experience mental health issues as compared to males. Poverty is a primary cause to increase unsatisfactory life, have chronic illnesses, and have fewer career options—all of which are known risk factors for major mental disorders (Reddy, 2019).

Previous research has shown that the authoritative parenting style is negatively linked with adolescents less likely to be engaged in substance abuse (Singh et al., 2017). While it positively linked with satisfaction of life and overall well-being and vice versa with the authoritarian parenting style (Singh et al., 2021). Positive parenting style and family relationships increase the self-esteem of an individual and all together this acts as a protective shield against depression and other mental disorders in adolescents and children (Singh et al., 2017).

2.5. Environment

An individual's relationship with his/ her environment can be positive or negative on their mental health (Baker et al., 2023). Positive mental health is often linked with the surrounding green spaces (Dzhambov et al., 2019) and blue spaces. Further, exposure to harmful gases and pollution is linked with negative mental health like anxiety and depression (Baker et al., 2023). In 30 years, more than half the population will live in urban areas (Gruebner et al., 2017). Clean environment is worthy to increase the psychopathology to learn advanced things for children in their livelihood (Pinto et al., 2015). The urban areas are characterised by numerous benefits but also living in closed settings, and low greenery (Callaghan, 2020), the more potentiality of drug abuse and stressful lives (Morgan & Mall, 2019).

Urbanization would be caused to increase pollution, risk of stress, anxiety, and depression, and mental health (Gruebner et al., 2017). Numerous studies reported that urban areas are significantly linked with mental disorders like addictive disorder, PTSD, anger and paranoia, schizophrenia, and psychotic disorder (Peen et al., 2009). The sensitivity in the environment can be positive or negative and it is influenced by personality traits and genetic makeup (Belsky & Pluess, 2009). For example, a person with a genetic index of depression has negative experiences with his/her environment that put him/her at high risk of depression and or addictive disorder (Andersen et al. 2017).

Moreover, pollution is one of the key factors that have a strong connection with mental disorders. A study based on air pollution in India states that air pollution harms the cognitive and emotional health of an individual. Air pollution is linked with various mental disorders like anxiety disorders, depressive disorders, and cognitive decline. The prevalence of Nitrogen oxide is correlated with the alteration of brain chemistry therefore leading to neurological disorders and high levels of anxiety. Persistent exposure to air pollution is associated with cognitive declination for example air pollution leads to increased low memory, inattention and poor decision-making processes along with behaviour and personality (Kapoor et al., 2024).

2.6. Climate Change and Natural Disasters

A disaster is described as a severe disruption to a community's or society's routine operations that causes substantial damage to individuals, goods, money, or the environment that beyond what the impacted population or society can cope on its own. Post-traumatic stress disorder (PTSD) includes flashbacks to the incident, elevated alertness, and avoiding reminders of the incident, depression, and anxiety are common mental disorders a population may experience after a disaster (Makwana, 2019; Negi et al., 2025). Recurring floods and drought, bushfires and hurricanes are related to climate change and are linked to the poor mental health of the victims (Padhy et al., 2015; Negi et al., 2025). In India, some districts in states like Uttar Pradesh and Bihar are more prone to occurrence of floods. Uttar Pradesh and Bihar are both agricultural states of India. Therefore, climate variability is caused to increase mental disorder in farming communities.

The changing climate is anticipated to have a significant influence on agriculturally reliant societies. The expansion of agricultural support industries, which employ manual labourers throughout the crop season, is also impeded by diminishing agricultural output. These may result in financial troubles, and contributing to an increase in mental health disorders. Drought-prone locations have higher rates of despair and helplessness, as well as poorer socioeconomic status. Prolonged droughts have been linked to worsening economic situations, which have been linked to dejection and depression (Padhy et al., 2015). Wind et al. (2013) perceived that seasonal floods have an adverse and devastating effect on the victim's mental health. Recurring floods or disasters desolate the agricultural lands into barren lands and homes along with mental health among affected individuals. When a person loses their home, surroundings, social networks, and loved ones, they may experience depression or bereavement (Padhy et al., 2015). Victims of recurrent floods are in survivor mode and these devastating circumstances impair their ability to function normally.

2.7. Technology Addiction

Recently, technology addiction is characterised by a reliance on the use of technology, leading to mental, neurological and physical consequences. Like any other dependencies, it includes mood tolerance, withdrawal, urges, conflict and relapse. Nowadays, the Internet has become a central component of life of the people (Tater & John, 2024). The primary causes of technology addiction are the ease and comfort of using the internet. The condition is caused by several factors, including mental anguish, loneliness, excessive social media use, and the desire to escape reality. When socialising online as opposed to in person, those with social anxiety reported feeling more at ease and disclosing more personal information (Das et al., 2017). Social media platforms' addictive traits are leading to increase mental and physical health problems among the youths (Taddi et al., 2024).

Adolescents with immature cognitive functioning are less able to evaluate information effectively than those with impulsive processing. Humanity is vulnerable due to inaccurate information and negative emotions (Siste et al., 2021). Research has reported that approximately 20-30% of internet users are involved in online erotic activities. Most online gamers miss out on at least one aspect of their lives, including sleep, employment, schooling, interacting with friends and family, and interacting with a significant other (Das et al., 2017). Anxiety and despair can lead to an increase in an obsession with social means and gaming as a way to cope with these unpleasant emotions. An excessive amount of Internet use might result from a maladaptive coping strategy, and raising the possibility of Internet addiction (Siste et al., 2021). These problems are made worse by continuous exposure to this information, especially for female adolescents (Taddi et al., 2024).

The epidemic of coronavirus disease 2019 (COVID-19) has hurt everyone in society. The spike in internet usage during the lockdown, and social distancing causes notable behavioural and social changes, particularly in adolescents. Physical distance encourages adolescents to spend more time at home, which lengthens their Internet usage for social media and video game playing in addition to academic purposes (Siste et al., 2021). Furthermore, cyberbullying is one of the emerging crimes globally and with technology addiction it is rising rapidly.

3. METHODOLOGY

3.1 Area of Research

This chapter includes India and SAC as research areas. While data and findings of other countries related to this research are also included in this chapter.

3.2. Selection and Inclusion Criteria of Research Articles

A total of 72 research articles has been finalized as per the objectives of this chapter. This study includes articles that are published in English-language. Except for the theories (Maslow and Lazarus & Folkman), the core published articles during 2000 – 2025. The core articles are in the domain of mental health, mental disorders, determinants of mental health, and the prevalence of mental disorders. These articles are taken from Google Scholar, ResearchGate and PubMed.

3.3. Source of Data

It used secondary data to explore the determinants and measurement of mental health in India and SAC. The required data is taken from the World Health Organization (WHO), Global Burden of Disease (GBD), and Global Health Estimation (GHE).

3.4. Statistical Analysis

Simple time trend analysis is used to explore the comparative performance of the mental health of India and SAC. A graphical presentation of collected data is presented to measure the comparative performance of India's mental health in SAC and global level.

4. RESULTS AND DISCUSSION

4.1. The Current State of Mental Health in the World and India

Mental Health in the World

Around 970 million individuals suffer from a mental disorder like anxiety and depression worldwide (WHO, 2019; WHO, 2024c). Mental illness is subdivided into two sub-groups based on severity: Any Mental Illness (AMI) and Serious Mental Illness (SMI) (NIMH, 2010). Around 23.1% and 6% of the adult population of the US suffer from AMI and SMI, respectively (NIMH, 2010). The prevalence of mental illness is more in females than males. Further, it is reported that the prevalence of mental illness is much higher in young adults (18-25 years) than in adults of age more than 25 years.

Mental health in Adolescents (10-19 years old)

Adolescence is an age group of drastic changes. Due to these changes, adolescents are more prone to develop mental health problems. Approximately 14% of adolescents globally experience mental health conditions (WHO, 2024d). Among them emotional disorders like anxiety (4.4 - 5.5%) and depression (1.4% to 3.5%), behavioural disorders like ADHD (2.2% - 2.9%) and Conduct disorder (1.9% - 3.5%) and eating disorders (0.1% - 0.5 5) are the most occurring disorders in adolescents worldwide (WHO, 2024d).

Mental health in older adults (60 and above)

It is estimated that by 2030, 1.4 billion people would be in an age group of 60 and above globally. It represents that one in every six people would be old adults. Among them, approximately 14% of older adult's experience mental disorders that affect 10.6% of DALYs. Social isolation, chronic illness, and abuse would be responsible for depression, anxiety and substance use disorders among the adults. Around 27.2% older adults are prone to commit suicide at global level (WHO, 2024e). In India, a survey conducted by NMHS in 2015-16 found that 10.6% of the adult population suffered from mental disorders. Lately, in a survey conducted by Jayasankar et al. (2022) with NMHS found the prevalence rate of common mental disorders is 5.1%

in India. Among them, the prevalence in females is much higher than in males. Furthermore, according to WHO, India has 2443 DALYs per population of one million, with an age-adjusted suicide rate of 21.1 per one million people (WHO, 2024). Approximately 160 million people are suffering from mental and substance use disorders globally (GHE, 2019). The most prevalent mental illnesses include alcohol and drug use disorders, schizophrenia, depression and anxiety.

Figure 1. Mental and substance use disorders globally (2010)

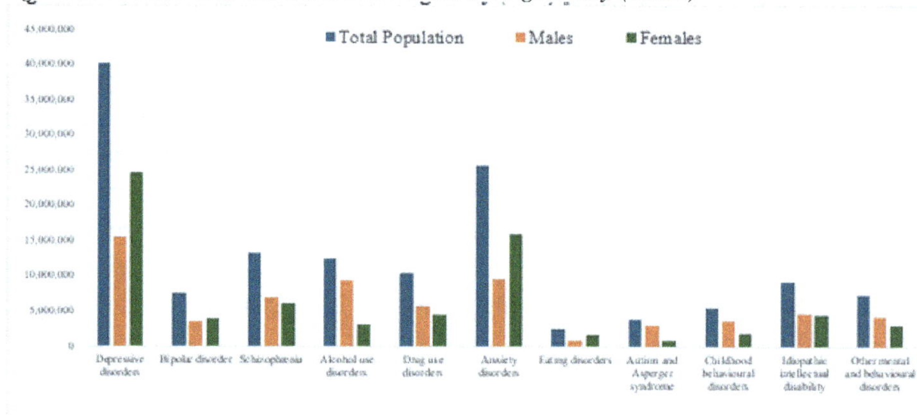

Source: *GHE (2025).*

Figure 2. Mental and Substance use Disorders at global level (2019)

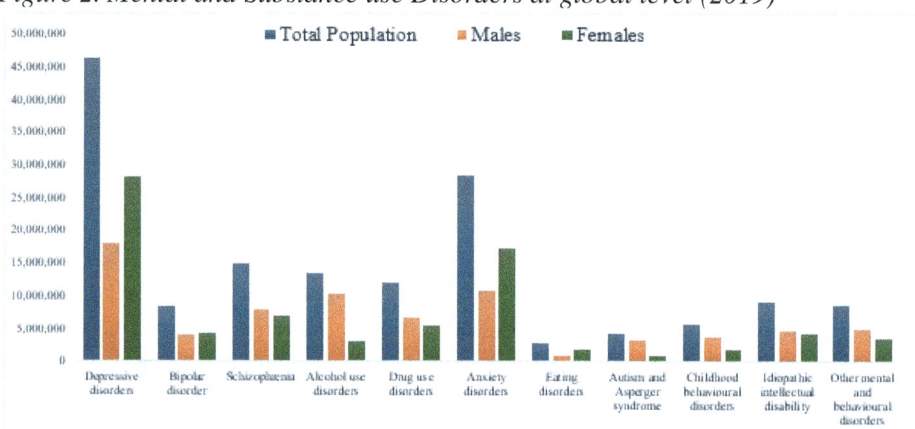

Source: *GHE (2025).*

Figures 1 and 2 indicate the burden of mental health disorders from the WHO Global Health Estimates (GHE) 2010 and 2019 data. In 2010, more than 130 million people suffered from mental health disorders that is increased to approximately 150 million people in 2019. Among them depression and anxiety disorders are the highest frequent mental disorders (approximately 50%). The prevalence of depression, bipolar, and eating disorders is observed higher in females than males in the world. The prevalence of schizophrenia, alcohol and drug use disorder, autism and Asperger syndrome, and childhood behaviour disorder are found higher among males than females in the world.

Prevalence of Schizophrenia

Figure 3. The prevalence of Schizophrenia in India and the world

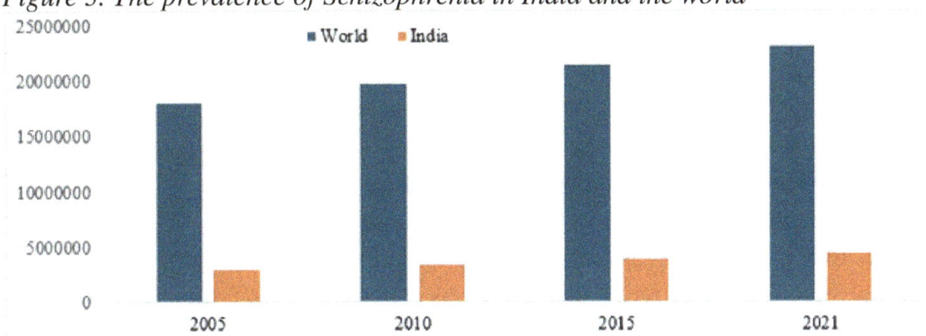

Source: *GBD (2021).*

Figure 3 indicates the prevalence of schizophrenia in India as compared to the global population (GBD, 2021). In 2005, the frequency of schizophrenia in India was observed 16.52%. In 2010, 16.9% of the global schizophrenic population were designated in India. The latest data (2021) indicates that the prevalence of schizophrenia in India is 18.8% of the global schizophrenic population. During 2005 – 2021, the global prevalence of schizophrenia increased by approximately 28.96% globally. The prevalence of schizophrenia among people has also increased consistently in India during 2005 – 2021.

Depressive Disorders

Figure 4. The prevalence of depressive disorders in India and the world

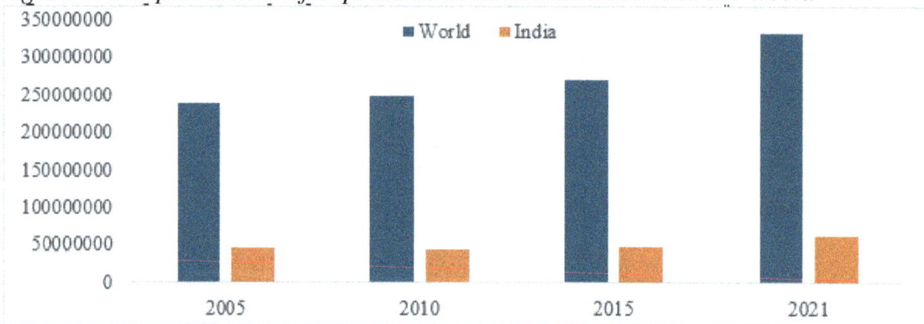

Source: *GBD (2021).*

The frequency of depressive disorders in India has escalated from 46 million (approximately) in 2005 to 62 million (approximately) in 2021 (Figure 4). In 2005, depressive disorder patients were approximately 46 million in India and 230 million globally. India has 19.42% of the global population who has depressive disorder. In 2010, the depressive disorder population of India (approximately 43 million) was 17.35% of the global depressive disorder population (approximately 240 million). The prevalence of depressive disorders was reported 17.82% (approximately 48 million) in 2015 in India as compared to the world depressive disorders population (approximately 270 million). In 2021, more than 62 million Indians are suffering from depressive disorders i.e., 18.79% of the global depressive disorder population.

Anxiety Disorders

Figure 5. The prevalence of anxiety disorders in India and the world

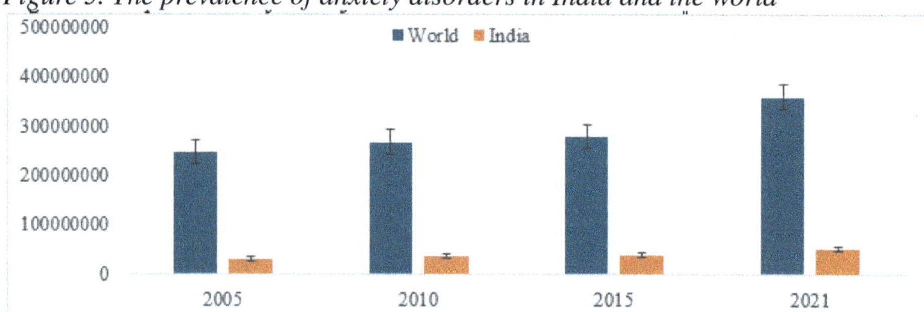

Source: *GBD (2021).*

Figure 5 indicates the prevalence of anxiety disorders in India as compared to the global population (GBD, 2021). The occurrence of anxiety disorders in India has amplified from 29 million (approximately) in 2005 to 51 million (approximately) in 2021. In 2005, anxiety disorder patients were approximately 29 million in India and 246 million globally. That is 12.06% as compared to the global anxiety disorders population. In 2010, the anxiety disorder population of India (approximately 35 million) was 13.33% of the global anxiety disorder population (approximately 267 million). The prevalence of anxiety disorders was 14.24% (approximately 398 million) in 2015 in India as compared to the world anxiety disorders population (approximately 278 million). In 2021, more than 51 million Indians are suffering from anxiety disorders i.e. 14.47% of the global anxiety disorder population.

Bipolar Disorders

Figure 6. The prevalence of bipolar disorders in India and the world

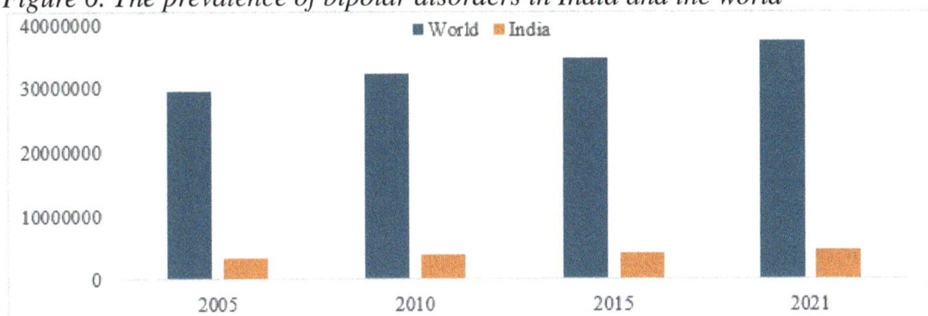

Source: *GBD (2021).*

Figure 6 indicates the prevalence of bipolar disorder in India as compared to the global population (GBD, 2021). In 2005, the frequency of bipolar disorder in India was observed as 11.41% of the global bipolar population. In 2010, 11.81% of the population had bipolar disorder. The constant increase in 2015 was approximately 3.8 million (12.27%) of the global bipolar disorder population of approximately 32 million. In 2021, the prevalence of bipolar disorder in India is 12.75% (more than 4.7 million) of the global bipolar disorder population (more than 37 million).

Autism Spectrum Disorders

Figure 7 indicates the occurrence of autism spectrum disorders in India as compared to the global population (GBD, 2021). The frequency of autism spectrum disorders in India has increased from 8.2 million (approximately) in 2005 to 10 million (approximately) in 2021. In 2005, the autism spectrum disorders patients were more than 8.2 million in India and 51 million globally. That is 16.08% as compared to the global autism spectrum disorders population. In 2015, more than 9.5 million patients had autism spectrum disorders in India. India has around 16.43% of the global autism spectrum disorders population. In 2021, it is estimated more than 10 million prevalence of autism spectrum disorders in India as compared to the global autism spectrum disorders population (more than 61 million). It indicates that autism spectrum disorders patients are consistently increasing in India and the world.

Figure 7. The prevalence of autism spectrum disorders in India and the world

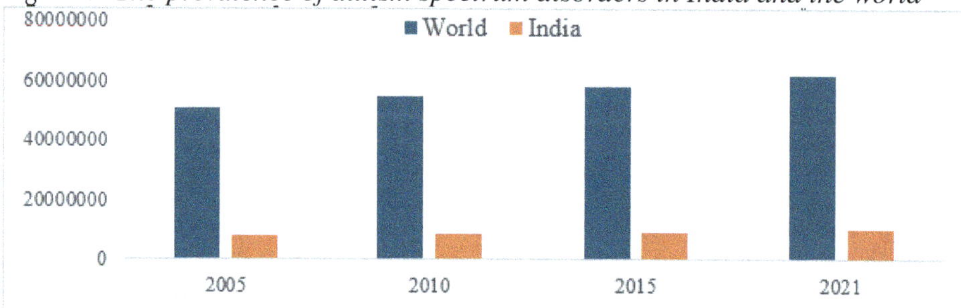

Source: *GBD (2021).*

Attention-deficit hyperactivity disorder (ADHD)

Figure 8. The prevalence of ADHD in India and the world

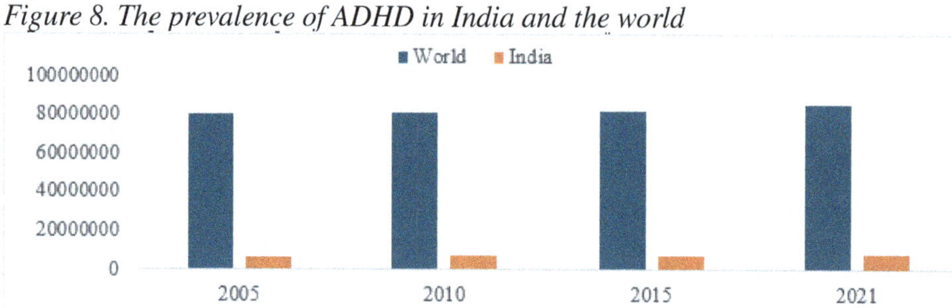

Source: *GBD (2021).*

Figure 8 indicates the prevalence of ADHD in India as compared to the global population (GBD, 2021). The frequency of ADHD in India has increased from 6.3 million (approximately) in 2005 to 7.7 million (approximately) in 2021. In 2005, the population of ADHD was estimated at more than 6.3 million in India and 80 million globally. India has a 7.93% global population who are suffering from ADHD. It is noticed that the ADHD population has significantly increased in India and the world during the mentioned time period. In 2015, more than 7.4 million (9.11%) patients had ADHD in India. In 2021, more than 7.7 million people had ADHD in India as compared to the global ADHD population (more than 84 million), i.e. 9.09%.

Conduct Disorder

Figure 9. The prevalence of Conduct disorder in India and the world

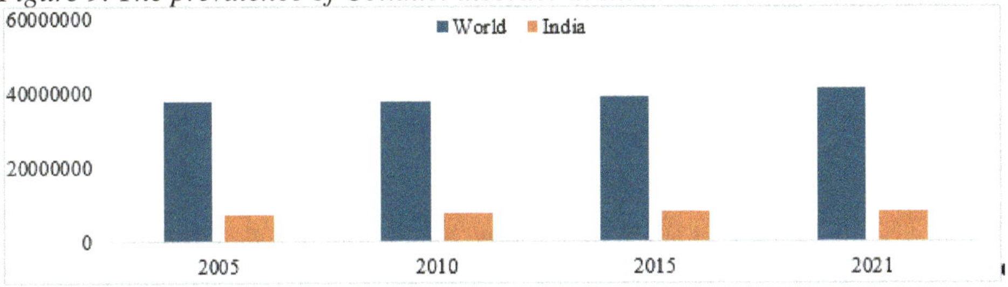

Source: *GBD (2021).*

In 2005, the population of conduct disorder in India was observed 16.52% of the global conduct disorder population (Figure 9). In 2010, the conduct disorder population of India (approximately 3.3 million) was 16.92% of the global conduct disorder population (approximately 19 million). In 2015, more than 3.8 million (18.08%) patients were suffering from conduct disorder in India. In 2021, the prevalence of conduct disorder in India is 18.86% (more than 4.3 million) of the global conduct disorder population (more than 23 million).

Idiopathic Developmental Intellectual Disability (IDID)

Figure 10. The prevalence of IDID in India and the world

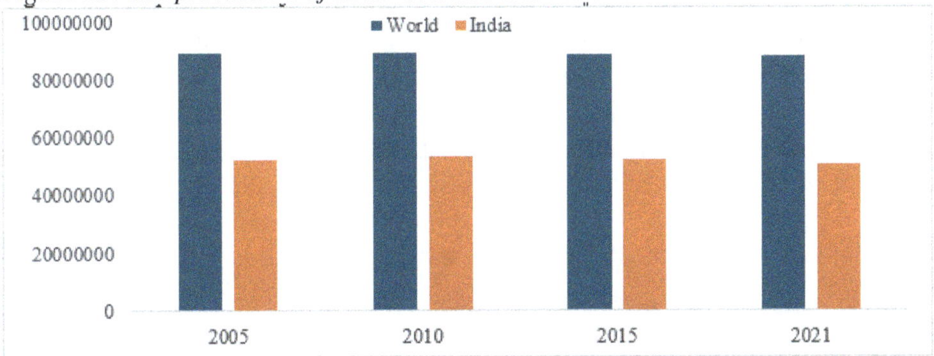

Source: *GBD (2021).*

Figure 10 indicates the prevalence of IDID in India as compared to the global population (GBD, 2021). In 2005, the prevalence of IDID in India was observed 58.48% of the global IDID population (more than 89 million). That is more than half of the IDID population in India (more than 52 million). In 2015, a million drop was observed from approximately 53 million (2005) to approximately 52 million (2015) in India. In 2021, the prevalence of IDID in India is 57.50% of the global IDID population. During 2005 – 2021, the global prevalence of IDID decreased by approximately 0.95% (more than 89 million (2005) more than 88 million (2021). Similarly, the prevalence of IDID among the people decreased by approximately 2.6%.

Eating Disorders

Figure 11. The prevalence of eating disorders in India and the world

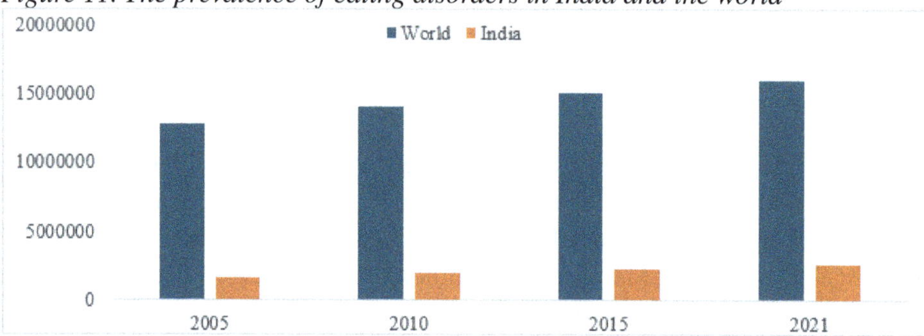

Source: *GBD (2021).*

Figure 11 indicates the prevalence of eating disorders in India as compared to the global population (GBD, 2021). In 2005, the occurrence of eating disorders in India was observed 12.62% of the global eating disorders population (more than 12 million). In 2010, the prevalence of eating disorders was estimated at 13.68% of the global eating disorders population. In 2015, the prevalence of eating disorders was approximately 1.9 million in India. The figure counts 15.02% of the eating disorders population of the world. In 2021, the population of eating disorders in India was 16.50% of the global eating disorders population.

Other Mental Disorders

Figure 12. The prevalence of other mental disorders in India and the world

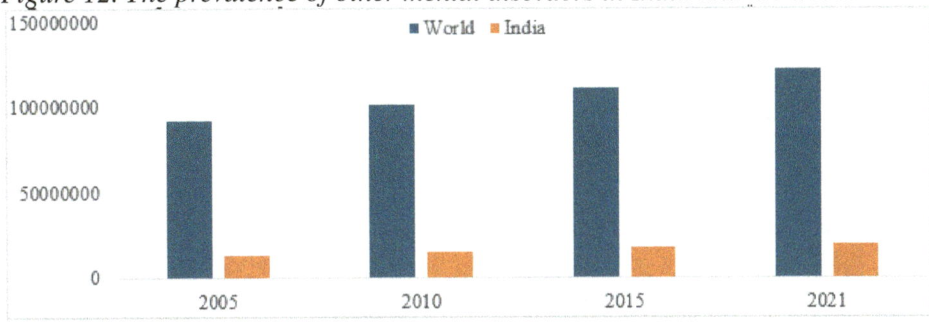

Source: *GBD (2021).*

Figure 12 indicates the prevalence of the other mental disorders in India as compared to the global population (GBD, 2021). The occurrence of other mental disorders in India was increased from 12 million (approximately) in 2005 to 19 million (approximately) in 2021. In 2005, the number of other mental disorder patients was more than 13 million in India and 91 million globally. India counted 14.56% patients suffering from other mental illnesses in the world. It is noted a constant increase in the number of patients suffering from other mental disorders in India and the world after 2010. In 2015, more than 17 million patients were suffering from other mental disorders in India. The figure counts 15.48% patients globally. In 2021, the prevalence of other mental disorders was in 19 million people in India. India has more patients suffering from other mental disorders as compared to global level.

4.2. Prevalence of Mental Disorders in SAC

Mental Disorder

Figure 13. Prevalence of mental disorders

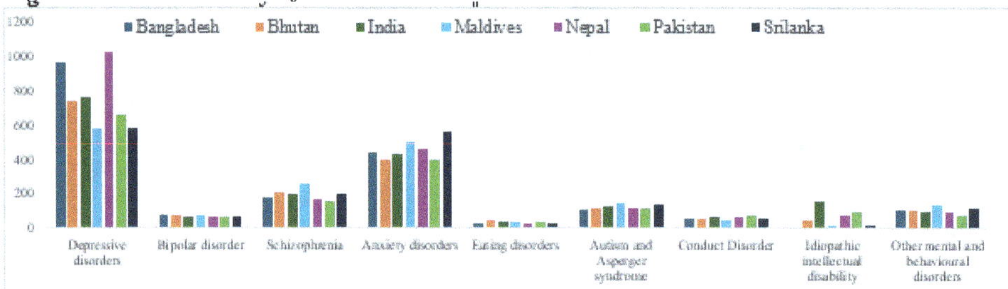

Source: *GBD (2021).*

Figure 13 shows the Years Lost to Disabilities (YLDs) per one million population in SAC (GBD, 2021). In 2021, there were estimated 1949.71 YLDs per million population with mental disorders in SAC. The frequency of depression is observed higher in Nepal, Bangladesh and India as compared to other SAC. Depressive disorder and anxiety disorder are much higher with comparison to the other mental conditions in all SAC. There are 1971.93 YLDs per million in India in 2021. The prevalence of depressive disorder, anxiety disorder and eating disorder is higher in Indian females. The prevalence of schizophrenia, autism and asperger syndrome, and conduct disorder is higher in Indian males.

Schizophrenia

Figure 14. The prevalence of schizophrenia

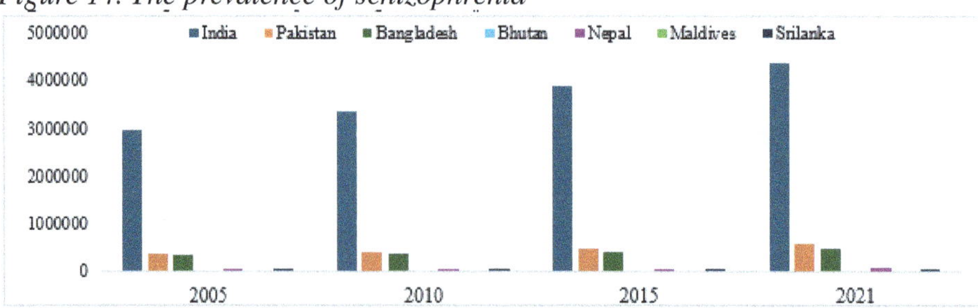

Source: *GBD (2021).*

Figure 14 indicates the occurrence of schizophrenia in SAC (GBD, 2021). India has the maximum number of schizophrenic populations in SAC. Maldives and Bhutan have the lowest number of schizophrenic populations in SAC. Schizophrenia is a continuously growing mental disorder in SAC. During 2005 – 2021, the prevalence of schizophrenia increased by approximately 47.17%, 66.43%, 40.39% and 37.87% in India, Pakistan, Bangladesh and Nepal, respectively. In Sri Lanka and Bhutan, the prevalence of schizophrenia decreased in 2021 as compared to previous years.

Depressive Disorders

Figure 15. The prevalence of depressive disorders

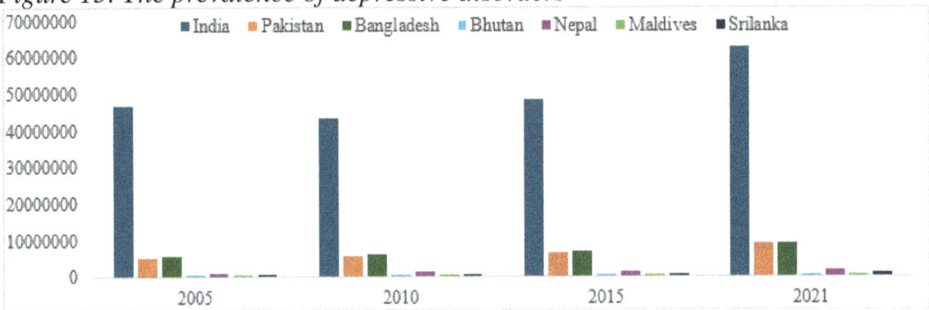

Source: *GBD (2021).*

India has a larger number of populations suffering from depressive disorders in SAC (Figure 15). Pakistan and Bangladesh also have a significant number of people who have a prevalence of depressive disorder. Nepal, Sri Lanka, Bhutan and Maldives have low populations. Hence, these countries have a low number of depressive disorder patients in South Asia. Maldives and Bhutan have the lowest number of depressive order people in SAC.

Anxiety Disorders

Figure 16. The prevalence of anxiety disorders

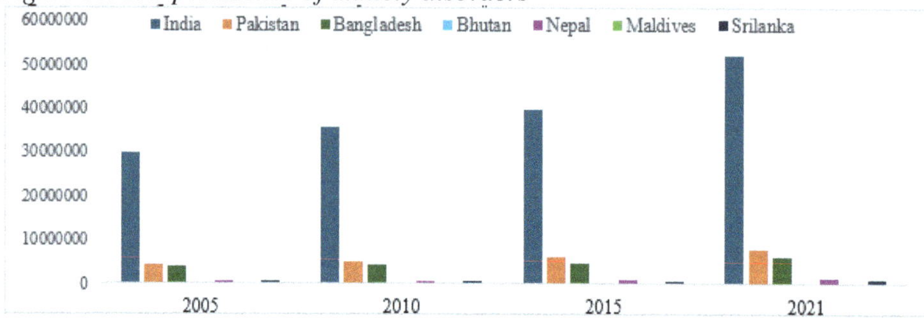

Source: *GBD (2021).*

Figure 16 indicates the occurrence of anxiety disorders in SAC in 2005, 2010 and 2021 (GBD, 2021). India's position on anxiety disorders is relatively higher than the other SAC. The prevalence of anxiety disorder has consistently increased in South Asia after 2005. Pakistan has the second highest rate of anxiety disorder patients. Nepal, Bhutan and Maldives are at the bottom of the occurrence of anxiety disorders among SAC. Anxiety disorders are ascending in all SAC.

Bipolar Disorders

Figure 17. The prevalence of bipolar disorders

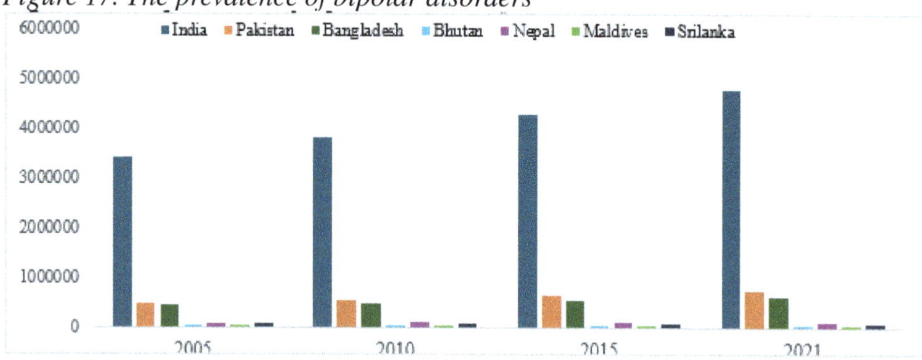

Source: *GBD (2021).*

Figure 17 indicates the occurrence of bipolar disorder among the people in SAC in 2005, 2010 and 2021 (GBD, 2021). India's strength in the prevalence of bipolar disorder is highest in comparison to other SAC. Followed by Pakistan, Bangladesh, Nepal, and Sri Lanka. Maldives and Bhutan have the least number of bipolar disorder populations in comparison to other SAC. The strength of bipolar disorder in India was 41.32% during 2005 – 2021.

Autism Spectrum Disorders

Figure 18. The prevalence of autism spectrum disorders

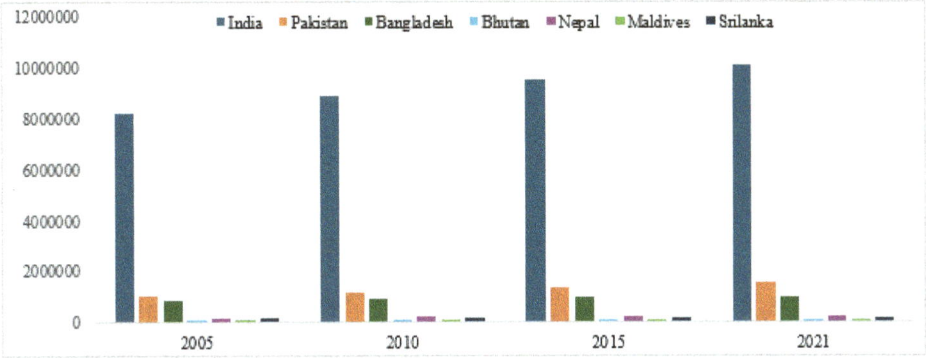

Source: *GBD (2021).*

Figure 18 indicates the occurrence of autism spectrum disorders in SAC in 2005, 2010 and 2021 (GBD, 2021). India has the highest population of autism spectrum disorders patients in SAC. While patients of autism spectrum disorders are approximately 23% increase in India during 2005-2021. Pakistan has the second highest patients of autism spectrum disorders in SAC. In Pakistan, the prevalence of autism spectrum disorders increased 49% during 2005 – 2021. In Bangladesh, the prevalence of autism spectrum disorders increased 16.27% during 2005 - 2021. Nepal holds the fourth position in the prevalence of autism spectrum disorders in SAC. There is an increase of 12.7% of autism spectrum disorders in Sri Lanka during 2005 - 2021. Bhutan and Maldives have the lowest populations of autism spectrum disorders among SAC.

Attention-deficit Hyperactivity Disorder (ADHD)

Figure 19. The prevalence of ADHD

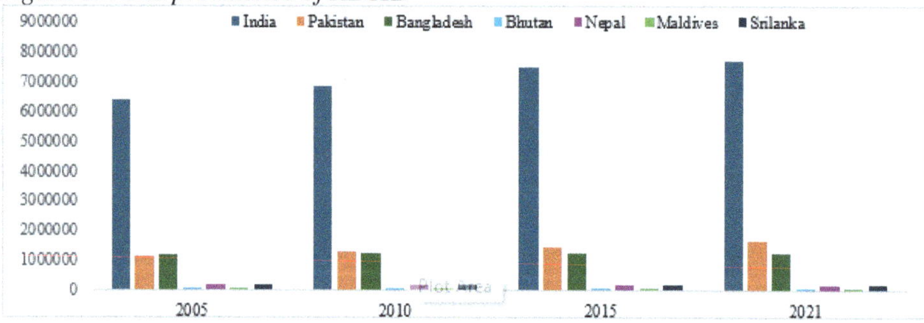

Source: *GBD (2021).*

Figure 19 indicates the occurrence of attention-deficit hyperactivity disorder in SAC in 2005, 2010 and 2021 (GBD, 2021). The population of ADHD was observed higher in India as compared to other SAC. The prevalence rate of ADHD in India has increased at the rate of 21.11% during 2005 – 2021. Pakistan has the second-highest prevalence of ADHD in SAC. While the ADHD increased at the rate of 4.40%, 10.44% and 4.9% in Bangladesh, Nepal and Sri Lanka, respectively during 2005 – 2021. Bhutan and Maldives have the lowest prevalence of ADHD in SAC. The prevalence of ADHD has decreased by 1.02% in Bhutan.

Conduct Disorder

Figure 20. The prevalence of conduct disorder

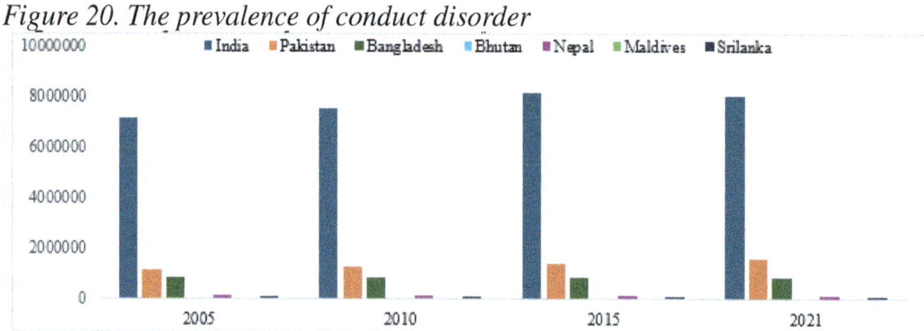

Source: *GBD (2021).*

Figure 20 indicates the prevalence of conduct disorder in SAC in 2005, 2010 and 2021 (GBD, 2021). India has the highest prevalence of conduct disorder population as compared to other SAC. During 2005 – 2021, the prevalence of conduct disorder increased by approximately 12.22%, 37.54%, 0.77% and 6.14% in India, Pakistan, Nepal and Sri Lanka, respectively. The prevalence of conduct disorder decreased by 1.8%, 16.17% and 13.21% in Bangladesh, Bhutan and Maldives, respectively during 2005 – 2021. The lowest prevalence of conduct disorder was observed in Maldives, Bhutan and Sri Lanka in 2021 in SAC.

Idiopathic Developmental Intellectual Disability (IDID)

Figure 21. The prevalence of IDID

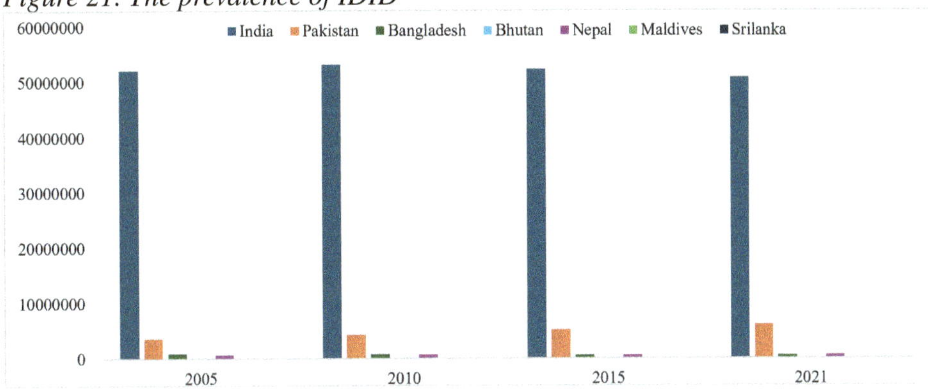

Source: *GBD (2021).*

Figure 21 indicates the prevalence of IDID in SAC in 2005, 2010 and 2021 (GBD, 2021). The prevalence of IDID is found highest in India as compared to other SAC. The prevalence of IDID has increased in Pakistan by 66.80% in 2021 with comparison to 2005. The prevalence of IDID decreased in the remaining SAC.

Eating Disorders

Figure 22. The prevalence of eating disorders

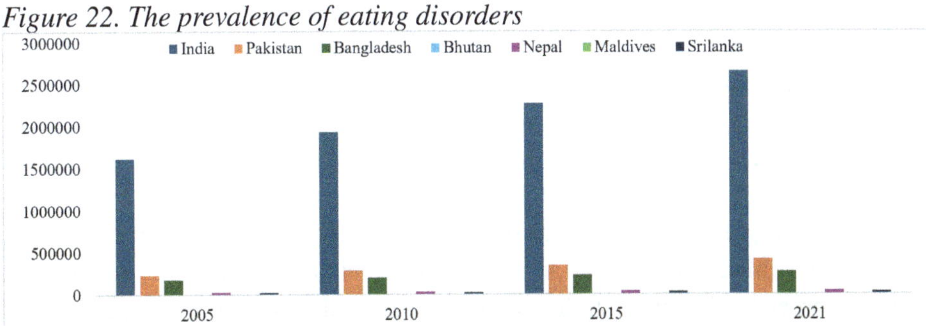

Source: *GBD (2021).*

Figure 22 indicates the rate of eating disorders in SAC in 2005, 2010 and 2021 (GBD, 2021). The population of eating disorders patients was observed highest in India in the mentioned time period as compared to other SAC. The eating disorder is consistently increasing in India in 2021 with comparison to 2005, 2010 and 2015. Pakistan has a second-highest frequency of eating disorders in SAC with an increased rate of around 76.72% from 2005-2021. The eating disorder has increased at a rate of 49.09%, 52.88% and 28.29% in Bangladesh, Nepal and Sri Lanka, respectively after 2005. Bhutan and Maldives have the lowest rate of eating disorders in SAC.

Other Mental Disorders

Figure 23. The prevalence of other mental disorders

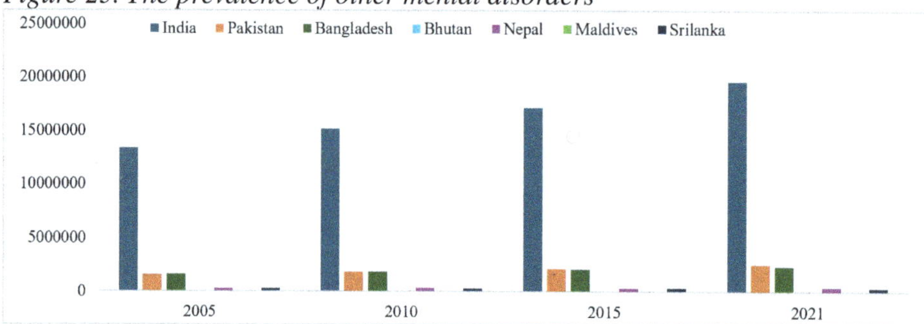

Source: *GBD (2021).*

Figure 23 indicates the dominance of other mental disorders in SAC in 2005, 2010 and 2021 (GBD, 2021). India has the highest population of other mental disorders patients in SAC. Pakistan has the second highest number of other mental disorders patients in SAC. The prevalence of other mental disorders increased at the rate of 67.04% in Pakistan from 2005 to 2021. Other mental disorders increased at the rate of 47.24% in Bangladesh from 2005 to 2021. The occurrence of other mental disorders has increased at the rate of 40.85% in Nepal after 2005. Sri Lanka has the third lowest-ranked in other mental disorder patients in SAC. Maldives and Bhutan have the lowest number of other mental disorders patients in SAC.

4.3. Policy Proposals for Improving Mental Health

Determinants of mental health can be used for policymaking and interventions for the target and vulnerable population to prevent, anticipate and cure the problems of mental disorder. For instance, studies found that a natural disaster-affected population often faces PTSD (Wind et al., 2013; Padhy et al., 2015). Although natural disasters are unavoidable, the repercussions on mental health which can be managed through interventions and mental health literacy programs among the affected masses. Similarly, intervention and educational programs on time management, negative impact of social media, smartphone addiction, and excessive reliance on smartphones can be implemented in schools, colleges and workspaces.

It is well known that lifestyle factors like appropriate sleeping, food intake, physical activities and social interaction can influence mental health (Song et al., 2015; Kim & Kim, 2017). While psychological stress can exacerbate mental disorders (Bhargav et al., 2022). Social awareness programs among the people must be initiated to increase the impact of a scientifically suggested time for sleeping and sleep hygiene, and food quality and nutrition intake can influence people to choose a better and healthier lifestyle (Dal & Bilici, 2024; Laishram et al., 2025). Ashtanga yoga techniques seek to balance lifestyle influences by bringing a person's biorhythm into harmony with nature. Yoga was thought to be the greatest way to start the integration process approach to mind-body healing (Bhargav et al., 2022).

4.4. Implications of Mental Health

Relationships: To establish healthy relationships with family and others is a key component of positive mental health. Positive relationship provides a healthier environment for a person to feel safe and secure to communicate and interact. Healthy relationships act as a protective layer from a non-favourable environment (Fusar-Poli, 2019). The first and foremost relationship of a child is with his/her parents. Research indicates that a positive parenting style (authoritative) is linked with positive emotion regulation and high satisfaction with life, therefore, positive mental health. However negative parenting style (authoritarian) is associated with negative emotion regulation and low satisfaction with life (Singh et al., 2021).

Healthy lifestyle: A healthy lifestyle refers to one's life choices to live a healthy life. Adequate amounts of sleep, healthy intake of food, physical activity, yoga and meditation are often linked with healthy habits for a positive healthy life. Enough amount of sleep helps in better cognitive function (Kim & Kim, 2017). Negative habits like tobacco addiction, alcohol addiction and smartphone addiction increase the risk of mental disorders by altering the neurotransmitters, breaking patterns of sleep, urges to scroll feed late at night on smartphones and deliberately choosing addiction over education, work and family (Das et al., 2017).

Self-esteem: Self-esteem is significant to increase well-being, resilience, and strong coping mechanisms of individuals. Low self-esteem is related to emotional distress and negative mental health that can lead to poor coping mechanisms and mental disorders like eating disorders and substance use disorders. Self-esteem increases the relationship of one with oneself and that also helps in other domains of life like relationships with others (Henriksen et al., 2017).

Resilience: It is ability of a person to recover from a traumatic and stressful incident and get past its negative effects of the situation (Dan et al., 2023). It displays emotional fortitude, the capacity to solve problems, and the adaptability to overcome obstacles. Resilient people use their inner resources and outside assistance to stay stable and develop constructively in the face of hardship or major life events (Tare et al., 2025). It is proactive toe reduce stressors, and non-favourable circumstances, and helps as a coping mechanism that leads to problem-solving skills, optimism, mindfulness and overall positive mental health and well-being. Low resilience is related to emotional distress and the likelihood of developing psychological problems (Tare et al., 2025). Additionally, resilience is suggested as a necessary component of therapeutic interventions and mental health activities, particularly in low-resource nations where stress-resilience training could improve the usefulness and success of treatment modalities (Dan et al., 2023).

Other Implications of Poor Mental Health: Young people and youth also committed to suicided due to poor mental health (Baluni et al., 2024). Youths face more problems due to mental disorders (NIH, 2010). Poor mental health is also negatively associated with the poor academic performance of students in higher educational institutions. Poor mental health of the people also reduces their social and economic responsibilities. There are many activities that are also negatively affected due to poor mental health of people.

5. CONCLUSION AND POLICY SUGGESTIONS

This study highlights the different definitions of mental health, common mental disorders, assessment tools for types of disorders, the prevalence of mental disorders in India compared to SAC and globally, and the implications of mental health. Mental health is defined by many researchers and organisations, and it can be concluded that mental health is an essential part of a person's overall health. So, the cruciality of this subject has been explored with the help of existing literature. It is also observed that prevalence of schizophrenia, alcohol and drug use disorder, autism and asperger syndrome, and childhood behaviour disorder was higher in males than females at world level. The prevalence of depression is observed higher in Nepal, Bangladesh and India as compared to other SAC. Depressive disorder and anxiety disorder both are higher in India as compared to the other mental disorders in SAC. The prevalence of depressive disorder, anxiety disorder and eating disorder is higher in females. The prevalence of schizophrenia, autism and asperger syndrome, conduct disorder is found higher in males. India is found unable to increase the mental health of people in SAC. Hence, India should take effective measures to increase its positions in mental health across SAC.

The prevalence of anxiety and depressive disorders was highest in India. Depressive disorders were among the top 20 diseases that are causing more deaths of people (GHE, 2019). Further, the strength of mental disorders into 2021 was most prevalent in India as compared to other SAC, followed by Pakistan and Bangladesh. In 2021, India's position in depressive disorders was 18.79%, anxiety disorders were 14.47%, bipolar disorder was 12.75%, eating disorders were 16.50%, conduct disorder was 18.86%, schizophrenia was 18.8%, ADHD was 9.09%, autism spectrum disorders were 16.67% and idiopathic developmental intellectual disability 0.95%. Idiopathic developmental intellectual disability is the only disorder whose prevalence has decreased in India and the world after 2005 (GBD, 2021). The determinants of mental disorders are thoroughly explored as per the existing literature. Lifestyle, environment, biology, social factors, and technology addiction have the most impact on mental health, and the negative impact of these factors can lead to an increase in several mental disorders. Moreover, the implication of positive mental health can lead to increased healthy relationships among family, friends, spouse and social relationships, healthy lifestyle, resilience, and high self-esteem.

Mental health literacy, accessible and affordable care, promoting mental health education and coping skills in schools, colleges and workplaces must be prompted to increase positive mental health. Further, appropriate counselling for youth in schools and workplaces would also enhance mental health of people. Moreover, mental disabilities among the youth are a global challenge. The prevalence of mental disabilities is also increasing suicide cases, depression, anxiety, and psychological disorders. While mental disabilities are also found in different forms (Baluni et al., 2024). Accordingly, it also increases economic, social, cultural, and mental vulnerability of the people. Hence, it must be resolved through effective policy mechanisms in India and other countries. For instance, social and economic factors are highly accountable for different mental health issues. Poor environmental and climatic conditions are also challenges for people to increase mental health security. Hence, a green environment is essential to increase mental health. Food habit change, quality of food, nutritional contents in food also determine mental health security. Therefore, the government should ensure the above-mentioned issues to reduce the problem of mental health. Education institutions should provide and organize more training programs to the students to sustain their health. Also, health literacy is necessary to increase quality of life and mental health. Employers should also take significant initiatives to increase mental health in different organizations in India and other countries. Mental health care must be promoted to reduce mental disorder among the people (Haugen et al., 2017).

6. INNOVATION OF THE RESEARCH

This chapter explores the determinants of mental health as per the existing literature. It also provides the current state of India's mental health as per the availability of data. It provides the global perspectives of mental health and its causing factors in different landscapes. It also describes various forms of mental health. Thereupon, implications of mental health are also highlighted in detail. Various measures of mental health are also provided in this chapter. The trend in mental health of India with comparison to SAC is also given. Therefore, it found a research area for considering further empirical research. Most specifically, this study provides a deeper understanding of the determinants and implications of mental health in India. It includes different definitions of mental health, the most prevalent mental disorder all over the world. The prevalence of mental disorders in India, SAC and globally are provided in detail. This study concludes all the prominent factors of mental health from different definitions, measurements, important determinants of mental disorders and mental health and the impact of mental health in an individual's life. Further, the occurrence of the most prominent mental disorders in India, SAC and the World are thoroughly discussed in this research.

7. LIMITATIONS AND SCOPE OF FURTHER RESEARCH

This chapter is based on existing literature and availability of secondary data that are taken from various sources. Hence, it does not develop an empirical model to assess the implications of different social, economic, environmental and other factors on mental health. Therefore, researchers can collect the primary data to get an insightful idea about mental health and its affecting factors. Accordingly, existing researchers can develop robust statistical and empirical models to check the validity of the findings of this chapter. This chapter explores the overall mental health of people in India and SAC. While mental health among male, female, children, youth and old aged people varies. However, this research could not include the variation in mental health among the male, female, children, youth and old aged person. The study explores the determinants and implications of mental health with reference to India. This study includes statistical data for related indicators during 2005 – 2021. Therefore, it is not updated because of the unavailability of the data. Further, the prevalence of mental disorders based on gender (males and females) is not explained in this chapter.

REFERENCES

Acoba, E. F. (2024). Social support and mental health: The mediating role of perceived stress. *Frontiers in Psychology, 15*(1), 1–10. DOI: 10.3389/fpsyg.2024.1330720 PMID: 38449744

American Psychiatric Association (APA). (2022). *Diagnostic and statistical manual of mental disorders* (5th ed., text rev.)., DOI: 10.1176/appi.books.9780890425787

American Psychological Association (APA). (2011). *Beck Depression Inventory (BDI).* [online]. https://www.apa.org/pi/about/publications/caregivers/practice-settings/assessment/tools/beck-depression

Andersen, A. M., Pietrzak, R. H., Kranzler, H. R., Ma, L., Zhou, H., Liu, X., Kramer, J., Kuperman, S., Edenberg, H. J., Nurnberger, J. I.Jr, Rice, J. P., Tischfield, J. A., Goate, A., Foroud, T. M., Meyers, J. L., Porjesz, B., Dick, D. M., Hesselbrock, V., Boerwinkle, E., & Han, S. (2017). Polygenic scores for major depressive disorder and risk of alcohol dependence. *JAMA Psychiatry, 74*(11), 1153. DOI: 10.1001/jamapsychiatry.2017.2269 PMID: 28813562

Assary, E., Oginni, O. A., Morneau-Vaillancourt, G., Krebs, G., Peel, A. J., Palaiologou, E., Lockhart, C., Ronald, A., & Eley, T. C. (2024). Genetics of environmental sensitivity and its association with variations in emotional problems, autistic traits, and wellbeing. *Molecular Psychiatry, 29*(8), 2438–2446. DOI: 10.1038/s41380-024-02508-6 PMID: 38499655

Baker, E., Barlow, C. F., Daniel, L., Morey, C., Bentley, R., & Taylor, M. P. (2023). Mental health impacts of environmental exposures: A scoping review of evaluative instruments. *The Science of the Total Environment, 912*(1), 1–10. DOI: 10.1016/j.scitotenv.2023.169063 PMID: 38048998

Baldassano, C. F. (2005). Assessment tools for screening and monitoring bipolar disorder. *Bipolar Disorders, 7*(1), 8–15. DOI: 10.1111/j.1399-5618.2005.00189.x PMID: 15762864

Baluni, P., Bhutani, R., Singh, R., & Singh, A. K. (2024). A systematic literature review for identifying the factors causing prevalences of suicide among youths in India. In Aloka, P. (Ed.), *Student Well-Being in Higher Education Institutions* (pp. 237–266). IGI Global., DOI: 10.4018/979-8-3693-4417-0.ch010

Barua, A., Ghosh, M. K., Kar, N., & Basilio, M. A. (2010). Socio-demographic factors of geriatric depression. *Indian Journal of Psychological Medicine, 32*(2), 87–92. DOI: 10.4103/0253-7176.78503 PMID: 21716860

Beck, A. T., Ward, C. H., Mendelson, M., Mock, J., & Erbaugh, J. (1961). An inventory for measuring depression. *Archives of General Psychiatry*, *4*(1), 561–571. DOI: 10.1001/archpsyc.1961.01710120031004 PMID: 13688369

Bedaso, A., Adams, J., Peng, W., & Sibbritt, D. (2021). The relationship between social support and mental health problems during pregnancy: A systematic review and meta-analysis. *Reproductive Health*, *18*(1), 1–9. DOI: 10.1186/s12978-021-01209-5 PMID: 34321040

Beilharz, J., Maniam, J., & Morris, M. (2015). Diet-induced cognitive deficits: The role of fat and sugar, potential mechanisms and nutritional interventions. *Nutrients*, *7*(8), 6719–6738. DOI: 10.3390/nu7085307 PMID: 26274972

Belsky, J., & Pluess, M. (2009). Beyond diathesis stress: Differential susceptibility to environmental influences. *Psychological Bulletin*, *135*(6), 885–908. DOI: 10.1037/a0017376 PMID: 19883141

Bhargav, H., Holla, B., Ramakrishna, K. K., Shivakumar, V., Gokulakrishnan, K., Varambally, S., & Gangadhar, B. N. (2022). Yoga and integrative healthcare. *International Journal of Yoga*, *15*(2), 150–157. DOI: 10.4103/ijoy.ijoy_56_22 PMID: 36329771

Bhugra, D., Till, A., & Sartorius, N. (2013). What is mental health? *The International Journal of Social Psychiatry*, *59*(1), 3–4. DOI: 10.1177/0020764012463315 PMID: 23349505

Buser, M. C., & Scinicariello, F. (2017). Cadmium, lead, and depressive symptoms: Analysis of national health and nutrition examination survey 2011-2012. *The Journal of Clinical Psychiatry*, *78*(5), 515–521. DOI: 10.4088/JCP.15m10383 PMID: 27929609

Callaghan, A., McCombe, G., Harrold, A., McMeel, C., Mills, G., Moore-Cherry, N., & Cullen, W. (2020). The impact of green spaces on mental health in urban settings: A scoping review. *Journal of Mental Health (Abingdon, England)*, *30*(2), 179–193. DOI: 10.1080/09638237.2020.1755027 PMID: 32310728

Cohen, S., Underwood, L. G., & Gottlieb, B. H. (2000). Social relationships and health. In Cohen, S., Underwood, L. G., & Gottlieb, B. H. (Eds.), *Social Support Measurement and Intervention: A Guide for Health and Social Scientists* (pp. 3–26). Oxford Academic Press., DOI: 10.1093/med:psych/9780195126709.003.0001

Dal, N., & Bilici, S. (2024). An overview of the potential role of nutrition in mental disorders in the light of advances in nutripsychiatry. *Current Nutrition Reports*, *13*(2), 69–81. DOI: 10.1007/s13668-024-00520-4 PMID: 38329691

Dan, V. H., Ponnuchamy, L., Anand, N. K., Bhaskarapillai, B., & Sharma, M. K. (2023). Resilience and self-compassion among persons with depressive disorders: Prerequisite for a positive mental health approach. *Journal of Family Medicine and Primary Care, 12*(8), 1621–1628. DOI: 10.4103/jfmpc.jfmpc_2270_22 PMID: 37767454

Das, A., Sharma, M. K., Thamilselvan, P., & Marimuthu, P. (2017). Technology addiction among treatment seekers for psychological problems: Implication for screening in mental health setting. *Indian Journal of Psychological Medicine, 39*(1), 21–27. DOI: 10.4103/0253-7176.198939 PMID: 28250554

Degan, T. J., Kelly, P. J., Robinson, L. D., & Deane, F. P. (2018). Health literacy in substance use disorder treatment: A latent profile analysis. *Journal of Substance Abuse Treatment, 96*(1), 46–52. DOI: 10.1016/j.jsat.2018.10.009 PMID: 30466548

Dzhambov, A. M., Hartig, T., Tilov, B., Atanasova, V., Makakova, D. R., & Dimitrova, D. D. (2019). Residential greenspace is associated with mental health via intertwined capacity-building and capacity-restoring pathways. *Environmental Research, 178*(1), 1–13. DOI: 10.1016/j.envres.2019.108708 PMID: 31526908

Fusar-Poli, P., De Pablo, G. S., De Micheli, A., Nieman, D. H., Correll, C. U., Kessing, L. V., Pfennig, A., Bechdolf, A., Borgwardt, S., Arango, C., & Van Amelsvoort, T. (2019). What is good mental health? A scoping review. *European Neuropsychopharmacology, 31*(1), 33–46. DOI: 10.1016/j.euroneuro.2019.12.105 PMID: 31901337

Galderisi, S., Heinz, A., Kastrup, M., Beezhold, J., & Sartorius, N. (2015). Toward a new definition of mental health. *World Psychiatry; Official Journal of the World Psychiatric Association (WPA), 14*(2), 231–233. DOI: 10.1002/wps.20231 PMID: 26043341

Grajek, M., Krupa-Kotara, K., Białek-Dratwa, A., Sobczyk, K., Grot, M., Kowalski, O., & Staśkiewicz, W. (2022). Nutrition and mental health: A review of current knowledge about the impact of diet on mental health. *Frontiers in Nutrition, 9*, 943998. Advance online publication. DOI: 10.3389/fnut.2022.943998 PMID: 36071944

Gruebner, O., Rapp, M. A., Adli, M., Kluge, U., Galea, S., & Heinz, A. (2017). Cities and mental health. *Deutsches Ärzteblatt International, 114*(1), 121–127. DOI: 10.3238/arztebl.2017.0121 PMID: 28302261

Hamilton, M. (1960). Hamilton depression rating scale (HDRS). *Journal of Neurology, Neurosurgery, and Psychiatry, 23*(1), 56–62. DOI: 10.1136/jnnp.23.1.56 PMID: 14399272

Haugen, P. T., McCrillis, A. M., Smid, G. E., & Nijdam, M. J. (2017). Mental health stigma and barriers to mental health care for first responders: A systematic review and meta-analysis. *Journal of Psychiatric Research*, *94*(1), 218–229. DOI: 10.1016/j.jpsychires.2017.08.001 PMID: 28800529

Henriksen, I. O., Ranøyen, I., Indredavik, M. S., & Stenseng, F. (2017). The role of self-esteem in the development of psychiatric problems: A three-year prospective study in a clinical sample of adolescents. *Child and Adolescent Psychiatry and Mental Health*, *11*(1), 1–13. DOI: 10.1186/s13034-017-0207-y PMID: 29299058

Huber, M., Knottnerus, J. A., Green, L., Horst, H. V. D., Jadad, A. R., Kromhout, D., Leonard, B., Lorig, K., Loureiro, M. I., Meer, J. W. M. V. D., Schnabel, P., Smith, R., Weel, C. V., & Smid, H. (2011). How should we define health? *BMJ (Clinical Research Ed.)*, *343*(2), 41–63. DOI: 10.1136/bmj.d4163 PMID: 21791490

Hwang, W., Myers, H., Abekim, J., & Ting, J. (2007). A conceptual paradigm for understanding culture's impact on mental health: The cultural influences on mental health (CIMH) model. *Clinical Psychology Review*, *28*(2), 211–227. DOI: 10.1016/j.cpr.2007.05.001 PMID: 17587473

Hyman, S. E. (2000). The genetics of mental illness: Implications for practice. *Bulletin of the World Health Organization*, *78*(4), 455–463. PMID: 10885164

Institute for Health Metrics and Evaluation (IHME). Global Burden of Disease (GBD). (2021). [Online]. https://vizhub.healthdata.org/gbd-results/

Jayasankar, P., Manjunatha, N., Rao, G. N., Gururaj, G., Varghese, M., & Benegal, V.NMHS India National Collaborator Group. (2022). Epidemiology of common mental disorders: Results from "National Mental Health Survey" of India, 2016. *Indian Journal of Psychiatry*, *64*(1), 13–19. DOI: 10.4103/indianjpsychiatry.indianjpsychiatry_865_21 PMID: 35400745

Kapoor, A. R., Patel, A., & Nair, V. P. (2024). Exploring the neurobiological mechanisms mediating the impact of air pollution on cognitive and emotional health in urban residents of New Delhi. *Studies in Psychological Science*, *2*(2), 21–31. DOI: 10.56397/SPS.2024.06.03

Kawachi, I., & Berkman, L. F. (2001). Social Ties and Mental Health. *Journal of Urban Health*, *78*(3), 458–467. DOI: 10.1093/jurban/78.3.458 PMID: 11564849

Kay, S. R., Fiszbein, A., & Opler, L. A. (1987). The positive and negative syndrome scale (PANSS) for schizophrenia. *Schizophrenia Bulletin*, *13*(2), 261–276. DOI: 10.1093/schbul/13.2.261 PMID: 3616518

Kendler, K. S., Myers, J. M., Maes, H. H., & Keyes, C. L. M. (2011). The relationship between the genetic and environmental influences on common internalizing psychiatric disorders and mental well-being. *Behavior Genetics*, *41*(5), 641–650. DOI: 10.1007/s10519-011-9466-1 PMID: 21451959

Kim, J., & Kim, H. (2017). Demographic and environmental factors associated with mental health: A cross-sectional study. *International Journal of Environmental Research and Public Health*, *14*(4), 1–12. DOI: 10.3390/ijerph14040431 PMID: 28420189

Kumari, S., Malik, M., Florival, C., Manalai, P., & Sonje, S. (2018). An Assessment of Five (PANSS, SAPS, SANS, NSA-16, CGI-SCH) commonly used Symptoms Rating Scales in Schizophrenia and Comparison to Newer Scales (CAINS, BNSS). *Journal of Addiction Research & Therapy*, *8*(3), 1–14. DOI: 10.4172/2155-6105.1000324 PMID: 29430333

Laishram, J., Fernandez, S., Devi, P. A., Bhowmick, M. R., Heigrujam, R., & Devi, H. S. (2025). Sleep quality and mental health among medical students in Imphal, Manipur: A cross-sectional study. *Journal of Family Medicine and Primary Care*, *14*(1), 276–282. DOI: 10.4103/jfmpc.jfmpc_1160_24 PMID: 39989537

Lakhan, S. E., & Vieira, K. F. (2008). Nutritional therapies for mental disorders. *Nutrition Journal*, *7*(2), 1–11. DOI: 10.1186/1475-2891-7-2 PMID: 18208598

Lee, M. S., Shin, J. S., Lee, J., Lee, Y. J., Kim, M. R., Park, K. B., Shin, D., Cho, J. H., & Ha, I. H. (2015). The association between mental health, chronic disease and sleep duration in Koreans: A cross-sectional study. *BMC Public Health*, *15*(1), 1–13. DOI: 10.1186/s12889-015-2542-3 PMID: 26627637

Lim, S. Y., Kim, E. J., Kim, A., Lee, H. J., Choi, H. J., & Yang, S. J. (2016). Nutritional factors affecting mental health. *Clinical Nutrition Research*, *5*(3), 1–15. DOI: 10.7762/cnr.2016.5.3.143 PMID: 27482518

Makwana, N. (2019). Disaster and its impact on mental health: A narrative review. *Journal of Family Medicine and Primary Care*, *8*(10), 1–9. DOI: 10.4103/jfmpc.jfmpc_893_19 PMID: 31742125

Manwell, L. A., Barbic, S. P., Roberts, K., Durisko, Z., Lee, C., Ware, E., & McKenzie, K. (2015). What is mental health? Evidence towards a new definition from a mixed methods multidisciplinary international survey. *BMJ Open*, *5*(6), 1–12. DOI: 10.1136/bmjopen-2014-007079 PMID: 26038353

Maslow, A. H. (1958). A dynamic theory of human motivation. In Stacey, C. L., & DeMartino, M. (Eds.), *Understanding human motivation* (pp. 26–47). Howard Allen Publishers., DOI: 10.1037/11305-004

McKenzie, K., Murray, G., Murray, A., Delahunty, L., Hutton, L., Murray, K., & O'Hare, A. (2018). Child and adolescent intellectual disability screening questionnaire to identify children with intellectual disability. *Developmental Medicine and Child Neurology*, *61*(4), 444–450. DOI: 10.1111/dmcn.13998 PMID: 30146754

Mental Health Foundation (MHF). (2008). What works for you? London. [online]. https://www.mentalhealth.org.uk/sites/default/files/2022-09/MHF-What-Works-For-You-study.pdf

Mohd, T. A. M. T., Yunus, R. M., Hairi, F., Hairi, N. N., & Choo, W. Y. (2019). Social support and depression among community dwelling older adults in Asia: A systematic review. *BMJ Open*, *9*(7), 1–10. DOI: 10.1136/bmjopen-2018-026667 PMID: 31320348

Morgan, N., & Mall, S. (2019). Pathways between urbanization and harmful substance use. *Current Opinion in Psychiatry*, *32*(3), 218–223. DOI: 10.1097/YCO.0000000000000488 PMID: 30695003

National Mental Health (NMH). (2010). *National survey confirms that youth are disproportionately affected by mental disorders*. [online]. https://www.nimh.nih.gov/health/statistics/mental-illness

Negi, S., Singh, R., & Singh, A. K. (2025). Natural disaster: prevalence of post-traumatic stress and psychological outcome of survivors in Joshimath, Uttarakhand, India. In Kurebwa, J., & Makwerere, D. (Eds.), *Managing the Health Risks of Climate Change* (pp. 107–134). IGI Global Scientific Publishing., DOI: 10.4018/979-8-3693-4183-4.ch005

Padhy, S., Sarkar, S., Panigrahi, M., & Paul, S. (2015). Mental health effects of climate change. *Indian Journal of Occupational and Environmental Medicine*, *19*(1), 3–13. DOI: 10.4103/0019-5278.156997 PMID: 26023264

Peen, J., Schoevers, R. A., Beekman, A. T., & Dekker, J. (2009). The current status of urban-rural differences in psychiatric disorders. *Acta Psychiatrica Scandinavica*, *121*(2), 84–93. DOI: 10.1111/j.1600-0447.2009.01438.x PMID: 19624573

Penberthy, J. K., Cox, D., Breton, M., Robeva, R., Kalbfleisch, M. L., Loboschefski, T., & Kovatchev, B. (2005). Calibration of ADHD Assessments across studies: A meta-analysis tool. *Applied Psychophysiology and Biofeedback*, *30*(1), 31–51. DOI: 10.1007/s10484-005-2172-0 PMID: 15889584

Pinto, R. Q., Soares, I., Carvalho-Correia, E., & Mesquita, A. R. (2015). Gene–environment interactions in psychopathology throughout early childhood. *Psychiatric Genetics, 25*(6), 223–233. DOI: 10.1097/YPG.0000000000000106 PMID: 26313931

Raine, A., Ling, S., Streicher, W., & Liu, J. (2022). The conduct and oppositional defiant disorder scales (CODDS) for disruptive behaviour disorders. *Psychiatry Research, 316*(1), 1–15. DOI: 10.1016/j.psychres.2022.114744 PMID: 35961152

Rao, T. S. (2008). Understanding nutrition, depression and mental illnesses. *Indian Journal of Psychiatry, 50*(2), 77–88. DOI: 10.4103/0019-5545.42391 PMID: 19742217

Rauf, T., & Freese, J. (2024). Genetic influences on depression and selection into adverse life experiences. *Social Science & Medicine, 344*(1), 1–11. DOI: 10.1016/j.socscimed.2024.116633 PMID: 38324978

Reddy, V. (2019). Mental health issues and challenges in India: A review. [IJSSME]. *International Journal of Social Sciences Management and Entrepreneurship, 3*(2), 1–11.

Rose, M., & Devine, J. (2014). Assessment of patient-reported symptoms of anxiety. *Dialogues in Clinical Neuroscience, 16*(2), 197–211. DOI: 10.31887/DCNS.2014.16.2/mrose PMID: 25152658

Sappok, T., Heinrich, M., & Underwood, L. (2015). Screening tools for autism spectrum disorders. *Advances in Autism, 1*(1), 12–29. DOI: 10.1108/AIA-03-2015-0001

Singh, A., Singh, R., & Singh, A. K. (2025). A review-based theoretical analysis on somatization of psychological symptoms and physical manifestation of trauma in youths. In Sofologi, M., Katsarou, D., & Efthymiou, E. (Eds.), *Exploring Cognitive and Psychosocial Dynamics Across Childhood and Adolescence* (pp. 273–294). IGI Global., DOI: 10.4018/979-8-3693-4022-6.ch014

Singh, K., Junnarkar, M., & Jain, A. (2017). Factors affecting mental health of north Indian adolescents. *Psychological Studies, 62*(2), 168–177. DOI: 10.1007/s12646-017-0398-6

Singh, R., Thapliyal, C., & Chowdhury, K. (2021). Emotion regulation, parenting style, and satisfaction with life in adult. *Webology, 1*(1), 1441–1448. DOI: 10.29121/WEB/V18I1/25

Siste, K., Hanafi, E., Sen, L. T., Murtani, B. J., Christian, H., Limawan, A. P., Siswidiani, L. P., & Adrian, N. (2021). Implications of COVID-19 and lockdown on internet addiction among adolescents: Data from a developing country. *Frontiers in Psychiatry, 12*(1), 1–13. DOI: 10.3389/fpsyt.2021.665675 PMID: 34054619

Song, H. T., Sun, X. Y., Yang, T. S., Zhang, L. Y., Yang, J. L., & Bai, J. (2015). Effects of sleep deprivation on serum cortisol level and mental health in servicemen. *International Journal of Psychophysiology*, *96*(3), 169–175. DOI: 10.1016/j.ijpsycho.2015.04.008 PMID: 25913092

Soto-Icaza, P., Aboitiz, F., & Billeke, P. (2015). Development of social skills in children: Neural and behavioral evidence for the elaboration of cognitive models. *Frontiers in Neuroscience*, *9*(1), 1–12. DOI: 10.3389/fnins.2015.00333 PMID: 26483621

Stoewen, D. L. (2022). Nature, nurture, and mental health Part 1: The influence of genetics, psychology, and biology. *The Canadian Veterinary Journal = La Revue Vétérinaire Canadienne*, *63*(4), 427–430. PMID: 35368400

Sundquist, K., Johansson, L., DeMarinis, V., Johansson, S., & Sundquist, J. (2005). Posttraumatic stress disorder and psychiatric co-morbidity: Symptoms in a random sample of female Bosnian refugees. *European Psychiatry : the Journal of the Association of European Psychiatrists*, *20*(2), 158–164. DOI: 10.1016/j.eurpsy.2004.12.001 PMID: 15797701

Taddi, V. V., Kohli, R. K., & Puri, P. (2024). Perception, use of social media, and its impact on the mental health of Indian adolescents: A qualitative study. *World Journal of Clinical Pediatrics*, *13*(3), 1–9. DOI: 10.5409/wjcp.v13.i3.97501 PMID: 39350908

Tare, S., Verma, H., & Jahagirdar, D. (2025). A Correlation Between Resilience and Positive Mental Health. *International Journal of Indian Psychology*, *3*(1), 1–13. DOI: 10.25215/1301.017

Tater, B., & John, K. (2024). Effects of smartphone addiction on the physical and mental well-being of Indian students. *Indian Journal of Science and Technology*, *17*(25), 2622–2634. DOI: 10.17485/IJST/v17i25.1355

Tikka, S. K., Garg, S., & Siddiqui, M. A. (2020). Prescribing Physical Activity in Mental Health: A focused review on the latest evidence, recommendations, challenges, and relevance to India. *Indian Journal of Psychological Medicine*, *43*(6), 535–541. DOI: 10.1177/0253717620972330 PMID: 35210683

Túry, F., Güleç, H., & Kohls, E. (2009). Assessment methods for eating disorders and body image disorders. *Journal of Psychosomatic Research*, *69*(6), 601–611. DOI: 10.1016/j.jpsychores.2009.05.012 PMID: 21109049

Wind, T. R., Joshi, P. C., Kleber, R. J., & Komproe, I. H. (2013). The impact of recurrent disasters on mental health: A study on seasonal floods in northern India. *Prehospital and Disaster Medicine*, *28*(3), 279–285. DOI: 10.1017/S1049023X13000290 PMID: 23611652

World Health Organisation (WHO). Global Health Estimation (GHE). (2019). [Online]. https://www.who.int/data/gho/data/themes/mortality-and-global-health-estimates

World Health Organization (WHO). (1992). *The ICD-10 classification of mental and behavioural disorders: Diagnostic criteria for research.* [Online]. https://www.who.int/publications/i/item/9241544554

World Health Organization (WHO). (2024a). Health and Well-being. [Online]. https://www.who.int/data/gho/data/major-themes/health-and-well-being

World Health Organization (WHO). (2024b). Mental health [Online]. https://www.who.int/india/health-topics/mental-health

World Health Organization (WHO). (2024c). Mental health Impact [Online]. https://www.who.int/health-topics/mental-health#tab=tab_2

World Health Organization (WHO). (2024d). Mental health of adolescents [Online]. https://www.who.int/news-room/fact-sheets/detail/adolescent-mental-health

World Health Organization (WHO). (2024e). Mental health of adolescents [Online]. https://www.who.int/news-room/fact-sheets/detail/mental-health-of-older-adults

KEY TERMS AND DEFINITIONS

Dementia: Mental disorder is a neurocognitive disorder linked with memory loss and cognitive abilities (problem-solving and thinking).

Emotion Regulation: Ability to know the emotions as well as regulate, manage and respond to maintain emotional and overall well-being

Genetic factors: Inherited qualities, characteristics, traits, and diseases from the parents as well as ancestors.

Mental Health Literacy: Education about mental health conditions, disorders, and providing information to access professional support and treatment.

Obesity: A health condition with an excessive amount of body fat and body weight.

Parenting style: The Approaches parents take to rear their children by creating an environment of demandingness and responsiveness to interact and raise their children.

Phobia: A type of anxiety disorder that is linked with extreme and persistent fear of an object or situation.

Post-Traumatic Stress Disorder: A type of Mental disorder, can be developed by experiencing or witnessing a traumatic event (Physical, emotional and/or sexual), causing extreme stress.

Chapter 8
Ethical Considerations in Health Psychology Practice and Research

Vijeta Sharma
Chandigarh University, India

P. Selvakumar
http://orcid.org/0000-0002-3650-4548
Department of Science and Humanities, Nehru Institute of Technology, Coimbatore, India

Rajshri Chalakh
http://orcid.org/0009-0003-4576-0847
MSS Law College, Hyderabad, India

Seema Jaidas Mulmule
http://orcid.org/0009-0001-9465-4544
Marwadi Siksha Samiti, India

Lalitha Saipogu
http://orcid.org/0009-0004-0245-4222
CVR College of Engineering, India

P. Radhika
SRM Institute of Science and Technology, India

ABSTRACT

Ethics plays a foundational and indispensable role in health psychology practice, shaping how professionals interact with clients, conduct research, design interventions, and contribute to public health. Health psychology, as an interdisciplinary field concerned with the relationships among biological, psychological, and social factors in health and illness, deals with sensitive aspects of human life such as physical well-being, mental health, cultural values, coping with illness, adherence to treatment, and end-of-life care. In this context, ethical principles act as guiding frameworks to ensure that practices are fair, respectful, and beneficial to clients, while minimizing harm and protecting vulnerable populations. Without strong ethical grounding, For example, pushing a patient toward behavior change without respect-

DOI: 10.4018/979-8-3373-6294-6.ch008

ing their readiness or cultural context could lead to resistance, guilt, or distress. Ethical practice therefore involves striking a delicate balance between supporting growth and avoiding unnecessary harm.

THE IMPORTANCE OF ETHICS IN HEALTH PSYCHOLOGY PRACTICE

Ethics plays a foundational and indispensable role in health psychology practice, shaping how professionals interact with clients, conduct research, design interventions, and contribute to public health. Health psychology, as an interdisciplinary field concerned with the relationships among biological, psychological, and social factors in health and illness, deals with sensitive aspects of human life such as physical well-being, mental health, cultural values, coping with illness, adherence to treatment, and end-of-life care. In this context, ethical principles act as guiding frameworks to ensure that practices are fair, respectful, and beneficial to clients, while minimizing harm and protecting vulnerable populations. Without strong ethical grounding, For example, pushing a patient toward behavior change without respecting their readiness or cultural context could lead to resistance, guilt, or distress. Ethical practice therefore involves striking a delicate balance between supporting growth and avoiding unnecessary harm.psychologists often work with clients navigating complex medical systems or making choices about lifestyle changes that can profoundly affect their lives. Upholding autonomy requires practitioners to provide clear, honest, and accessible information about psychological interventions, potential outcomes, and alternative options, empowering clients to participate actively in decision-making. `(Aboujaoude, 2018)This principle also highlights the importance of informed consent, which is more than a legal requirement; it is an ethical commitment to transparency, respect, and shared decision-making.

At the same time, ethical practice recognizes that confidentiality is not absolute. Situations may arise where disclosure is necessary to protect the client or others from harm—for example, in cases of suicidal ideation, abuse, or threats of violence. Navigating these ethical dilemmas requires judgment, sensitivity, and adherence to professional guidelines that balance the duty of confidentiality with the duty to protect life and safety. Health psychologists must clearly communicate the boundaries of confidentiality at the outset of their professional relationships so clients understand the conditions under which information might be shared. equity in access to care, treatment, and research participation. Health psychology practice often intersects with broader social determinants of health, such as socioeconomic status, race, gender, and geography, which can create disparities in healthcare outcomes. Ethical practitioners must strive to ensure that psychological services are accessible and non-discriminatory, actively working against systemic barriers that prevent marginalized groups from receiving equitable care. (Aboujaoude et al., 2020)For instance, providing culturally adapted interventions, advocating for underserved populations, and addressing health inequities are ethical imperatives that extend beyond individual client interactions into the realm of public health advocacy. Justice also plays a crucial role in research ethics, where health psychologists must ensure that participants are treated fairly, that vulnerable groups are not exploited, and that the benefits and burdens of research are equitably distributed across society.their work, including clinical practice, teaching, and research. Misrepresentation of credentials, exaggeration of treatment effectiveness, or selective reporting of research findings not only violates ethical codes but also undermines public trust in psychology as a discipline. Ethical integrity also extends to managing conflicts of interest, such as avoiding dual relationships where personal and professional roles overlap in ways that could compromise objectivity or client welfare.

ETHICAL PRINCIPLES IN HEALTH PSYCHOLOGY RESEARCH AND PRACTICE

Ethical principles are the cornerstone of health psychology research and practice, providing a framework for ensuring that the pursuit of scientific knowledge and the delivery of psychological interventions are conducted with fairness, compassion, respect, and integrity. Health psychology, as a discipline at the intersection of psychology, medicine, and public health, deals with issues that directly influence human well-being—ranging from stress management and behavior change to chronic disease adjustment, pain management, and coping with terminal illness (Bagarić & Jokić-Begić, 2020). Because of its profound impact on human lives, the field requires careful adherence to ethical standards that safeguard the dignity, autonomy, and rights of individuals while also promoting societal health and justice. Ethical principles act as both preventive and proactive measures, preventing harm and exploitation on one hand and encouraging the cultivation of trust, equity, and beneficence on the other. By grounding their work in ethical guidelines, health psychologists protect vulnerable populations, ensure responsible use of psychological knowledge, and uphold the credibility of psychology as a science and a profession.psychologists to act in ways that enhance the well-being of clients, patients, and participants. In both research and practice, this requires that interventions, counseling techniques, or health promotion strategies are designed to maximize potential benefits—whether these benefits are psychological relief, improved coping, better adherence to medical regimens, or enhanced quality of life.

Informed decisions about their health, treatment, and participation in research. In practice, autonomy requires health psychologists to seek informed consent before implementing interventions, providing clients with accurate, comprehensive, and understandable information about the nature, purpose, risks, and benefits of treatment. Consent is not merely a bureaucratic formality but a process of dialogue that fosters respect, trust, and collaboration between psychologist and client. In research, autonomy similarly necessitates voluntary participation, where individuals are free to withdraw at any time without penalty. Special attention must be paid to vulnerable populations—such as children, elderly patients, or individuals with cognitive impairments—who may lack full decision-making capacity. In such cases, ethical practice demands surrogate decision-making, assent where possible, and heightened vigilance to ensure protection of participants' rights and dignity (Balcombe & De Leo, 2021). Respect for autonomy also entails cultural sensitivity, acknowledging that values around independence, authority, and family decision-making vary across cultures. Ethical health psychology thus requires practitioners to honor cultural contexts. The rise of digital health technologies, such as online therapy platforms, wearable devices, and mobile health apps, presents new challenges for confidentiality. Health psychologists must ensure that data privacy protections keep pace with technological advances, safeguarding clients' and participants' information from misuse, unauthorized access, or exploitation. Clear communication about the limits of confidentiality is equally important, enabling individuals to understand when their information may need to be shared for safety reasons.

OBTAINING INFORMED CONSENT IN HEALTH PSYCHOLOGY RESEARCH

Informed consent represents one of the most fundamental ethical requirements in health psychology research, serving as a mechanism through which respect for individual autonomy, dignity, and rights is safeguarded. Health psychology, as a field that examines the complex interplay between psychological, behavioral, and biological factors in health and illness, often requires researchers to work with sensitive populations, gather deeply personal health-related data, and implement interventions that may influence physical and psychological well-being. Within this context, obtaining informed consent is not merely a procedural step or a legal obligation but an ongoing ethical commitment to transparency, respect, and partnership between researcher and participant. The principle of informed consent ensures that individuals are not coerced or deceived into participation and that they retain agency over their involvement in research projects. It embodies the ethical ideals of autonomy and justice while also serving as a cornerstone of beneficence and non-maleficence by protecting participants from harm and exploitation. (Charan et al., 2025a). Without robust informed consent procedures, the credibility of health psychology research would be undermined, trust in researchers eroded, and participants exposed to risks they neither anticipated nor agreed to accept.potential participants with complete and accurate information regarding the study's purpose, procedures, risks, benefits, confidentiality measures, and their rights, including the right to withdraw at any time without penalty. This information must be presented in clear and accessible language, avoiding technical jargon or ambiguous phrasing that could obscure understanding. In health psychology, where research often addresses issues such as coping with chronic illness, stress management, lifestyle interventions, or mental health, disclosure is understand the information provided.

Researchers are ethically obligated to ensure that participants grasp what participation entails, which may require adapting consent materials manipulation, particularly when participants may feel pressure due to hierarchical dynamics possess the mental and legal capacity to provide valid consent; where capacity is compromised, researchers must obtain surrogate consent while still seeking the assent of the updated about new findings, changes in procedures, or emerging risks, with the option to reaffirm or withdraw their consent throughout the study(Charan et al., 2025b). The principle of autonomy is at the heart of informed consent, and in health psychology research this becomes particularly significant because studies often engage populations who may feel vulnerable or disempowered. Patients managing chronic diseases, individuals with mental health conditions, children, elderly participants, and those from marginalized communities may experience diminished control over health-related decisions in their daily lives, making the protection of autonomy in research settings all the more critical. Respecting autonomy through informed consent empowers participants to reclaim agency, allowing them to make choices that align with their values, preferences, and cultural frameworks. This requires sensitivity on the part of researchers, who must avoid paternalistic assumptions about what is "best" for participants and instead foster an environment of dialogue and respect. Informed consent thus functions as a practical expression of respect for persons, ensuring that research participants are treated not merely as data sources but as individuals with rights and inherent dignity.

In health psychology research, obtaining informed consent also intersects with the principle of beneficence, as participants must be made aware of potential benefits arising from their involvement. These may include psychological support, access to new health interventions, or contributions to scientific knowledge that could improve healthcare for others. At the same time, informed consent embodies non-maleficence by requiring that potential risks—such as psychological distress from discussing sensitive topics, discomfort from experimental procedures, or breaches of confidentiality—are clearly communicated and minimized. By disclosing both risks and benefits honestly, researchers respect participants' right to make decisions aligned with their personal thresholds for risk tolerance. (Department of Health and Aged Care, 2021). This balance is particularly delicate in research involving vulnerable populations, where even minimal risks may carry disproportionate consequences.further underscores the importance of transparency regarding digital privacy and data security. Ethical researchers must ensure that participants are not only told about these risks but also provided with reassurances about the steps being taken to protect their data in an evolving technological landscape. Cultural and contextual considerations play a significant role in obtaining informed consent in health psychology research.

Concepts such as autonomy, authority, and individual decision-making may vary across cultural settings. In some cultures, health-related decisions are made collectively within families or communities rather than by individuals alone, requiring researchers to adapt consent procedures to honor these norms while still safeguarding the rights of individual participants. Language barriers also pose challenges, making it essential for consent forms to be translated into local languages and for interpreters or cultural mediators to be involved in the consent process. Furthermore, literacy levels may vary widely, necessitating the use of verbal explanations, visual aids, or interactive consent processes to ensure comprehension. Without attention to these cultural and contextual factors, informed consent risks becoming a superficial exercise rather than a meaningful ethical practice.legal and developmental considerations. Studies with individuals experiencing cognitive impairments, such as dementia, demand careful assessment of decision-making capacity and reliance on surrogate consent while respecting the person's preferences to the greatest extent possible. (Dijksman et al., 2017)In research with economically disadvantaged populations, it is vital to ensure that compensation for participation does not become coercive, creating undue influence that undermines voluntariness. Similarly, in clinical settings where patients may perceive participation as linked to their medical care, researchers must take additional steps to clarify that participation is voluntary and independent of treatment outcomes.

RESPECTING PATIENT AUTONOMY IN HEALTH PSYCHOLOGY PRACTICE

Respecting patient autonomy is a central ethical obligation in health psychology practice, reflecting a broader commitment to human dignity, individual rights, and self-determination in matters of health and well-being. Patient autonomy refers to the right of individuals to make informed, voluntary decisions about their own health, treatment, and participation in psychological or medical interventions, free from coercion or undue influence. Within health psychology, where practitioners often work with individuals managing chronic illness, mental health conditions, lifestyle changes, or complex healthcare decisions, respecting autonomy is both ethically and practically significant. Autonomy recognizes patients as active agents in their care, rather than passive recipients of professional authority, and affirms their capacity to shape their health trajectories in accordance with personal values, cultural traditions, and life goals. Respecting autonomy requires practitioners to engage in transparent communication, provide accessible information about treatment options, honor diverse perspectives, and support informed decision-making even when patients' choices diverge from professional recommendations. By grounding practice in respect for autonomy, health psychologists not only uphold ethical standards but also foster trust, strengthen therapeutic relationships, and empower patients Patients must be provided with accurate, comprehensive, and comprehensible information about their condition, the nature and purpose of proposed interventions, potential risks and benefits, alternatives, and the likely consequences of declining treatment. (Erbe et al., 2017)Information must be conveyed in a manner sensitive to patients' literacy levels, cognitive capacities, and cultural backgrounds, avoiding technical jargon that could hinder understanding.

Cultural diversity adds another critical layer to the ethical imperative of respecting patient autonomy. Concepts of autonomy and decision-making are not universal but are shaped by cultural values, social structures, and collective traditions. In some cultural contexts, health-related decisions are made collectively within families or communities rather than by individuals alone. For instance, patients from collectivist cultures may prefer to involve family members in treatment decisions or defer to elders or community leaders. Health psychologists must be sensitive to these cultural frameworks, adapting their practices to respect collective approaches to autonomy while still safeguarding the individual's rights and dignity. Culturally competent care involves recognizing and valuing these diverse expressions of autonomy rather than imposing a Western individualistic model of decision-making. By embracing cultural sensitivity, health psychologists demonstrate respect not only for individual autonomy but also for the broader social and cultural contexts that shape health behaviors and choices.those with severe mental illness. (Feijt et al., 2018)Respecting confidentiality empowers patients to disclose sensitive information without fear of stigma, discrimination, or unwanted intrusion, thereby strengthening their ability to make authentic health-related decisions. However, ethical practice also requires clear communication about the limits of confidentiality, such as when disclosure is necessary to prevent harm to the patient or others.

CULTURAL SENSITIVITY AND INFORMED CONSENT

Cultural sensitivity is a crucial dimension of obtaining informed consent in health psychology research and practice, ensuring that the ethical principles of autonomy, beneficence, non-maleficence, and justice are upheld in ways that are respectful of diverse cultural frameworks and lived experiences. Informed consent, at its core, is an ethical process that guarantees individuals the right to make voluntary and informed decisions about their participation in research or engagement in therapeutic interventions. (Gun et al., 2011)However, this process cannot be meaningfully achieved without acknowledging the profound influence of cultural norms, languages, traditions, and values on how individuals perceive health, illness, authority, and decision-making. Cultural sensitivity in informed consent requires researchers and practitioners to go beyond standardized procedures and legalistic documentation, instead cultivating an ethical practice rooted in respect, dialogue, and adaptability. By integrating cultural sensitivity into informed consent, health psychologists can prevent misunderstandings, reduce power imbalances, and foster genuine autonomy, thereby ensuring that participants and patients are not merely compliant signatories on consent forms but active agents whose voices and values shape their engagement with health-related research and care One of the central challenges in obtaining informed consent across diverse cultural contexts is the variation in how are conceptualized. In Western traditions, informed consent often reflects an individualistic model, where the patient or research participant is seen as the sole authority in making health-related choices.This dynamic can undermine voluntariness, as individuals may agree to participate not because they genuinely consent but because they feel obliged to comply.

Different cultural groups may evaluate risks and benefits through distinct lenses. For example, in some cultures, potential harm may be interpreted not only in physical or psychological terms but also in spiritual or communal terms. Likewise, the benefits of participation may be seen less as individual gains and more as contributions to family, community, or collective well-being. Health psychologists must adapt their explanations of risks and benefits to reflect these cultural perspectives, ensuring that participants can make decisions consistent with their values. This requires moving beyond standardized biomedical definitions of risk to embrace a more holistic and culturally inclusive understanding of what participation entails. as refugees, migrants, (Guru Basava Aradhya et al., 2025)Indigenous peoples, or individuals from economically disadvantaged backgrounds may face additional barriers to informed consent due to limited education, systemic discrimination, or precarious social positions. These factors increase the risk of exploitation or coercion in research. This may involve hybrid approaches that combine digital tools with in-person explanations, or community-based consent models that integrate local cultural practices with international ethical standards.

MAINTAINING CONFIDENTIALITY IN HEALTH PSYCHOLOGY PRACTICE

Confidentiality is one of the most fundamental ethical principles in health psychology practice, serving as the cornerstone of trust, respect, and professional integrity in the therapeutic and research relationship. It refers to the obligation of health psychologists to protect personal, sensitive, and private information shared by patients or participants and to ensure that such information is not disclosed to unauthorized individuals. The promise of confidentiality provides a secure environment where individuals feel safe enough to disclose intimate details about their psychological, emotional, and physical health without fear of judgment, stigma, or unwanted consequences. In health psychology, where practitioners often deal with deeply personal issues such as chronic illness, pain management, lifestyle behaviors, addiction, trauma, and mental health concerns, maintaining confidentiality is not only a matter of professional ethics but also an essential requirement for fostering therapeutic alliance and empowering patients to engage openly in their care. By ensuring confidentiality, health psychologists uphold the principles of respect for autonomy, beneficence, non-maleficence, and justice, thereby aligning their practice with broader ethical standards that safeguard human dignity and well-being.(Harmanpreet et al., 2025)The importance of confidentiality becomes especially clear when considering the nature of the information patients and participants disclose in health psychology. Unlike general medical consultations that may focus primarily on biological symptoms, health psychology often involves exploring the psychological and social dimensions of health.

Electronic health records, online therapy platforms, and digital communication channels raise significant risks related to privacy breaches, hacking, or inadvertent sharing of data. Ethical practice requires robust cybersecurity measures, secure data storage protocols, and strict adherence to privacy regulations such as HIPAA in the United States or GDPR in Europe. Psychologists must also be cautious when communicating with patients via email, text messages, or telehealth platforms, ensuring that these communications are encrypted and confidential. Furthermore, in research contexts, confidentiality requires anonymizing data, using pseudonyms, and ensuring that research findings cannot inadvertently identify participants. By adopting rigorous safeguards in both clinical and research settings, psychologists demonstrate their commitment to maintaining confidentiality in a rapidly evolving digital landscape.for example, health-related information may traditionally be shared among family members or community leaders, rather than being considered strictly private. Health psychologists must therefore balance respect for cultural norms with the ethical obligation to protect the individual's confidentiality. (Hilvert-Bruce et al., 2012)This may involve negotiating consent around information sharing with families or communities, while ensuring that the patient's rights and preferences are not compromised. In multicultural contexts, maintaining confidentiality also involves being sensitive to how stigma varies across cultures. By safeguarding confidentiality in research, health psychologists honor participants' trust and contribute to ethically sound and socially responsible scholarship. Psychologists must continuously update their knowledge of legal and regulatory frameworks governing confidentiality and stay informed about emerging challenges, such as those posed by artificial intelligence in healthcare or genetic testing that reveals sensitive information about individuals and families. Professional organizations such as the American Psychological Association (APA) or the British Psychological Society (BPS) provide guidelines that serve as ethical anchors, but practitioners must also cultivate reflexivity to navigate the gray areas where ethical codes provide limited direction. Supervision, peer consultation, and ongoing ethics training are essential tools for strengthening professional capacity to uphold confidentiality in diverse and complex contexts.

PROTECTING PATIENT PRIVACY IN RESEARCH AND PRACTICE

Protecting patient privacy is one of the most vital ethical responsibilities in health psychology research and clinical practice, as it safeguards the dignity, autonomy, and trust of individuals who share deeply personal information in vulnerable contexts. Privacy extends beyond the principle of confidentiality, encompassing the broader right of individuals to control access to their personal, psychological, and health-related information, and to determine the conditions under which this information is collected, stored, used, or shared. In both therapeutic and research settings, patients disclose sensitive data about their emotional states, coping mechanisms, cultural backgrounds, social relationships, medical conditions, and behavioral choices, often in ways that expose their identities and vulnerabilities. Without strong protections for privacy, individuals may be reluctant to seek help, avoid participating in research, or withhold important information, undermining the quality of care and the validity of scientific inquiry.(Johansson et al., 2013) Therefore, health psychologists must adopt rigorous ethical, professional, and legal safeguards to ensure that patient privacy is respected at every stage of practice, from the initial encounter to record-keeping, data analysis, and dissemination of findings. Protecting privacy not only fulfills ethical obligations but also strengthens therapeutic alliance, encourages transparency, and enhances the credibility of health psychology as a discipline committed to social responsibility and human well-being.In clinical practice, patient privacy begins with the recognition that the therapeutic space is an environment of trust where individuals share information they may not disclose anywhere else.

Figure 1. Ethical Considerations in Qualitative Research

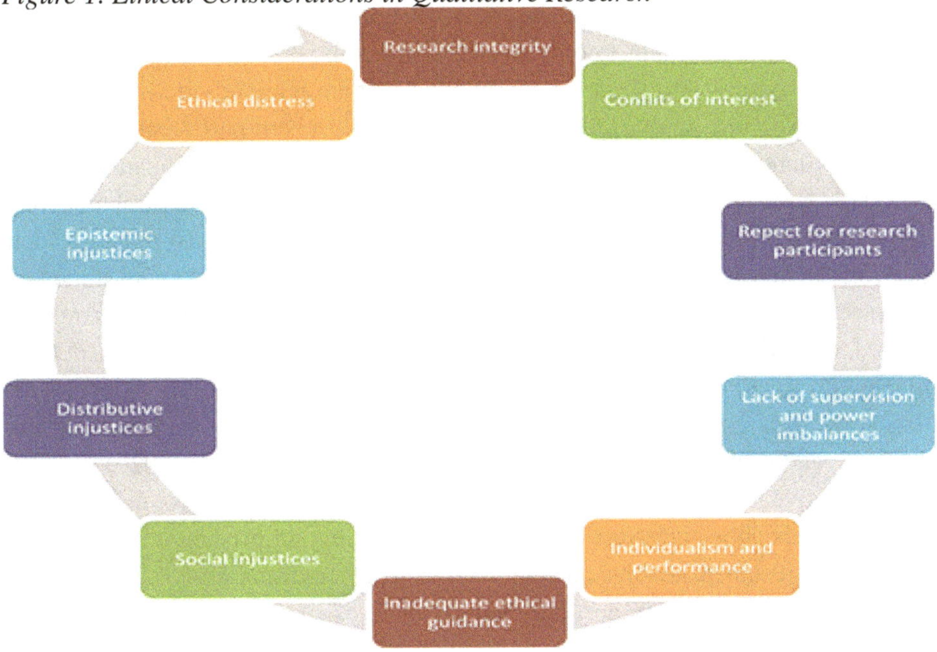

Research integrity
Conflits of interest
Repect for research participants
Lack of supervision and power imbalances
Individualism and performance
Inadequate ethical guidance
Social injustices
Distributive injustices
Epistemic injustices
Ethical distress

Health psychologists must therefore be vigilant about the physical and procedural dimensions of privacy, such as conducting sessions in private settings, ensuring that conversations cannot be overheard, and safeguarding clinical notes from unauthorized access. For example, in hospital or community clinic settings, patients may be reluctant to speak openly if sessions are conducted in shared spaces or if staff members move in and out of rooms without clear boundaries. Ethical practice requires creating conditions that protect the confidentiality of conversations and reassure patients that their disclosures will remain private. Beyond the physical setting, protecting privacy involves carefully managing clinical records, whether in paper or electronic form, and ensuring that these records are only accessible to authorized personnel directly involved in the patient's care.can enhance the accessibility and efficiency of healthcare, they also introduce risks such as data theft, hacking, unauthorized surveillance, or inadvertent data sharing across platforms. (Kemmeren et al., 2019) Health psychologists using telehealth must ensure that communication platforms are encrypted, secure, and compliant with relevant data protection regulations, such as HIPAA in the United States or GDPR in Europe. Furthermore, patients must be informed about the potential risks of digital communication, including the possibility of interception or data leaks, so that they can make informed decisions about their participation. Protecting privacy in the digital age requires ongoing vigilance, investment in cybersecurity measures, and transparency with patients regarding how their data are protected in technologically mediated contexts.

.This often involves anonymizing data, assigning pseudonyms or codes, and limiting access to raw data to only essential research personnel. Ethical research design also requires careful consideration of how findings are reported, particularly in studies involving small or close-knit communities where participants could be indirectly identified through demographic details or contextual information. For example, reporting the experiences of a small group of patients in a rural area may inadvertently reveal identities, even if names are not disclosed. To mitigate such risks, researchers must balance the need for rich, contextualized data with strategies to protect privacy, such as aggregating findings or obtaining explicit consent will be used, who will have access to it, and what measures will be taken to protect their privacy. Informed consent must be more than a formal signature on a document; it must be an ongoing dialogue that allows individuals to ask questions, express concerns, and exercise control over their information.(Knott et al., 2020) Patients should be given clear explanations aboutty as different cultural groups may hold distinct beliefs about information sharing, disclosure, and privacy. In collectivist societies, for instance, health-related information may traditionally be shared within families or communities rather than being treated as strictly private. Health psychologists must balance respect for cultural practices with the ethical obligation to protect individual rights. This may involve carefully negotiating with patients and their families to determine what information can be shared, while ensuring that the individual's autonomy is not compromised. In some cultural contexts, disclosure of sensitive health conditions such as HIV/AIDS, infertility, or mental illness may lead to severe stigma, discrimination, or social exclusion, making privacy protections even more critical.

Culturally competent practice therefore requires not only technical measures to secure data but also sensitivity to the social consequences of disclosure in specific Health psychologists must therefore engage in continuous ethical reflection, professional training, and advocacy to ensure that emerging technologies serve patients' interests without compromising their privacy.Many individuals may feel pressured to disclose information or to consent to the use of their data because they view health professionals as authority figures. Ethical practice requires creating an environment where patients and participants feel empowered to withhold or withdraw consent without fear of judgment, denial of services, or negative repercussions.

Health psychologists must emphasize that participation in research is voluntary, that patients retain ownership of their personal information, and that privacy protections are designed to safeguard their rights rather than to serve institutional convenience. Respecting patients' and participants' agency in this way strengthens trust and reinforces the collaborative nature of both clinical care and research.

BALANCING CONFIDENTIALITY WITH DUTY TO WARN

One of the most ethically complex dilemmas in health psychology practice lies in balancing the principle of confidentiality with the duty to warn, a responsibility that requires practitioners to breach confidentiality under specific circumstances where an individual poses a serious and foreseeable risk of harm to themselves or others. Confidentiality is foundational to the therapeutic and research relationship, offering patients and participants the assurance that sensitive disclosures will remain private and thereby fostering openness, trust, and therapeutic progress. However, the principle of non-maleficence—the obligation to prevent harm—sometimes conflicts with confidentiality, placing psychologists in difficult positions where protecting privacy must yield to protecting life or safety. . Here, the psychologist's responsibility involves balancing respect for patient autonomy and confidentiality with the ethical imperative to preserve life. While patients may fear stigmatization, hospitalization, or loss of control if their disclosures about self-harm are shared, psychologists must weigh these concerns against the potentially irreversible harm of inaction.(Lal & Adair, 2014) Intervening may involve contacting family members, crisis teams, or emergency services, depending on the severity of the risk. Ethical practice requires psychologists to handle such situations with sensitivity, involving patients in safety planning whenever possible and explaining the reasons for breaching confidentiality in a compassionate and transparent manner.in many countries require health professionals to disclose information about suspected child abuse, elder abuse, or domestic violence, even if the patient has not consented. These legal requirements override confidentiality in the interest of protecting individuals who may be unable to protect themselves. For example, if a patient discloses during therapy that they are abusing a child, the psychologist is legally obligated to report this information to child protection services. Similarly, in cases of domestic violence, psychologists may face dilemmas about whether to report threats to protect victims while also considering the potential risks of escalation or retaliation. Balancing confidentiality with duty to warn in these contexts requires not only adherence to legal mandates but also careful ethical reasoning to minimize harm and respect the dignity of all involved.

Cultural sensitivity plays an important role in managing the balance between confidentiality and duty to warn, as cultural norms shape how patients communicate distress, express anger, and interpret confidentiality. In some cultures, discussing violent thoughts may be considered taboo or symbolic rather than literal, requiring psychologists to carefully interpret whether such disclosures indicate actual risk. Similarly, in collectivist cultures where family involvement is central, disclosing threats to family members may be seen as acceptable or even expected, while in individualistic cultures, patients may perceive such disclosures as a serious breach of privacy. Health psychologists must therefore exercise cultural competence in interpreting threats and in communicating the limits of confidentiality to patients. This includes explaining from the outset that confidentiality may be breached if safety is at risk, but doing so in a way that acknowledges cultural understandings of privacy, family roles, and authority. psychologists may face difficulties identifying or locating patients who make threats in online settings, especially if they live in different jurisdictions.(LaMonica et al., 2019) Ethical practice requires that psychologists establish clear protocols for handling disclosures of harm in digital contexts, including obtaining emergency contact information during intake, clarifying the limits of confidentiality in online sessions, and being prepared to involve local emergency services when necessary. Protecting patient privacy in digital contexts while fulfilling duty to warn obligations highlights the need for ongoing adaptation of ethical practices to new technologies.From a research perspective, balancing confidentiality with duty to warn is also critical. Participants in studies involving sensitive topics such as violence, trauma, or mental illness may disclose information that suggests imminent risk of harm. Researchers must establish protocols for handling such, ethical review by institutional review boards (IRBs), and training for research staff are essential to ensure that duty to warn obligations are met without compromising participant trust unnecessarily.

ETHICAL REVIEW BOARDS AND HEALTH PSYCHOLOGY RESEARCH

Ethical review boards, often referred to as Institutional Review Boards (IRBs) or Research Ethics Committees (RECs), play a critical role in overseeing health psychology research by safeguarding the rights, welfare, and dignity of participants while promoting responsible scientific inquiry. In a field as sensitive as health psychology, where research often involves individuals dealing with illness, psychological distress, or vulnerable circumstances, the oversight of ethical review boards ensures that scientific progress does not come at the expense of human well-being. These boards serve as independent evaluators of research protocols, tasked with determining whether proposed studies respect fundamental ethical principles such as autonomy, beneficence, non-maleficence, justice, and respect for persons. Their function goes beyond procedural compliance, embodying a broader commitment to fostering trust between researchers and the public, ensuring that participants can contribute to knowledge generation without being exposed to unnecessary risks or exploitation. By requiring that research protocols undergo ethical review, institutions demonstrate a commitment to balancing the pursuit of knowledge with the protection of individuals whose lives and health may be directly affected by the research process.The origins of ethical review boards can be traced to historical abuses in biomedical and behavioral research, such as the Tuskegee Syphilis Study and unethical wartime experiments, which revealed the devastating consequences of conducting research without proper oversight. In response to such violations, international guidelines such as the Nuremberg Code, the Declaration of Helsinki, and the Belmont Report articulated principles that now serve as the ethical foundation for human research. These documents emphasized the importance of informed consent, the minimization of risk, and the equitable distribution of research benefits and burdens. Ethical review boards operationalize these principles by scrutinizing study designs to ensure compliance with both international standards and local laws. In health psychology, this is particularly significant because research often involves exploring deeply personal issues—such as coping with chronic illness, trauma recovery, or mental health challenges—that could expose participants to emotional distress or stigma if not handled carefully. Thus, the existence of ethical review boards reflects the lessons of history, ensuring that the mistakes of the past are not repeated in contemporary health research.

This is particularly important in health psychology, where participants may be in vulnerable states due to illness, mental health conditions, or socio-economic disadvantages that could compromise their decision-making capacity. (Ojha & Syed, 2020)Boards often require that informed consent documents be written in accessible language, avoiding overly technical terms that could confuse or mislead participants. By requiring such measures, boards ensure that the pursuit of knowledge does not compromise participants' mental health or well-being.Confidentiality and privacy are also central concerns for ethical review boards in health psychology research. Because participants often disclose highly sensitive personal information—such as health histories, coping strategies, family dynamics, or mental health struggles—ethical review boards rigorously examine data handling procedures to ensure that confidentiality is protected. This includes reviewing how data will be stored, whether identifiers will be removed, who will have access to the information, and how results will be reported. In the era of digital research, where data is often collected and stored electronically, review boards place increasing emphasis on cybersecurity measures, such as encryption, password protection, and secure servers, to protect participant privacy. They may also evaluate how researchers plan to handle incidental findings—such as the disclosure of suicidal ideation during an interview—which may require breaching confidentiality to protect participant safety. In these ways, ethical review boards help researchers balance the duty of confidentiality with other ethical imperatives like duty to warn or duty to protect.burdened or exploited. In health psychology, there is often a temptation to recruit participants from easily accessible groups, such as patients in clinics, students, or individuals from marginalized communities who may have fewer resources to resist participation. Review boards scrutinize recruitment methods to ensure that participants are not being targeted simply because they are convenient or vulnerable. At the same time, boards encourage inclusive research practices that ensure marginalized groups are not excluded from the potential benefits of research findings. For example, excluding non-English speakers from health psychology studies might simplify data collection but would limit the generalizability of findings and perpetuate inequities in health research. Ethical review boards, therefore, require researchers to justify inclusion and exclusion criteria, promoting both fairness and scientific rigor.

PROTECTING VULNERABLE POPULATIONS IN HEALTH PSYCHOLOGY RESEARCH

Protecting vulnerable populations in health psychology research is a central ethical responsibility that underscores the discipline's commitment to justice, respect, and beneficence. Vulnerable populations refer to groups who, due to personal, social, cultural, or medical circumstances, may face an increased risk of exploitation, harm, or diminished capacity to provide fully informed and voluntary consent. Such groups often include children, older adults, individuals with cognitive impairments, people living with chronic illness or mental health conditions, economically disadvantaged communities, refugees, and marginalized or stigmatized groups. (Sivanand et al., 2025)In the context of health psychology, where research frequently explores sensitive topics such as coping with illness, trauma, behavioral change, or healthcare disparities, participants from these populations are not only essential to generating inclusive knowledge but also especially susceptible to coercion, misunderstanding, and harm. Thus, researchers have a heightened obligation to ensure that these individuals are recruited ethically, protected throughout the research process, and empowered to participate in ways that respect their dignity, autonomy, and rights.The need for special protections for vulnerable populations stems from historical instances where these groups were exploited in the name of scientific advancement. (Orman & O'Dea, 2018)In cases involving individuals with impaired decision-making capacity, surrogate decision-makers may provide consent, but researchers are ethically obliged to involve the participant as much as possible in the decision-making process. Ethical review boards play a crucial role in evaluating these consent procedures, ensuring that vulnerable populations are not merely signed into studies without a genuine understanding of their participation.To minimize such risks, researchers are encouraged to use trauma-informed practices, provide access to counseling or debriefing, and build in protocols for responding to participant distress during data collection. They must also consider the broader implications of participation, such as the potential for stigma if sensitive information about mental cultural norms, and design studies that respect local traditions and values. Culturally sensitive approaches not only protect participants but also enhance the validity and applicability of research findings by ensuring that they reflect the lived realities of diverse populations.

CULTURAL COMPETENCE IN HEALTH PSYCHOLOGY PRACTICE

Cultural competence in health psychology practice represents a foundational ethical and professional commitment to providing care and conducting research that acknowledges, respects, and integrates the diverse cultural identities, values, and experiences of patients and communities. Defined broadly, cultural competence refers to the ability of practitioners to work effectively across cultural differences, recognizing that health, illness, and psychological well-being are shaped by deeply embedded social, historical, and cultural contexts. In health psychology, where practitioners address the interplay of psychological processes with physical health, cultural competence becomes particularly crucial because individuals' perceptions of illness, coping strategies, treatment adherence, and health behaviors are profoundly influenced by their cultural backgrounds. Without cultural competence, health psychology risks imposing narrow, culturally biased models of care that may alienate patients, exacerbate disparities, and ultimately compromise therapeutic outcomes. Conversely, culturally competent practice fosters trust, strengthens therapeutic alliances, enhances patient engagement, and ensures that interventions are relevant, respectful, and effective across diverse populations.The need for cultural competence arises from the growing diversity of societies worldwide, where globalization, migration, and demographic changes bring together individuals from a wide range of cultural, linguistic, and religious backgrounds. Health psychologists increasingly encounter patients whose worldviews differ from their own or from dominant healthcare paradigms, necessitating an openness to learning, adaptation, and humility. (Sanjari et al., 2014)For instance, while Western biomedical models often emphasize individual responsibility for health behaviors, collectivist cultures may interpret health as a family or community matter, requiring interventions that engage social networks rather than focusing solely on individual change.

Similarly, beliefs about mental health vary widely: in some cultures, psychological distress is primarily expressed through somatic symptoms such as headaches or fatigue rather than emotional language, meaning that clinicians who are culturally unaware may misdiagnose or misunderstand patient concerns. Recognizing these differences is essential to providing equitable care that avoids stereotyping, pathologizing, or overlooking culturally shaped experiences of illness(Park et al., 2019). Awareness involves recognizing one's own cultural identity, values, and biases, as well as understanding how these factors may influence clinical interactions. Knowledge refers to familiarity with the cultural practices, health beliefs, and social determinants that shape patients' experiences. Skills include the ability to communicate effectively across language and cultural barriers, adapt assessment tools, and design interventions that are responsive to cultural contexts. Attitudes involve cultivating respect, openness, and cultural humility, acknowledging that no practitioner can ever achieve complete mastery of another culture and that learning must be continuous. Together, these dimensions form a dynamic process rather than a static achievement, requiring practitioners to remain reflective and adaptable throughout their careers.

For example, measures of depression or anxiety that emphasize individual emotional states may fail to capture culturally normative expressions of distress that manifest in physical or relational terms. Culturally competent practitioners critically evaluate the tools they use, seeking validated translations, culturally adapted measures, or qualitative methods that capture participants' lived experiences more accurately. They also remain attentive to language barriers, using trained interpreters rather than family members to ensure accuracy and confidentiality, and adapting health education materials to reflect culturally relevant metaphors, symbols, and narratives. By tailoring interventions to cultural contexts, health psychologists increase the likelihood of positive outcomes and reduce the risk of treatment dropout.include an understanding of how structural factors—such as racism, poverty, discrimination, and unequal access to healthcare—shape health outcomes for marginalized populations. Health psychologists who adopt a culturally competent lens recognize that patient behaviors cannot be understood in isolation from these broader determinants. For example, low medication adherence among economically disadvantaged groups may reflect financial barriers rather than lack of motivation, requiring interventions that address affordability, access, and systemic discrimination. By incorporating advocacy into their practice, culturally competent health psychologists not only support individual patients but also contribute to efforts aimed at reducing health inequities at the community and policy levels.

THE IMPACT OF BIAS AND STEREOTYPING ON HEALTH PSYCHOLOGY PRACTICE

Bias and stereotyping represent profound challenges within health psychology practice, shaping not only how practitioners perceive and interact with patients but also how patients experience and respond to healthcare systems. Bias, whether conscious or unconscious, refers to the tendency to favor or disadvantage individuals based on preconceived notions, while stereotyping involves assigning generalized characteristics to individuals based on their membership in a social group. Both processes are deeply embedded in human cognition, yet when left unchecked in healthcare contexts, they can produce harmful consequences for patient outcomes, therapeutic relationships, and the broader pursuit of health equity. In health psychology, which emphasizes the relationship between psychological processes, health behaviors, and physical well-being, the presence of bias and stereotyping undermines the field's mission to provide ethical, evidence-based, and culturally competent care.(Warale et al., 2025) By reinforcing disparities, eroding trust, and distorting clinical judgment, bias and stereotyping act as hidden barriers to effective intervention and research, necessitating ongoing reflection, education, and structural reform to mitigate their impact.may overlook important symptoms or dismiss patient concerns. Test (IAT) has shown that even well-intentioned healthcare providers often hold unconscious associations linking certain racial groups with negative traits, which subtly influences clinical decision-making. In health psychology practice, this may manifest in shorter consultation times, less empathetic communication, or lower expectations for treatment adherence when interacting with marginalized patients. These subtle biases accumulate over time, contributing to systemic disparities in healthcare quality and outcomes. Addressing implicit bias requires not only self-awareness but also institutional commitment to training, reflection, and accountability.

For instance, low-income patients may be assumed to lack the willpower or resources to adhere to health regimens, leading providers to withhold more complex interventions. Similarly, stereotypes about gender may shape assumptions regarding coping styles, with women being perceived as more emotional and men as more stoic, influencing the type of psychological support offered. (Werner-Seidler et al., 2019)These biases create self-fulfilling prophecies: when patients sense lowered expectations or dismissive attitudes, they may disengage from treatment, reinforcing the very stereotypes that prompted the biased behavior in the first place. Health psychologists, therefore, must actively counteract these dynamics by setting equitable standards of care, fostering open dialogue, and emphasizing collaborative treatment planning that recognizes patients as active agents in their health journey.s problem-solving or emotion regulation, neglecting collectivist approaches that prioritize family or community support. Similarly, measures of mental health that privilege emotional self-disclosure may underrepresent distress in cultures where stoicism or somatic expressions are the norm. These oversights perpetuate stereotypes about what constitutes "normal" or "healthy" behavior, marginalizing non-dominant groups and limiting the generalizability of research findings. Culturally competent research design requires critically interrogating these biases, engaging with diverse populations, and ensuring that interventions are relevant, respectful, and inclusive.

THE IMPORTANCE OF CONTINUING EDUCATION AND PROFESSIONAL DEVELOPMENT

Continuing education and professional development represent critical pillars in the field of health psychology and the broader health professions, serving as mechanisms that ensure practitioners remain competent, ethical, and effective in their practice. Unlike professions where a single degree or certification may suffice for a lifetime career, health psychology operates in a dynamic environment shaped by evolving scientific knowledge, technological innovations, shifting cultural norms, changing health care policies, and increasingly complex patient needs. Continuing education is not merely an optional pursuit but a professional obligation tied directly to patient welfare, public trust, and the advancement of the discipline. Health psychologists, as both clinicians and researchers, must continually refine their knowledge base, update their skill sets, and reflect on their ethical responsibilities in light of new challenges. The importance of professional development lies in its ability to enhance clinical competence, reinforce ethical decision-making, foster cultural sensitivity, reduce professional isolation, and prepare practitioners to address emerging issues such as digital health, telepsychology, and the integration of artificial intelligence in New findings in behavioral medicine, neuroscience, genetics, and health disparities frequently reshape our understanding of illness, resilience, and treatment. Continuing education workshops, online seminars, and professional conferences often incorporate case-based learning, enabling psychologists to explore complex ethical dilemmas and develop nuanced reasoning skills. By investing in ongoing training, practitioners demonstrate their commitment to ethical responsibility, thereby maintaining the trust of patients and the broader public.socioeconomic backgrounds. Continuing education programs often provide specialized training in cross-cultural communication, the impact of cultural beliefs on health behaviors, and strategies for reducing health disparities.(Topooco et al., 2017) For example, understanding how cultural values shape perceptions of mental illness or health interventions allows practitioners to tailor treatment in ways that are both respectful and effective. Cultural competence is not a skill that can be mastered once and for all; it requires lifelong learning, exposure to diverse perspectives, and reflective practice. Professional development thus enables psychologists to continually refine their ability to serve diverse populations while promoting equity and inclusion in health care.

Health psychologists must be trained not only to use these tools effectively but also to critically evaluate their appropriateness for different patients. Continuing education opportunities in digital health, data security, and technology-assisted interventions prepare practitioners to navigate these changes responsibly, ensuring that technology enhances rather than undermines patient care.psychologists are vulnerable to burnout, compassion fatigue, and reduced clinical effectiveness. Professional development programs often include training on resilience-building, mindfulness, stress management, and work-life balance. They also provide opportunities for peer networking, mentorship, and collaborative learning, which reduce professional isolation and foster a sense of community. In this way, continuing education not only enhances technical competence but also sustains the personal and professional well-being of practitioners, enabling them to provide long-term, high-quality care.patients and for the discipline, psychologists must possess skills in leadership, organizational behavior, public communication, and policy analysis. Professional development programs often include training in these areas, equipping practitioners to contribute beyond the therapy room. By engaging in continuing education, health psychologists can amplify their impact by shaping health policy, advancing research agendas, and leading interdisciplinary teams.a specified number of continuing education hours to maintain their credentials. (Titzler et al., 2018) These requirements underscore the recognition, at the institutional level, that lifelong learning is essential to professional competence. While some practitioners may view these mandates as bureaucratic, they reflect a deeper ethical and social contract: professionals entrusted with the health and well-being of others must demonstrate an ongoing commitment to excellence. Continuing education requirements provide accountability mechanisms that protect patients and reinforce the credibility of the profession.(Reynolds et al., 2015)Continuing education and professional development further serve the advancement of the In conclusion, the importance of continuing education and professional development in health psychology cannot be overstated. It ensures that practitioners remain aligned with current scientific evidence, uphold evolving ethical standards, and meet the diverse and complex needs of patients. It fosters cultural competence, prepares psychologists to harness new technologies, supports practitioner well-being, and equips professionals to take on leadership and advocacy roles. It also reflects a broader professional commitment to accountability, public trust, and the collective advancement of the discipline.(Raman et al., 2025) In a rapidly changing health care environment, where new challenges emerge alongside new opportunities, continuing education and professional development serve as the foundation for sustainable, ethical, and effective practice. By embracing lifelong learning, health psychologists not only enhance their own competence but also contribute to the creation of a health care system that is responsive, equitable, and grounded in excellence.

CONCLUSION

Navigating dual relationships and conflicts of interest is a central ethical challenge in health psychology practice, as these situations involve the delicate management of overlapping roles, responsibilities, and interests that can compromise professional objectivity, patient trust, and therapeutic effectiveness. A dual relationship occurs when a psychologist engages with a patient in more than one context, whether personal, social, financial, academic, or professional, beyond the primary therapeutic role. For example, a health psychologist treating a patient might also be their neighbor, colleague, teacher, or research participant. Similarly, a rises when the practitioner's personal, financial, or professional interests interfere—or appear to interfere—with their ability to act in the best interest of the patient. While dual relationships and conflicts of interest are sometimes unavoidable, especially in small or close-knit communities, their improper management can blur professional boundaries, create role confusion, undermine therapeutic neutrality, and even lead to exploitation or harm. Thus, health psychologists must approach these situations with vigilance, ethical reasoning, and transparency, ensuring that patient welfare always remains the highest priority.create vulnerabilities when professional roles intersect with personal ones. For example, engaging in a business relationship with a patient could unintentionally exploit the patient's trust or dependency. Even when intentions are benign, dual relationships can compromise objectivity, as the psychologist may struggle to balance personal and professional roles. A common example in health psychology involves rural or small communities where the practitioner may inevitably encounter patients in social settings or community organizations. In such contexts, total avoidance of dual relationships may not be possible, but careful management—including transparency, informed consent, and consultation with peers or supervisors—is essential to minimize risks.

Psychologists should document their reasoning, actions taken to minimize risks, and any consent obtained from patients. Finally, peer consultation and institutional support help practitioners navigate difficult situations with accountability and shared wisdom.he consequences of poorly managed dual relationships and conflicts of interest can be severe. Patients may experience confusion, loss of trust, or even psychological harm when roles are blurred. Practitioners who engage in exploitative or unethical relationships risk disciplinary action, loss of licensure, reputational damage, and legal liability. Beyond individual cases, such breaches erode public trust in the profession as a whole, making it essential for health psychologists to demonstrate vigilance and accountability in boundary management. By contrast, when managed transparently and ethically, dual relationships can sometimes strengthen therapeutic alliances, particularly in culturally specific contexts. The key lies in distinguishing situations where overlaps enhance trust and access to care from those where they compromise objectivity and patient welfare.In conclusion, navigating dual relationships and conflicts of interest in health psychology requires a careful balance of professional integrity, cultural sensitivity, and practical judgment. While some overlaps in roles are inevitable, particularly in small communities or multicultural contexts, psychologists must remain committed to ethical principles that prioritize patient welfare, autonomy, and justice. This involves ongoing reflection, transparency, consultation, and proactive communication about boundaries. Conflicts of interest, whether financial, professional, or personal, must be identified, disclosed, and managed in ways that preserve trust and impartiality. As health psychology continues to evolve in response to technological innovations, global interconnectedness, and expanding professional roles, the challenges of dual relationships and conflicts of interest will only become more complex. Ultimately, ethical navigation of these dilemmas is not about rigidly avoiding all potential overlaps but about maintaining clarity, fairness, and accountability in ways that protect patients and uphold the integrity of the profession.

REFERENCES

Aboujaoude, E. (2018). Telemental health: Why the revolution has not arrived. *World Psychiatry; Official Journal of the World Psychiatric Association (WPA), 17*(3), 277–278. DOI: 10.1002/wps.20551 PMID: 30192097

Aboujaoude, E., Gega, L., Parish, M. B., & Hilty, D. M. (2020). Editorial: Digital interventions in mental health: Current status and future directions [Editorial]. *Frontiers in Psychiatry, 11*, 111. Advance online publication. DOI: 10.3389/fpsyt.2020.00111 PMID: 32174858

Bagarić, B., & Jokić-Begić, N. (2020). Measuring therapists' attitudes toward integration of technology in psychotherapy and predicting their use of technology. *Journal of Clinical Psychology, 76*(6), 1151–1172. DOI: 10.1002/jclp.22967 PMID: 32410312

Balcombe, L., & De Leo, D. (2021). Digital mental health challenges and the horizon ahead for solutions. *JMIR Mental Health, 8*(3), e26811. DOI: 10.2196/26811 PMID: 33779570

Charan, J. K., Chandra, S., Vaissnave, V., Ragupathi, T., Satyanarayana, P., & Manjunath, T. C. (2025). Impact of Generative AI on Industries and Organizations. In Zhao, J., Kumar, V., Katina, P., & Richards, J. (Eds.), *Humans and Generative AI Tools for Collaborative Intelligence* (pp. 509–528). I Global Scientific Publishing., DOI: 10.4018/979-8-3693-8332-2.ch022

Charan, J. K., Meera, K. L., Sudheer, P., Gopalakrishnan, G., Sharma, M., & Manjunath, T. C. (2025). Applications of Generative AI and Human-AI Collaboration. In Zhao, J., Kumar, V., Katina, P., & Richards, J. (Eds.), *Humans and Generative AI Tools for Collaborative Intelligence* (pp. 423–440). IGI Global Scientific Publishing., DOI: 10.4018/979-8-3693-8332-2.ch018

Department of Health and Aged Care. (2021). National digital mental health framework. Retrieved from https://www.health.gov.au/resources/publications/national-digital-mental-health-framework

Dijksman, I., Dinant, G., & Spigt, M. (2017). The perception and needs of psychologists toward blended care. *Telemedicine Journal and e-Health, 23*(12), 983–995. DOI: 10.1089/tmj.2017.0031 PMID: 28556693

Erbe, D., Eichert, H., Riper, H., & Ebert, D. (2017). Blending face-to-face and internet-based interventions for the treatment of mental disorders in adults: Systematic review. *Journal of Medical Internet Research, 19*(9), e306. DOI: 10.2196/jmir.6588 PMID: 28916506

Feijt, M., de Kort, Y., Bongers, I., & IJsselsteijn, W. (2018). Perceived drivers and barriers to the adoption of eMental health by psychologists: The construction of the levels of adoption of eMental health model. *Journal of Medical Internet Research, 20*(4), e153. DOI: 10.2196/jmir.9485 PMID: 29691215

Gun, S., Titov, N., & Andrews, G. (2011). Acceptability of internet treatment of anxiety and depression. *Australasian Psychiatry, 19*(3), 259–264. DOI: 10.3109/10398562.2011.562295 PMID: 21682626

Guru Basava Aradhya, S., Chithambar Gupta, V., Raman, M. S., Singh, J., Manjunath, T. C., & Sharma, M. (2025). Health Crises and Digitalization: Digital Health. In Yıldırım, D., Yıldırım, S., & Kandpal, V. (Eds.), *Sustainable Digitalization Strategies in Business and Healthcare* (pp. 171–198). IGI Global Scientific Publishing., DOI: 10.4018/979-8-3373-5087-5.ch007

Harmanpreet, C. S., Kalshetti, P., Satyanarayana, P., Sharma, M., & Manjunath, T. C. (2025). Digital Transformation in the Public Sector Entities. In A. Santos Ferreira & C. Lourenço dos Santos (Eds.), Enhancing Public Sector Accountability and Services Through Digital Innovation (pp. 353-380). IGI Global Scientific Publishing. DOI: 10.4018/979-8-3693-9251-5.ch011

Hilvert-Bruce, Z., Rossouw, P., Wong, N., Sunderland, M., & Andrews, G. (2012). Adherence as a determinant of effectiveness of internet cognitive behavioural therapy for anxiety and depressive disorders. *Behaviour Research and Therapy, 50*(7–8), 463–468. DOI: 10.1016/j.brat.2012.04.001 PMID: 22659155

Johansson, R., Björklund, M., Hornborg, C., Karlsson, S., Hesser, H., Ljótsson, B., Rousseau, A., Frederick, R. J., & Andersson, G. (2013). Affect-focused psychodynamic psychotherapy for depression and anxiety through the Internet: A randomized controlled trial. *PeerJ, 1*, e102. DOI: 10.7717/peerj.102 PMID: 23862104

Kemmeren, L. L., van Schaik, A., Smit, J. H., Ruwaard, J., Rocha, A., Henriques, M., Ebert, D. D., Titzler, I., Hazo, J.-B., Dorsey, M., Zukowska, K., & Riper, H. (2019). Unraveling the black box: Exploring usage patterns of a blended treatment for depression in a multicenter study. *JMIR Mental Health, 6*(7), e12707. DOI: 10.2196/12707 PMID: 31344670

Knott, V., Habota, T., & Mallan, K. (2020). Attitudes of Australian psychologists towards the delivery of therapy via video conferencing technology. *Australian Psychologist, 55*(6), 606–617. Advance online publication. DOI: 10.1111/ap.12464

Lal, S., & Adair, C. (2014). E-Mental health: A rapid review of the literature. *Psychiatric Services (Washington, D.C.), 65*(1), 24–32. DOI: 10.1176/appi.ps.201300009 PMID: 24081188

LaMonica, H., Davenport, T., Braunstein, K., Ottavio, A., Piper, S., Martin, C., Hickie, I. B., & Cross, S. (2019). Technology-enabled person-centered mental health services reform: Strategy for implementation science. *JMIR Mental Health, 6*(9), e14719. DOI: 10.2196/14719 PMID: 31538938

Ojha, R., & Syed, S. (2020). Challenges faced by mental health providers and patients during the coronavirus 2019 pandemic due to technological barriers. *Internet Interventions : the Application of Information Technology in Mental and Behavioural Health, 21*, 100330. DOI: 10.1016/j.invent.2020.100330 PMID: 32542180

Orman, J., & O'Dea, B. (2018). e-Therapy in primary care mental health. *Australian Journal of General Practice, 47*(4), 168–172. DOI: 10.31128/AJGP-11-17-4410 PMID: 29621855

Park, M., Kim, D., Lee, U., Na, E., & Jeon, H. (2019). A literature overview of virtual reality (VR) in treatment of psychiatric disorders: Recent advances and limitations. *Frontiers in Psychiatry, 10*, 505. Advance online publication. DOI: 10.3389/fpsyt.2019.00505 PMID: 31379623

Raman, M. S., Koppa, K. B., Chithambar Gupta, V., Bhat, V. A., & Guru Basava Aradhya, S. (2025). Digital Transformation and Sustainability Artificial Intelligence and Sustainable Development. In Yıldırım, D., Yıldırım, S., & Kandpal, V. (Eds.), *Effects of Digitalization and Circular Economy on Sustainable Policy and Climate Change Prevention* (pp. 69–96). IGI Global Scientific Publishing., DOI: 10.4018/979-8-3693-9909-5.ch003

Reynolds, J., Griffiths, K., Cunningham, J., Bennett, K., & Bennett, A. (2015). Clinical practice models for the use of E-Mental health resources in primary health care by health professionals and peer workers: A conceptual framework. *JMIR Mental Health, 2*(1), e6. DOI: 10.2196/mental.4200 PMID: 26543912

Sanjari, M., Bahramnezhad, F., Fomani, F. K., Shoghi, M., & Cheraghi, M. A. (2014). Ethical challenges of researchers in qualitative studies: The necessity to develop a specific guideline. *Journal of Medical Ethics and History of Medicine, 7*, 14. PMID: 25512833

Sivanand, R., Selvakumar, P., & Sharma, N. (2025). Nanotechnology Applications in Cancer Drug Delivery Systems: A Review. *Journal of Environmental Nanotechnology, 14*(2), 458–470. DOI: 10.13074/jent.2025.06.2511221

Titzler, I., Saruhanjan, K., Berking, M., Riper, H., & Ebert, D. D. (2018). Barriers and facilitators for the implementation of blended psychotherapy for depression: A qualitative pilot study of therapists' perspective. *Internet Interventions : the Application of Information Technology in Mental and Behavioural Health, 12*, 150–164. DOI: 10.1016/j.invent.2018.01.002 PMID: 30135779

Topooco, N., Riper, H., Araya, R., Berking, M., Brunn, M., Chevreul, K., Cieslak, R., Ebert, D. D., Etchmendy, E., Herrero, R., Kleiboer, A., Krieger, T., García-Palacios, A., Cerga-Pashoja, A., Smoktunowicz, E., Urech, A., Vis, C., & Andersson, G. (2017). Attitudes towards digital treatment for depression: A European stakeholder survey. *Internet Interventions : the Application of Information Technology in Mental and Behavioural Health, 8*, 1–9. DOI: 10.1016/j.invent.2017.01.001 PMID: 30135823

Warale, P. N., Limbore, N. V., Anute, N., Ahluwalia, G. K., & Raut, A. (2025). AI-Enhanced Customer Engagement and Experience: Chatbots, Virtual Assistants, and AI-Powered Customer Interactions. In Hussain, Z., Khan, A., Uzir, M., Sharipudin, M., & Shaheen, A. (Eds.), *Impacts of AI-Generated Content on Brand Reputation* (pp. 335–362). IGI Global Scientific Publishing., DOI: 10.4018/979-8-3373-4327-3.ch014

Werner-Seidler, A., Wong, Q., Johnston, L., O'Dea, B., Torok, M., & Christensen, H. (2019). Pilot evaluation of the Sleep Ninja: A smartphone application for adolescent insomnia symptoms. *BMJ Open, 9*(5), e026502. DOI: 10.1136/bmjopen-2018-026502 PMID: 31133584

Chapter 9
From Illness to Flourishing:
Positive Psychology Interventions in Health Promotion

Avani Manjunath
http://orcid.org/0009-0008-6274-4036
PES University, India

Shreya Ghosh
http://orcid.org/0009-0008-9309-3424
PES University, India

ABSTRACT

This chapter integrates Positive Psychology Interventions (PPIs) into health psychology shifts the focus from pathogenesis to salutogenesis. Rooted in frameworks like SOC, Broaden-and-Build, and PERMA, PPIs build resilience and well-being. Evidence shows they reduce anxiety and depression, supported by neurobiology (e.g., vagal tone). The chapter discusses their application across settings, addresses methodological issues, the "tyranny of the positive," and the need for rigorous, culturally adapted research using EMA, providing a roadmap for a holistic, well-being-centered health model.

CHAPTER INTRODUCTION AND OBJECTIVES

This chapter explores the theoretical necessity and empirical efficacy of integrating Positive Psychology Interventions (PPIs) within the field of health psychology. The core argument rests on reframing health from a traditional disease-avoidance

DOI: 10.4018/979-8-3373-6294-6.ch009

paradigm (pathogenesis) to a strengths-based, flourishing-oriented model (salutogenesis). The limitations of a purely pathogenic approach, which focuses primarily on eliminating disease and identifying risk factors, are addressed by advocating for the proactive cultivation of psychological resources that enable individuals to maintain health and thrive even in the face of significant stressors. The field of health psychology must evolve from asking "How do we fix what is broken?" to asking, "How do we cultivate what is already strong and make it stronger?"

For over a century, the dominant paradigm in both medicine and health psychology has been pathogenesis. This strategy, which focuses on illness origins, has historically proven extremely useful in delivering huge public health gains in infectious disease control, sanitation, and acute care. Pathogenesis has supplied the framework for antibiotics, vaccinations, and enhanced surgical methods, resulting in a remarkable improvement in human life expectancy worldwide. However, when confronted with 21st-century health concerns, the pathogenic model is structurally flawed. The disease burden has switched dramatically from acute infectious infections to complicated, slow-onset chronic ailments including cardiovascular disease (CVD), type 2 diabetes, metabolic syndrome, and increased rates of anxiety and depression. These symptoms are seldom due to a single disease. Diseases are instead caused by a combination of persistent psychosocial stress, lifestyle choices, environmental circumstances, and self-regulation failures.

The key drawback of the pathogenic approach is its restrictive definition of health: health is only the absence of sickness. This deficit-focused paradigm unavoidably presents the individual as a passive recipient of external risk factors or a collection of internal, curable disorders. It encourages a purely reactive approach to health, with interventions occurring only after illness has begun. For health psychology, this translates to a research focus primarily on coping mechanisms for existing stressors (e.g., pain management, adherence to post-diagnosis regimens) and identifying psychological risk factors that lead to illness.

This leads to a fundamental conceptual gap: the pathogenic model cannot explain the phenomenon of the hardy survivor—the individual who, despite facing significant adversity (e.g., chronic illness, poverty, trauma), maintains high levels of vitality, psychological resilience, and subjective well-being. If health is solely determined by the absence of risk factors, these individuals should be perpetually unwell. Their thriving state demonstrates that there must be powerful, protective mechanisms rooted in the active presence of psychological and social resources.

To address this profound conceptual gap, the field of health psychology must undergo a paradigm shift toward salutogenesis, a model conceptualized by medical sociologist Aaron Antonovsky (1979). Salutogenesis, derived from the Latin salus (health) and Greek genesis (origin), asks a transformative question: What are the origins of health, well-being, and successful human functioning? This model posits that health and disease are not distinct categories but occupy a dynamic continuum, and every individual is perpetually exposed to stressors. The objective of salutogenesis is not the unattainable removal of stresses, but rather the proactive growth of the internal and external resources required to successfully navigate the chaos and sustain moving toward the health pole of the spectrum.

This model's key concept is the Sense of Coherence (SOC). SOC is described as a broad, long-term attitude that conveys the amount to which one considers their life and surroundings as ordered, predictable, and controllable, resulting in the confident feeling that one's resources are sufficient to handle life's demands. A robust SOC serves as a powerful, all-encompassing psychological buffer, significantly impacting how external dangers are perceived and absorbed. PPIs are especially created as actionable tools for building and strengthening the SOC's three pillars: Comprehensibility (the idea that the world makes cognitive sense), Manageability (the belief that one has the means to face obstacles), and Meaningfulness (the profound conviction that life's demands are worthy of investment and commitment, which is the motivational core). By stressing General Resistance Resources (GRRs), which include psychological assets like as optimism, self-efficacy, and a strong sense of purpose, the salutogenic viewpoint provides the critical theoretical foundation for integrating Positive Psychology Interventions. PPIs are, by definition, focused approaches to producing, installing, and maintaining these critical GRRs.

Positive psychology interventions (PPIs) are practical applications of salutogenic theory. They are planned, evidence-based exercises, such as gratitude journaling, recognizing and developing trademark strengths, or practicing loving-kindness meditation, that aim to actively nurture the psychological resources that support resilience and thriving rather than treat mental illness. They explicitly address the pathogenic model's inadequacy by emphasizing strengths over deficiencies. PPIs are effective because they are based on strong, observable psychological hypotheses. Fredrickson's extend-and-Build Theory describes how positive affect develops resources over time, demonstrating that pleasant emotions temporarily extend cognitive and behavioral repertoires, resulting in the long-term accumulation of intellectual, social, and physical capital. Meanwhile, Seligman's PERMA Model offers the what: a precise, five-component framework of flourishing (Positive Emotion, Engagement, Relationships, Meaning, and Accomplishment) that serves both the blueprint for PPI creation and the standard for assessing their effectiveness.

The rising corpus of research proving that PPIs' psychological effects transfer into concrete, protective physiological changes provides the most persuasive case for incorporating them into health psychology. The development of good affect and psychological resources is more than just a subjective sensation; it is a technique for lowering the body's allostatic load, or the cumulative wear and tear caused by chronic stress.

This chapter will detail the precise neurobiological pathways through which PPIs modulate critical regulatory systems. For instance, interventions like loving-kindness meditation have been shown to increase vagal tone, an objective measure of the body's capacity for rapid emotional regulation controlled by the parasympathetic nervous system (PNS). Furthermore, by mitigating perceived stress, PPIs help to dampen the chronic, harmful activation of the HPA axis, thereby normalizing cortisol levels, reducing systemic inflammation, and protecting against cardiovascular risk. By providing the necessary psychological capital (SOC, GRRs, PERMA components) that translates directly into physiological resilience (HRV, HPA modulation), Positive Psychology Interventions are not merely a valuable addition to health psychology—they are an essential component of any model that aims to promote genuine, long-term well-being and thriving, rather than simply managing disease. This conceptual foundation sets the stage for the systematic exploration of PPIs within this chapter, moving from theoretical necessity to empirical application and critical evaluation.

CHAPTER OBJECTIVES AND ROADMAP

The chapter's six objectives form a conceptual roadmap, moving logically from theoretical justification to empirical validation, practical application, and critical analysis, ensuring a comprehensive exploration of Positive Psychology Interventions (PPIs) in health psychology.

To establish the conceptual shift from the pathogenic model of health to the salutogenic model, introducing the core construct of the Sense of Coherence (SOC) and detailing the role and interaction of General Resistance Resources (GRRs):

This foundational objective initiates the critical analysis by structurally defining the limitations of the pathogenic model in addressing modern chronic diseases, which are heavily influenced by lifestyle and stress. We fully articulate the salutogenic model as the necessary complement, shifting focus from disease origins to the origins of health and resilience. Central to this is the Sense of Coherence (SOC)—Comprehensibility, Manageability, and Meaningfulness—which acts as the overarching psychological buffer against life's stressors. We categorize General Resistance Resources (GRRs), highlighting the psychological assets (e.g., optimism, self-efficacy) that PPIs are specifically designed to cultivate, thereby establishing the theoretical necessity of these interventions for fostering enduring health.

To outline the foundational theoretical frameworks underpinning PPIs, including the Broaden-and-Build Theory and the PERMA model of flourishing, detailing their psychological and physiological mechanisms:

This section provides the scientific backbone for PPI efficacy. We dissect Fredrickson's Broaden-and-Build Theory to explain the micro-level mechanism of change, showing how positive emotions momentarily broaden thought and action repertoires, leading to the long-term building of durable personal and social resources. Concurrently, Seligman's PERMA model (Positive Emotion, Engagement, Relationships, Meaning, Accomplishment) is presented as the macro-level blueprint, ensuring that interventions target the complete five-component definition of human flourishing. This paradigm guarantees that PPIs are recognized as scientifically derived instruments for promoting overall well-being.

To introduce and elaborate upon the neurobiological and physiological pathways through which positive affect and PPIs exert their influence on physical health, including the autonomic and endocrine systems:

This aim grounds the psychological advantages in objective, quantifiable science. We examine the bidirectional relationship between positive affect and the Autonomic Nervous System (ANS), describing how interventions such as Loving-Kindness Meditation (LKM) improve vagal tone, an objective measure of the body's capacity for emotional regulation and resilience that is frequently measured using Heart Rate Variability (HRV).

Furthermore, we investigate the endocrine effects of PPIs, explaining how they lower perceived stress and chronic hypothalamic-pituitary-adrenal (HPA) axis activity. This long-term regulation reduces the synthesis of cortisol and other stress hormones, resulting in a significant reduction in allostatic load and inflammation.

To give a complete, comprehensive taxonomy of evidence-based PPIs (e.g., gratitude, strengths, meaning, loving-kindness, savoring) and highlight their quantitative influence on mental, physical, and behavioral health outcomes, accompanied by concrete clinical and public health application examples:

This key component shifts to empirical data. It provides a thorough taxonomy of the most effective, organized PPIs, including the "Three Good Things" gratitude exercise and the Best Possible Self (BPS) visualization. Importantly, we describe the quantitative impact of various therapies using reliable meta-analyses. We emphasize the considerable impact sizes on psychological distress, such as the reported 7.76% reduction in GAD-7 scores (anxiety) and 6.89% reduction in PHQ-9 scores (depression). Specific examples demonstrate how these strategies promote health behaviors such as exercise adherence, pain tolerance, and sleep quality in both clinical and general populations.

To contextualize the practical implementation of PPIs across multiple settings, including the specialized care of chronic illness (CVD, cancer), workplace well-being initiatives, and the potential and hazards inherent in digital health delivery, we propose best practice design principles.

The practical importance of PPIs is investigated by looking at their deployment throughout the health ecosystem. We investigate tertiary prevention in clinical settings, focusing on how meaning-making might help people cope with chronic illnesses (for example, post-traumatic growth).

We analyze primary prevention in workplace well-being programs, focusing on organizational interventions (e.g., Active Constructive Responding) to combat burnout. Finally, the section addresses the opportunities for scalable, personalized PPIs in Digital Health Delivery via apps and JITAI (Just-in-Time Adaptive Interventions), while simultaneously establishing ethical and design principles to maximize engagement and efficacy in a remote context.

To critically discuss the methodological challenges, emphasizing the need for Ecological Momentary Assessment (EMA), address ethical concerns (e.g., "tyranny of the positive"), and outline a rigorous future research agenda for the field, focusing on biomarkers, AI ethics, and cultural adaptation:

The final objective ensures the field's critical rigor. We address the pervasive methodological challenge of reliance on retrospective measures and argue for the necessity of Ecological Momentary Assessment (EMA) and wearable biosensors to establish definitive causality and dosage effects. Ethical scrutiny is applied to the "tyranny of the positive" critique, advocating for optimal emotional balance over forced happiness. The chapter concludes by setting a clear research agenda focused on large-scale longitudinal biomarker studies (e.g., cortisol, telomeres), establishing ethical guidelines for AI-driven PPI delivery, and prioritizing cultural adaptation to ensure global relevance and equity in positive health science.

CONCEPTUAL FRAMEWORK FOR POSITIVE HEALTH INTERVENTIONS

The transition from illness to flourishing requires a structured, multi-stage intervention model. Table 1 illustrates the proposed conceptual framework, showing how the positive psychology paradigm moves beyond merely addressing pathology to actively promoting full human flourishing.

Table 1. Conceptual Framework for Positive Health Interventions

Stage	Focus	Mechanisms / Interventions	Outputs / Results
Pathogenesis	Disease Focus, Risk Factors, Deficit Model	Stressors, Illness Diagnosis, Symptom Presentation	Disease/Dis-ease, Resource Depletion, Low Resilience
Salutogenesis	Resource Focus, Resilience Building	General Resistance Resources (GRRs), Sense of Coherence (SOC)	Comprehensibility, Manageability, Meaningfulness
Positive Psychology Intervention (PPI)	Intentional Resource Cultivation	Gratitude Practices, Signature Strengths Use, Meaning Interventions, LKM	Increased Positive Affect, Enhanced Coping Skills, Behavioral Adherence
Outcomes	Measurable Health Improvements	Reduced Symptoms (Anxiety/Depression), Stronger Immune Function, Greater Self-Efficacy	Well-being Reserve, Sustained Health Behaviors
Flourishing	Optimal Functioning	PERMA Elements (P, E, R, M, A)	Optimal Physical and Psychological Health, High Quality of Life

1. A PARADIGM SHIFT: FROM PATHOGENIC TO SALUTOGENIC HEALTH

The traditional focus of health psychology and medicine, termed the pathogenic orientation, is dominated by the scientific investigation into the etiology of disease and the identification of specific risk factors involved in disease generation (Antonovsky, 1996). This model often necessitates the use of external healing devices and interventions designed to eliminate pathogenic factors, positioning the individual as a passive recipient of treatment (Antonovsky, 1996). However, a growing body of research advocates for a fundamental shift in perspective toward a strengths-based, flourishing-oriented model known as salutogenesis (Antonovsky, 1996). This transition is crucial for addressing the multidimensional nature of chronic disease and achieving truly holistic health outcomes.

1.1 Reframing the Health Continuum: The Deficit Model vs. The Positive Health Model

Salutogenesis, a concept developed by Aaron Antonovsky, fundamentally challenges the pathogenic axiom by rejecting a binary definition of health (healthy or unwell) (Antonovsky, 1996). Instead, it views health as a dynamic continuum that runs from "ease" to "dis-ease" (Antonovsky, 1996). Within this framework, daily stressors constantly push the individual toward the disease end of the continuum, but the emphasis shifts to identifying and mobilizing salutary factors, known as General Resistance Resources (GRRs), that actively promote health and mitigate this downward movement (Antonovsky, 1996).

This resource-focused viewpoint supports the positive health paradigm, which focuses on optimum functioning, or what is right with individuals, allowing them to have satisfying lives and recover from trauma (Rashid & Ostermann, 2010). According to contemporary academic discourse, good health is a measured "reserve in capacities" of physiological, psychological, and social resources that an individual may draw on to preserve function and enhance outcomes when confronted with adversity (Peiro et al., 2023). This viewpoint entails a substantial conceptual shift: intervention aims should not end after symptoms are alleviated (the pathogenic goal), but rather be continued proactively to improve the patient's inherent potential to flourish (the salutogenic goal) (Antonovsky 1996).

1.2 General Resistance Resources (GRRs): The Building Blocks of Health

General Resistance Resources (GRRs) are any characteristics of a person, organization, or environment that allow for good stress management (Antonovsky, 1996). These materials serve as the raw material for developing a strong sense of coherence. PPIs are specifically intended to foster or utilize these resources. GRRs are extensively classified, demonstrating the multi-system aspect of salutogenic health:

1. Constitutional GRRs include biological and physical endowments including a strong immune system, physical fitness, and favorable genetics.
2. Material GRRs refer to tangible resources like secure income, excellent housing, transportation, and healthcare.
3. Psychosocial GRRs include internal qualities such as self-esteem, efficient coping methods, cognitive flexibility, self-efficacy, and a cohesive worldview. PPIs are mostly targeted at this category.
4. Cultural GRRs include belief systems, values, rituals, and cultural stability that shape meaning and identity.
5. Relational GRRs include robust social support networks, secure interpersonal relationships, and social integration.

By identifying the interaction of these resources, the salutogenic approach offers a comprehensive paradigm for health promotion that PPIs may directly implement. The purpose of a PPI is not only to make a patient "happier," but also to increase the number and quality of their accessible psychosocial and relational GRRs, making them more robust to future stresses.

1.3 Antonovsky's Sense of Coherence (SOC): The Motivational Core of Salutogenesis

The core construct underpinning the salutogenic model is the **Sense of Coherence (SOC)**, defined as a global orientation, a pervasive, enduring, yet dynamic feeling of confidence, that one's internal and external environments are predictable and that there is a high probability that things will work out as well as can reasonably be expected (Antonovsky, 1996). A strong sense of self is seen to be a critical survival resource, assisting individuals in navigating the endless number of stresses experienced in life and enhancing health-generating abilities (Antonovsky, 1996).

The SOC has three interacting aspects that constitute a synergistic system:

- **Comprehensibility (Cognitive):** Anatonovsky (1996) defines comprehension as the belief in the structure, order, consistency, and predictability of inputs and information from one's environment. A high comprehension level indicates that a health diagnostic or life stressor is perceived as a problem that can be comprehended and mentally mapped, rather than a chaotic, unpredictable, and frightening event. This cognitive clarity is necessary for making logical health decisions.

    Manageability (Behavioural): The idea that one possesses the skills, support structures, or General Resistance Resources (GRRs) necessary to cope with life's demands, viewing challenges as controllable and under one's control (Antonovsky, 1996). PPIs such as strengths-based exercises directly improve this dimension by confirming the individual's internal ability to act.
- **Meaningfulness (Motivational):** The amount to which one believes that life has emotional significance, perceiving at least some of life's obligations as tasks deserving of effort and dedication rather than just as responsibilities (Antonovsky, 1991). This is the volitional core; it is the willingness to expend the energy required to overcome obstacles. Without a strong feeling of Meaningfulness, Comprehensibility, and Manageability, there is no motivation to maintain healthy habits.

    Measuring the SOC and Predictive Validity: The SOC is typically measured using the 29-item or 13-item Orientation to Life Questionnaire (OLQ). Empirical research consistently validates the SOC as a powerful predictor of health. Longitudinal studies have shown that a high SOC is inversely correlated with mortality risk, chronic pain prevalence, and self-reported sickness. Crucially, the SOC is not merely a measure of perceived control or self-efficacy; it is a higher-order concept that reflects the individual's global disposition toward life's demands, making it a critical intermediary variable in the effects of PPIs on long-term health.

2. FOUNDATIONAL CONCEPTS AND THEORETICAL FRAMEWORKS

To understand the efficacy of PPIs in promoting holistic health, it is essential to review the key theoretical constructs that define and explain well-being and resource generation, providing the rationale for intervention design.

2.1 Defining Well-being: Hedonic vs. Eudaimonic Models

Well-being is a multifaceted concept that is typically differentiated into two primary forms that often underpin PPI design:

- **Subjective Well-being (SWB) / Hedonic Well-being:** SWB focuses on the individual's current affective state and cognitive evaluation of their life. Its components often include the existence of positive affect, the absence of negative affect, and overall life satisfaction. Hedonic well-being is a short-term outcome that is frequently examined soon after intervention.
- **Psychological Well-being (PWB) and Eudaimonic Well-being:** Carol Ryff established this concept, which focuses on optimal human functioning and reaching one's full potential (Ryff 1989). PWB is assessed using six factors: self-acceptance, positive relationships with others, autonomy, environmental mastery, life purpose, and personal growth. Eudaimonic well-being, specifically Purpose in Life, is a greater predictor of long-term health indicators such as decreased inflammation and lifespan, implying that it is the genuine, long-term focus of salutogenic therapies. PPIs strive to shift from brief hedonic advantages to long-term eudaimonic growth.

2.2 Mechanisms of Positive Emotions: The Broaden-and-Build Theory (B&B)

Barbara Fredrickson's Broaden-and-Build Theory provides the critical causal mechanism explaining how positive emotions generate long-term psychological and physical resources (Fredrickson, 2004). The theory posits that positive emotions, such as joy, interest, and contentment, broaden an individual's momentary thought-action repertoire, leading to more flexible, creative, and non-defensive thinking. In a health context, this broadening means a patient is more likely to consider a wider array of coping strategies or to view a diagnosis as a challenge rather than a catastrophic dead end.

Over time, these repeated broadened states build enduring personal resources, including physical, intellectual, social, and psychological capital (Fredrickson, 2004). These accrued resources function as reserves (Positive Health Reserve) that can be drawn upon later to improve coping and survival when facing stress or illness (Fredrickson, 2004). The B&B theory serves as the theoretical link between the acute effects of PPIs (eliciting a positive emotion) and their long-term salutogenic effect (building GRRs and strengthening SOC).

2.3 The PERMA Model of Flourishing: A Framework for Resource Optimization

Martin Seligman's PERMA model serves as a comprehensive, measurable, and actionable framework for understanding and promoting flourishing (Kern et al., 2014). As a multidimensional constructivist paradigm, it offers five unique routes, each of which contributes independently to overall well-being and guides the development of specific PPIs.

- Positive emotions include optimism, pleasure, and thankfulness. Targeted by appreciation and LKM.
- **Engagement (E)**: being fully immersed in activities and experiencing flow. Targeted by strengths-based treatments and hobby involvement.
- **Relationships (R):** The ability to build and sustain positive, mutually beneficial connections. Appreciation and social skills training are being used to target them. Strong connections are essential for Relational GRR (Uchino et al., 2003).
- **Meaning (M):** sense of belonging to something bigger than oneself. Clarifying values and volunteering with a purpose are the goals.

    Accomplishment (A): Working toward and mastering goals leads to a sense of accomplishment and self-efficacy. Goal-setting and strength application exercises directly promote SOC-Manageability.

2.4 Leveraging Character Strengths (VIA Classification) for Personal Agency

The **Values in Action (VIA) Classification of Character Strengths and Virtues** shifts the clinical focus from "what is wrong" to identifying and mobilizing "what is right" with an individual (Rashid & Ostermann, 2010). The VIA inventory organizes 24 positive traits (e.g., curiosity, kindness, honesty) into six core virtues.

The practical implementation involves helping individuals identify their signature strengths and intentionally applying them to achieve health goals, directly supporting the Manageability dimension of the Sense of Coherence. By focusing on intrinsic capabilities, this approach fosters self-determination and intrinsic motivation, which are essential for durable behavioural change.

3. THE NEUROBIOLOGICAL AND PHYSIOLOGICAL BASIS OF RESOURCE BUILDING

The enduring effects of PPIs on health cannot be fully understood without examining the underlying physiological pathways. The Broaden-and-Build Theory suggests that psychological resources are built by positive emotions; Section 3 demonstrates that these resources are biologically measurable, primarily through the autonomic and neuroendocrine systems.

3.1 Autonomic Nervous System Regulation and Vagal Tone

One of the most robust physiological markers influenced by PPIs is Vagal Tone, which is the activity of the vagus nerve (the tenth cranial nerve), the primary component of the parasympathetic nervous system (PNS). The vagus nerve is essential for maintaining homeostasis, controlling heart rate variability (HRV), and suppressing inflammatory reactions.

Mechanism: Positive emotions, including those created via Loving-Kindness Meditation (LKM), directly enhance High-Frequency Heart Rate Variability (HF-HRV), a non-invasive indicator of vagal tone. A greater resting vagal tone indicates a more flexible and resilient physiological system, or a detectable Constitutional GRR. This "physiological reserve in capacities" enables the body to recover faster from stress (Fredrickson et al., 2008).

Empirical Link: According to research, people who engage in LKM over time have significant improvements in vagal tone, which mediates the association between LKM practice and improved happy feelings and felt social connectivity (Kok and Fredrickson, 2010). This relationship gives actual scientific proof that PPIs do more than just make you feel happy; they fundamentally boost the body's ability to self-regulate and resist illness.

3.2 Modulation of the HPA Axis and Cortisol Levels

The Hypothalamic-Pituitary-Adrenal (HPA) axis is the body's central stress response system, responsible for releasing cortisol. Chronic activation of the HPA axis leads to sustained high levels of cortisol, which is immunosuppressive and contributes to allostatic load, insulin resistance, and cardiovascular risk.

- **Mechanism:** Positive emotions, engagement, and a strong sense of meaning (SOC-Meaningfulness) act as powerful psychological buffers that reduce the perceived threat of stressors. By changing the cognitive appraisal of a situation (Comprehensibility), PPIs reduce the initial triggering of the HPA axis.
- **Empirical Link:** Intervention studies involving mindfulness and meaning-making have demonstrated a measurable reduction in evening salivary cortisol levels in stressed populations. This downregulation of the HPA axis indicates a decrease in chronic stress exposure, directly preserving biological resources and supporting immune function, which is critical for disease management and recovery.

3.3 Neurotransmitters and Reward Circuitry

PPIs engage the brain's intrinsic reward pathways, strengthening behaviours associated with well-being and adherence.

- **Dopamine:** Practices that promote Accomplishment (goal setting) and Engagement (flow) release dopamine, reinforcing the behaviours that led to the positive feeling. This mechanism is key to promoting long-term health adherence, for instance, making exercise or diet compliance feel intrinsically rewarding rather than punitive.
- **Oxytocin:** Relational PPIs, such as expressing gratitude or engaging in LKM toward loved ones, promote the release of oxytocin, often called the "bonding hormone." Oxytocin enhances trust, reduces social anxiety, and reinforces social bonds, thereby strengthening a patient's **Relational GRRs** (Uchino et al., 2003) and providing a critical buffer against isolation during illness.

4. A COMPREHENSIVE TYPOLOGY OF POSITIVE PSYCHOLOGY INTERVENTIONS (PPIS) IN PRACTICE

This section provides an in-depth analysis of five core, evidence-based PPIs, detailing their specific mechanisms, clinical protocols, and quantified evidence across various health outcomes.

4.1 Gratitude Interventions: Shifting Attentional Bias

Gratitude is a positive emotional state and a moral virtue that involves recognizing and appreciating the benefits one has received. It is one of the most rigorously studied PPIs due to its simplicity and robust efficacy.

Mechanism and Protocol

- **Mechanism:** Gratitude operates primarily by shifting **attentional bias** and reducing **social comparison bias**. It forces the individual to focus their cognitive resources on existing external benefits and internal strengths, thereby directly enhancing SOC-Comprehensibility (by making the environment seem more orderly and beneficial) and SOC-Meaningfulness.
- **Clinical Protocol Example: Three Good Things:** Patients are instructed to spend 5-10 minutes each night writing down three things that went well that day and providing a causal explanation for why they happened. This is typically prescribed daily or three times per week for 4 to 6 weeks.
- **Quantified Evidence:** Analysis of 579 patients demonstrated that gratitude interventions resulted in a 7.76% lower Generalized Anxiety Disorder (GAD-7) score compared to control groups (Iodice et al., 2021). Similarly, analysis of 525 patients indicated a 6.89% lower Patient Health Questionnaire-9 (PHQ-9) score for depression symptoms (Iodice et al., 2021). Furthermore, research in chronic heart failure patients has linked gratitude journaling to improved sleep quality and a reduction in pro-inflammatory biomarkers, suggesting direct physical benefit.

4.2 Signature Strengths Interventions: Cultivating Manageability

Strength-based interventions focus on identifying and utilizing the client's signature strengths, derived from the VIA classification, to address problems and achieve goals.

Mechanism and Protocol

- **Mechanism:** By encouraging the patient to use a core strength (e.g., humour, creativity, perseverance) in a new way every day, the intervention directly boosts self-efficacy and personal agency, strongly reinforcing SOC-Manageability. The focus shifts the patient's identity from a "sick person" to a "person with strengths coping with illness."

- **Clinical Protocol Example: Strength Spotting and Application:** The intervention involves three stages: 1) Identification (using the VIA survey), 2) Narrative (discussing past successes tied to that strength), and 3) Novel Application (designing a specific task where the strength is used to overcome a current health barrier, e.g., using "Curiosity" to research and understand their medication regimen better).
- **Quantified Evidence:** Meta-analyses show that 62.9% of studies report effectiveness in enhancing overall well-being and reducing depressive symptoms (Schotanus-Dijkstra et al., 2024). In the context of cancer survivorship, using strengths like Hope and Bravery has been shown to mediate the relationship between trauma exposure and post-traumatic growth, transforming the illness experience into a vehicle for deeper personal development.

4.3 Meaning and Purpose Interventions: Anchoring Health Behaviours

Meaning interventions are designed to help individuals find or create purpose, particularly in the face of suffering or existential crises associated with illness.

Mechanism and Protocol

- **Mechanism:** These interventions address the existential void often precipitated by a chronic diagnosis, directly strengthening the SOC-Meaningfulness dimension. They provide a motivational core that makes challenging health behaviours (like a restrictive diet or painful therapy) seem worthwhile because they serve a greater life goal or value.
- **Clinical Protocol Example: Values Clarification and Purpose Narrative:** Patients are asked to identify their core life values (e.g., family, legacy, learning) and then develop a narrative linking their current health goals (e.g., adhering to an exercise plan) to the fulfilment of that value. For example, "I exercise not just to live longer, but to be able to actively teach my grandchildren" (linking exercise to the value of 'Legacy').
- **Quantified Evidence:** Meaning and purpose are critical for improved coping with chronic illness (Helgeson & Zajdel, 2022). High purpose in life has been consistently linked to reduced risk of stroke and myocardial infarction in older adults, even after controlling for traditional risk factors. This suggests a direct protective effect on cardiovascular health, possibly mediated by reduced HPA axis activity.

4.4 Loving-Kindness Meditation (LKM): Building Relational Resources

LKM is a contemplative practice aimed at cultivating feelings of warmth, benevolence, and connection toward oneself and others, starting with a neutral target and progressing outward.

Mechanism and Protocol

- **Mechanism:** LKM is a potent intervention for the **Broaden-and-Build Theory**. By intentionally generating positive emotions (unconditional love), it broadens thought-action repertoires and, crucially, builds Relational GRRs by enhancing the perceived availability and quality of social support (Fredrickson et al., 2008). Physiologically, it is a proven method for increasing Vagal Tone (Kok & Fredrickson, 2010).
- **Clinical Protocol Example: Metta Meditation:** The patient mentally or verbally repeats phrases wishing well to different groups: 1) Self, 2) Loved ones, 3) Neutral acquaintances, 4) Difficult people, and 5) All beings. Practice time is typically 10-20 minutes daily.
- **Quantified Evidence:** Beyond the measured increase in vagal tone, LKM interventions have been shown to effectively reduce negative bias and increase positive reappraisal skills in high-stress populations. In patients with high social anxiety, LKM significantly improves perceived social connection, which is a critical buffer against the immune-compromising effects of chronic loneliness.

4.5 Savouring Interventions: Maximizing Positive Affect Duration

Savouring is the capacity to attend to, appreciate, and enhance the positive emotions associated with events, whether past, present, or anticipated. It is distinct from gratitude (which is retrospective and focused on source) as savouring is focused on amplifying the *experience* itself.

Mechanism and Protocol

- **Mechanism:** Savouring works by extending the duration and intensity of positive emotional states, effectively optimizing the "P" (Positive Emotion) component of PERMA. By making positive moments more salient and memorable, it contributes to the overall pool of positive affective resources, which the Broaden-and-Build theory utilizes to build resilience.

- **Clinical Protocol Example: Mental Photography:** When a patient experiences a small positive moment (e.g., enjoying a cup of coffee, feeling relief from pain), they are instructed to "take a mental photograph" of the experience, noticing sights, sounds, smells, and internal sensations, and then revisit that image later in the day.
- **Quantified Evidence:** Savouring interventions have been successfully used to reduce depressive symptoms and anxiety by increasing the availability and accessibility of positive memories. In a health context, savouring small victories (e.g., a good night's sleep, a successful physical therapy session) reinforces the positive loop of the health behavior change, making sustained adherence more likely.

5. APPLICATION AND CONTEXTUALIZATION OF PPIS IN HEALTH SETTINGS

The efficacy of PPIs is realized when they are successfully translated and tailored across diverse practice settings. Successful implementation requires matching the chosen PPI to the specific setting's goals and target population.

5.1 Specialized Application in Chronic Disease Management

PPIs offer unique value in chronic disease management by moving beyond symptom control to address the psychological and existential impact of long-term illness.

5.1.1 Cardio-vascular disease (CVD)

CVD patients often experience high levels of stress, anxiety, and depression, which are themselves risk factors for adverse cardiac events.

- **Intervention Focus:** Stress reduction and social support.
- **Targeted PPIs:** LKM (to increase vagal tone and reduce physiological arousal) and Gratitude Interventions (to foster positive outlook and decrease hostility).
- **Impact:** Studies have shown that a strong SOC and PPI-enhanced social support are correlated with lower blood pressure and better long-term adherence to cardiac rehabilitation programs, as the intervention provides the patients with a stronger **GRR** to cope with the fear of recurrence.

5.1.2 Cancer Survivorship and Palliative Care

Cancer diagnosis and treatment frequently lead to post-traumatic stress, anxiety, and a profound loss of meaning.

- **Intervention Focus:** Meaning-making and post-traumatic growth (PTG).
- **Targeted PPIs:** Meaning/Values Clarification and Signature Strengths Application.
- **Impact:** Meaning-focused PPIs help patients re-author their life narratives, finding purpose not despite their illness, but often because of it. Applying strengths (e.g., using "Humor" to cope with treatment side effects) increases self-efficacy and shifts the focus toward PTG, where individuals report a greater appreciation for life and closer relationships post-diagnosis.

5.2 Workplace Well-being and Public Health

In the workplace, PPIs aim to reduce burnout (a state of emotional exhaustion directly opposed to Positive Emotion and Engagement) and improve organizational climate, acting as primary prevention (Table 2).

Table 2. Typology of Positive Psychology Interventions (PPIs) by Setting, Goal, and Outcome

Setting	Primary Goal	Target PPIs	Measured Outcome
Workplace (Public Health/Prevention)	Reduce burnout, enhance organizational commitment	PERMA-structured initiatives, strengths-based leadership training, positive feedback (Active Constructive Responding).	Increased job satisfaction, higher vitality, reduced burnout and psychological distress (Kern et al., 2014).
Educational Settings (Primary Prevention)	Develop resilience and emotional literacy in youth	Character Strengths assessments, Mindfulness programs, Growth Mindset training.	Improved academic engagement, lower incidence of internalizing problems, greater self-efficacy.

5.3 Digital Health Opportunities and Design Principles

Digital health tools, including mobile applications and conversational AI, offer unprecedented scalability for delivering PPIs (Donaldson et al., 2021). However, maximizing their salutogenic potential requires moving beyond simple automation to principles that mirror human-centered resource building.

The Challenge of Eudaimonic Delivery

As noted, current digital platforms struggle with the salutogenic goal (resource building and promoting flourishing) (Tielman et al., 2024). This is frequently owing to an overreliance on basic, isolated PPIs (such as daily check-ins), which lack the individualized, relational context essential for profound eudaimonic development.

Salutogenic Design Principles for Digital PPIs:

1. **Contextual Personalization (SOC-Comprehensibility):** AI should use user data to propose PPIs that are extremely relevant to the present life context (for example, recommending a "Kindness" strength test right after a reported disagreement).
2. **Relational Scaffolding (PERMA-R):** Digital technologies must enable human-to-human connections, not merely human-to-bot interactions. This includes prompts that urge the user to share their good experiences or strengths with others.
3. **Meaning and Value Integration (SOC-Meaningfulness):** The AI should constantly connect the micro-level PPI job (e.g., a thankfulness entry) to the user's macro-level basic beliefs and life goals, ensuring that the intervention feels meaningful rather than merely a compliance chore.
4. **Ethical Non-Maleficence:** Given the potential of AI-enabled damage (Haber et al., 2023), digital PPIs must closely adhere to safety rules, including prompt handoff to human crisis services when necessary and avoiding language that may be regarded as dismissive or toxic-positive.

5.4 Diverse Populations and Cultural Adaptations

PPIs' generalizability is hampered by their Western roots (Spahn et al., 2022). Cultural adaptation is necessary to ensure effectiveness and ethical practice.

- Adapt PPIs to target cultural patterns, meanings, and values. For example, in many collectivist societies, an intervention concentrating on individual Self-Acceptance (PWB) may be less effective than one focusing on Positive Relationships with Others (PERMA-R) and communal participation.
- The Importance of Relationality: Culturally appropriate, strengths-based PPIs emphasizing cultural connectivity, social support, and collective resilience have been demonstrated to enhance healing in communities that have endured historical and intergenerational trauma (Spahn et al., 2022). The Relational GRR is frequently the most important factor in these situations.

6. CHALLENGES, ETHICAL CONSIDERATIONS, AND FUTURE RESEARCH SCOPE

To cement its position as a fundamental contributor to overall health, positive psychology must thoroughly address persistent scientific and ethical concerns.

6.1 Methodological Rigor and the Need for Objective Measurement

A principal critique levelled against positive psychology involves issues with proper theorizing and problematic measurement of positive psychological constructs, primarily due to an over-reliance on self-report measures (Miron et al., 2023). This introduces significant methodological weaknesses, including susceptibility to social desirability bias, respondent reactivity, and consequently, challenges with generalizability and replicability (Miron et al., 2023).

Advancing Measurement Beyond Self-Report

Future research must commit to a multi-methodology approach:

1. **Ecological Momentary Assessment (EMA):** PPIs are dynamic and context-dependent. EMA involves collecting real-time data on emotions, behaviours, and context multiple times a day via a smartphone app. This drastically reduces recall bias and captures the true "in-the-moment" efficacy of a PPI (e.g., how the use of a strength immediately mitigated a stressor).
2. **Objective Behavioural and Physiological Measures:** Mandating the inclusion of objective physical health markers, such as Heart Rate Variability (HRV), inflammatory cytokines (C-Reactive Protein), and glycosylated haemoglobin (HbA1c) in diabetes studies, to definitively link PPIs to physical outcomes.
3. **Sophisticated Statistical Modelling:** Employing mediation and moderation analyses to test the theoretical model explicitly (e.g., does Gratitude (PPI) lead to increased SOC-Meaningfulness (Mediator), which in turn predicts better adherence (Outcome)?). This confirms the causal chain hypothesized by the salutogenic framework.
4. **Preregistration and Replication:** Adopting rigorous open science practices, including pre-registration of RCTs and transparent data sharing, to address replicability concerns and enhance the field's scientific credibility.

6.2 Ethical Imperatives: The "Tyranny of the Positive" and Justice

The most significant ethical challenge is the concept of the "tyranny of the positive attitude," or toxic positivity (Held, 2002). This societal pressure forces the repression of unpleasant emotions and the preservation of continual cheerfulness, which can have harmful psychological consequences by discrediting real pain and sorrow (Held, 2002).

- **Clinical Responsibility:** Clinicians must affirm negative experiences, acknowledging that anxiety, pain, and loss are natural parts of the human experience and are frequently crucial antecedents to personal growth and resilience (Held, 2002). PPIs must be positioned as resource-building tools to cope with challenging situations, not mandates to ignore them.
- **Justice and Equity:** A crucial ethical necessity is to address the possibility of using PPIs to "blame the victim" (Held, 2002). It is unfair to require people who are experiencing structural disadvantages, systematic injustice, or poverty (low Material GRRs) to be appreciative or find meaning. Future research should include PPIs into structural and systemic change initiatives, acknowledging that individual psychology cannot fix social problems. The emphasis must be on communal well-being and social justice as a source of meaning.

6.3 Future Research Suggestions for Holistic Health

The scientific agenda for positive health must prioritize several areas to fulfil the promise of holistic well-being:

- **PPI impact on biomarkers/inflammation:** Investigating the causality between specific PPIs and objective, biological markers of health (e.g., inflammatory cytokines, allostatic load) to conclusively determine their impact on physical health and disease progression, establishing true "positive health reserves."
- **AI + personalized PPI ethical framework:** Focusing on the ethical integration of positive psychology into technological domains, leveraging generative AI to create personalized, eudaimonic-focused PPIs while establishing strong ethical safeguards against bias, lack of empathy, and potential harm.
- **Cultural studies in non-Western contexts:** Directing research efforts toward extending PPIs to marginalized and historically ignored groups, ensuring the systematic development and rigorous evaluation of culturally adapted

interventions in non-Western contexts, prioritizing Relational and Communal GRRs.

- **Longitudinal studies on SOC-Meaningfulness:** Conducting long-term studies using EMA and objective markers to better understand the fluctuating hierarchy of the SOC components and determine which is the most critical for sustained health promotion across the lifespan, particularly focusing on the motivational role of Meaningfulness.

CONCLUSION AND FUTURE SCOPE

The evidence compiled herein firmly supports the conclusion that Positive Psychology Interventions offer a powerful, evidence-based roadmap for achieving holistic health. By intentionally shifting the paradigm from the reactive management of disease (pathogenesis) toward the proactive cultivation of human strengths and resources (salutogenesis), PPIs provide a necessary and empirically validated complement to traditional health psychology models.

The theoretical foundations of PPIs, resting on the Sense of Coherence (SOC), the Broaden-and-Build Theory, and the PERMA model, demonstrate that well-being can be actively built through tangible practices that modulate the neurobiological systems, particularly by enhancing Vagal Tone and downregulating the HPA axis. The empirical data confirms the therapeutic value of these practices, offering quantifiable effects on critical psychological comorbidities such as anxiety and depression (Iodice et al., 2021), and measurable improvements in long-term health adherence and physiological indicators, as supported by the in-depth typology and clinical applications. The emergence of scalable digital delivery methods promises broader access, provided the ethical challenges of the "tyranny of the positive" and AI safety are rigorously addressed.

Chapter Limitations and Contribution: While this chapter comprehensively reviews the shift from pathogenesis to salutogenesis and the efficacy of core PPIs, a key limitation is its necessary reliance on existing meta-analyses, some of which are based on self-report measures. The chapter's novel contribution lies in: 1) Explicitly linking the PERMA, B&B, and the Neurobiological pathways to the core dimensions of Antonovsky's SOC, showing how PPIs directly promote Comprehensibility, Manageability, and Meaningfulness; 2) Providing a robust, multi-methodological agenda that mandates the use of Ecological Momentary Assessment (EMA) and objective biomarkers; and 3) Offering detailed, salutogenic design principles for digital health applications.

By addressing the critical needs for methodological rigor, cultural adaptation, and social responsibility, positive psychology interventions can deliver on their profound potential: offering a person-centered model of health that is defined not merely by the absence of illness, but by the active, enduring presence of well-being, meaning, and resilience, a measurable and sustainable reserve in capacities.

REFERENCES

Antonovsky, A. (1991). The structural components of the sense of coherence: Meaningfulness, manageability, and comprehensibility. *The Global Perspective on Health and Illness*, *41*, 1–18.

Antonovsky, A. (1996). The salutogenic model of health. *American Journal of Health Promotion*, *10*(1), 5–18.

Donaldson, S. I.. (2021). Future perspectives on positive psychology: A research agenda. *Frontiers in Psychology*, *12*, 760088.

Fredrickson, B. L. (2004). The broaden-and-build theory of positive emotions: Resources for successful coping. *Psihologijske Teme*, *13*(2), 143–154.

Fredrickson, B. L., Cohn, M. A., Coffey, K. A., Pek, J., & Finkel, S. M. (2008). Open hearts build lives: Positive emotions, induced through loving-kindness meditation, build consequential personal resources. *Journal of Personality and Social Psychology*, *95*(5), 1045–1062. DOI: 10.1037/a0013262 PMID: 18954193

Haber, N.. (2023). Dangers of large language models in mental health care. *ACM Conference on Fairness, Accountability, and Transparency*.

Held, B. S. (2002). The tyranny of the positive attitude in America: Observation and speculation. *Journal of Clinical Psychology*, *58*(9), 965–991. DOI: 10.1002/jclp.10093 PMID: 12209859

Helgeson, V. S., & Zajdel, M. (2022). Psychosocial interventions for people newly diagnosed with a chronic disease. *Health Psychology Review*, *16*(3), 333–353.

Iodice, J. A., Malouff, J. M., & Schutte, N. S. (2021). The effects of gratitude interventions on anxiety and depression: A systematic review and meta-analysis. *Einstein (Sao Paulo, Brazil)*, *19*, eRW5887.

Kern, M. L.. (2014). A holistic approach to measuring well-being: The PERMA-Profiler. *The Journal of Positive Psychology*, *10*(3), 226–236. PMID: 25745508

Kok, B. E., & Fredrickson, B. L. (2010). Upward spirals of the heart: Vagal tone, positive emotions, and upward spirals of health. *Biological Psychology*, *84*(3), 432–436. DOI: 10.1016/j.biopsycho.2010.09.005 PMID: 20851735

Miron, A.. (2023). Theoretical and methodological critiques of positive psychology: Issues with measurement and self-report bias. *The Journal of Positive Psychology*, *18*(4), 501–518.

Peiro, P., et al. (2023). Defining positive health as a "reserve in capacities." *European Journal of Public Health, 33*(4), ckae144.834.

Rashid, T., & Ostermann, R. F. (2010). Strength-based assessment in clinical practice. *Journal of Clinical Psychology*, *66*(6), 488–498. PMID: 19294732

Ryff, C. D. (1989). Happiness is everything, or is it? Explorations on the meaning of psychological well-being. *Journal of Personality and Social Psychology*, *57*(6), 1069–1081. DOI: 10.1037/0022-3514.57.6.1069

Schotanus-Dijkstra, M.. (2024). Efficacy of strengths-based positive psychology interventions in enhancing well-being. *Applied Psychology. Health and Well-Being*.

Spahn, K. C.. (2022). Guidelines for the cultural adaptation of positive psychology interventions (PPIs) when working with non-Western populations. *Frontiers in Psychology*, *13*, 809362.

Tielman, M. L.. (2024). Efficacy of chatbot-delivered interventions for mental health and well-being: A meta-analysis. *JMIR Mental Health*, *1*(1), e59560.

Uchino, B. N.. (2003). Social support and health outcomes: A meta-analysis. *Psychological Bulletin*, *129*(2), 273–295.

Conclusion

The chapters presented across these volumes collectively demonstrate that health psychology has become an essential framework for understanding the complexity of contemporary human experience. Far beyond its traditional association with illness behavior or treatment adherence, the field now encompasses broader questions concerning resilience, emotional adaptation, social justice, caregiving, cultural identity, technology, education, creativity, and meaning-making. The diverse contributions included in this collection reveal the extent to which psychological well-being is deeply intertwined with personal, relational, societal, and structural realities.

A central conclusion emerging from the volume is that psychological health cannot be adequately understood through reductionist or exclusively biomedical perspectives. Across the chapters, health and illness are consistently portrayed as multidimensional phenomena shaped by emotional, cognitive, behavioral, interpersonal, sociocultural, and environmental factors. Whether examining chronic illness, trauma, caregiving, migration, educational stress, workplace dynamics, or digital environments, the contributors highlight that psychological experiences are always embedded within broader systems of meaning and social context. The concept of resilience appears repeatedly throughout the collection, though not as a simplistic narrative of strength or invulnerability. Instead, resilience is conceptualized as a fluid and evolving process that develops through relationships, coping strategies, emotional regulation, cultural resources, and access to social support. Importantly, many chapters emphasize that resilience does not eliminate suffering. Rather, it reflects the capacity to continue adapting, functioning, and reconstructing meaning despite adversity. This distinction is especially significant in contexts involving chronic illness, caregiving burden, trauma exposure, disability, and prolonged stress.

The findings and reflections presented in these volumes also underline the psychological importance of meaning-making processes. Human beings continuously attempt to interpret painful experiences in ways that preserve identity, coherence, and hope. Across different populations and settings, meaning emerges as a protective psychological mechanism that supports emotional adaptation and existential stability. The chapters focusing on forgiveness, coping, post-traumatic growth, chronic illness, and caregiving particularly demonstrate how individuals seek to maintain psychological continuity even under conditions of uncertainty and loss. Another major conclusion concerns the importance of emotional regulation and interpersonal support. Several contributors highlight that psychological distress is often intensified when individuals experience isolation, stigma, emotional invalidation, or lack of practical assistance. Conversely, supportive relationships, empathic communication, and psychologically safe environments appear to function as significant protective factors across educational, healthcare, familial, and organizational settings. This has important implications for mental health interventions, healthcare policy, and professional training programs.

The collection also demonstrates that caregivers constitute one of the most psychologically vulnerable populations within healthcare systems. The experiences described across multiple chapters reveal the profound emotional, physical, and social burden associated with long-term caregiving responsibilities. Caregivers frequently experience exhaustion, sleep disturbance, social withdrawal, anxiety, and emotional overload while simultaneously attempting to preserve dignity and quality of care for their loved ones. These findings reinforce the need for healthcare systems to move beyond patient-centered models alone and toward family-centered and caregiver-inclusive approaches.

Several chapters further illustrate the growing role of positive psychology within health-related interventions. Strengths-based approaches focusing on flourishing, emotional resources, engagement, and psychological flexibility appear increasingly relevant in both clinical and educational settings. However, the contributors also caution against overly individualistic interpretations of well-being that ignore structural inequalities or sociocultural realities. Psychological empowerment cannot be fully achieved without considering access to healthcare, social inclusion, economic security, and cultural sensitivity.

The impact of technological transformation emerges as another defining theme throughout the collection. Digital health interventions, telemedicine, artificial intelligence, and virtual communication platforms are reshaping healthcare delivery and psychological support worldwide. The contributors recognize the considerable opportunities associated with these innovations, including increased accessibility, personalized care, and expanded mental health outreach. At the same time, concerns regarding digital fatigue, ethical boundaries, privacy, depersonalization, and inequality remain highly relevant. The future of health psychology will likely depend on balancing technological advancement with the preservation of empathy, human connection, and ethical responsibility. The educational and creative dimensions of psychological well-being are also strongly represented within these volumes. The chapters exploring art therapy, creativity, mathematics anxiety, embodied learning, and neuroscience-informed educational practices demonstrate that emotional well-being can be supported through imaginative, experiential, and expressive processes. These approaches challenge purely symptom-focused models and encourage more holistic understandings of learning, adaptation, and psychological development. An additional contribution of this collection lies in its multicultural orientation. Mental health experiences vary considerably across cultural, social, and political contexts, and the chapters included here collectively reinforce the importance of culturally responsive approaches. Concepts such as resilience, suffering, coping, caregiving, and emotional expression are shaped by family systems, religious beliefs, social expectations, and cultural narratives. Consequently, interventions that ignore these contextual realities risk becoming ineffective or psychologically disconnected from the populations they intend to support.

The volume also highlights the importance of interdisciplinary collaboration. Many of the challenges discussed cannot be adequately addressed by psychology alone. Effective healthcare increasingly requires cooperation among psychologists, nurses, physicians, educators, social workers, policymakers, public health specialists, and community organizations. Integrated models of care that recognize the interaction between mental, physical, and social dimensions of health are likely to become increasingly important in future healthcare systems.

Despite the breadth of topics covered, several unresolved challenges remain evident. Significant gaps persist in mental health accessibility, caregiver support services, culturally adapted interventions, digital ethics frameworks, and trauma-informed healthcare implementation. Additionally, the rapid pace of social and technological change continues to create new psychological stressors that require ongoing research and adaptation.

Ultimately, the chapters gathered in these volumes collectively reaffirm a fundamental principle: health psychology is deeply concerned with the human capacity to adapt, connect, create meaning, and preserve dignity under difficult circumstances. Psychological well-being cannot be separated from relationships, culture, identity, community, and social structures. Understanding health therefore requires attention not only to symptoms and disorders but also to lived experience, emotional reality, resilience processes, and the broader conditions shaping everyday life.

The editors hope that this collection will contribute to ongoing dialogue, future research, reflective practice, and more compassionate models of healthcare and education. In a world increasingly characterized by uncertainty, fragmentation, and rapid change, the insights offered by health psychology remain essential for supporting both individual and collective well-being.

Agathi Argyriadi

American University, UAE

Alexandros Argyriadis
Hellenic Mediterranean University, Greece

Compilation of References

Aboujaoude, E. (2018). Telemental health: Why the revolution has not arrived. *World Psychiatry; Official Journal of the World Psychiatric Association (WPA)*, *17*(3), 277–278. DOI: 10.1002/wps.20551 PMID: 30192097

Aboujaoude, E., Gega, L., Parish, M. B., & Hilty, D. M. (2020). Editorial: Digital interventions in mental health: Current status and future directions [Editorial]. *Frontiers in Psychiatry*, *11*, 111. Advance online publication. DOI: 10.3389/fpsyt.2020.00111 PMID: 32174858

Acoba, E. F. (2024). Social support and mental health: The mediating role of perceived stress. *Frontiers in Psychology*, *15*(1), 1–10. DOI: 10.3389/fpsyg.2024.1330720

Ahirwar, G., Tiwari, G. K., & Rai, P. K. (2019). Exploring the nature, attributes and consequences of forgiveness in children: A qualitative study. *Psychological Thought*, *12*(2), 214–231. DOI: 10.5964/psyct.v12i2.347

Akhtar, S., & Barlow, J. (2018). Forgiveness therapy for the promotion of mental well-being: A systematic review and meta-analysis. *Trauma, Violence & Abuse*, *19*(1), 107–122. DOI: 10.1177/1524838016637079

Aldao, A., Nolen-Hoeksema, S., & Schweizer, S. (2010). Emotion-regulation strategies across psychopathology: A meta-analytic review. *Clinical Psychology Review*, *30*(2), 217–237. DOI: 10.1016/j.cpr.2009.11.004 PMID: 20015584

American Psychiatric Association (APA). (2022). *Diagnostic and statistical manual of mental disorders* (5th ed., text rev.)., DOI: 10.1176/appi.books.9780890425787

American Psychological Association (APA). (2011). *Beck Depression Inventory (BDI)*. [online]. https://www.apa.org/pi/about/publications/caregivers/practice-settings/assessment/tools/beck-depression

Ammerman, R. T., Cassisi, J. E., Hersen, M., & Van Hasselt, V. B. (1986). Consequences of physical abuse and neglect in children. *Clinical Psychology Review*, *6*(4), 291–310. DOI: 10.1016/0272-7358(86)90003-6

Andersen, A. M., Pietrzak, R. H., Kranzler, H. R., Ma, L., Zhou, H., Liu, X., Kramer, J., Kuperman, S., Edenberg, H. J., Nurnberger, J. I.Jr, Rice, J. P., Tischfield, J. A., Goate, A., Foroud, T. M., Meyers, J. L., Porjesz, B., Dick, D. M., Hesselbrock, V., Boerwinkle, E., & Han, S. (2017). Polygenic scores for major depressive disorder and risk of alcohol dependence. *JAMA Psychiatry*, *74*(11), 1153. DOI: 10.1001/jamapsychiatry.2017.2269

Anderson, A. P., Mayer, M. D., Fellows, A. M., Cowan, D. R., Hegel, M. T., & Buckey, J. C. (2017). Relaxation with Immersive Natural Scenes Presented Using Virtual Reality. *Aerospace Medicine and Human Performance*, *88*(6), 520–526. DOI: 10.3357/AMHP.4747.2017 PMID: 28539139

Antonovsky, A. (1991). The structural components of the sense of coherence: Meaningfulness, manageability, and comprehensibility. *The Global Perspective on Health and Illness*, *41*, 1–18.

Antonovsky, A. (1996). The salutogenic model of health. *American Journal of Health Promotion*, *10*(1), 5–18.

Argyriadi, A., Katsarou, D., Patelarou, A., Megari, K., Patelarou, E., Kotrotsiou, S., Giakoumidakis, K., Abdoola, S., Mantsos, E., Efthymiou, E., & Argyriadis, A. (2025). Digital Stress Scale (DSC): Development and Psychometric Validation of a Measure of Stress in the Digital Age. *International Journal of Environmental Research and Public Health*, *22*(7), 1080. DOI: 10.3390/ijerph22071080 PMID: 40724147

Assary, E., Oginni, O. A., Morneau-Vaillancourt, G., Krebs, G., Peel, A. J., Palaiologou, E., Lockhart, C., Ronald, A., & Eley, T. C. (2024). Genetics of environmental sensitivity and its association with variations in emotional problems, autistic traits, and wellbeing. *Molecular Psychiatry*, *29*(8), 2438–2446. DOI: 10.1038/s41380-024-02508-6

Athan, A. M. (2011). *Postpartum flourishing: Motherhood as opportunity for positive growth and self-development.* ProQuest Dissertations Publishing. https://search.proquest.com/openview/e31d26d93e356c201d593c371d69578c/1

Atienza-Carrasco, J., Linares-Abad, M., Padilla Ruiz, M., & Morales Gil, I. M. (2019). Experiences and outcomes following diagnosis of congenital foetal anomaly and medical termination of pregnancy: A phenomenological study. *Journal of Clinical Nursing*, *29*(1-2), 93–104. DOI: 10.1111/jocn.15162 PMID: 31887230

Bagarić, B., & Jokić-Begić, N. (2020). Measuring therapists' attitudes toward integration of technology in psychotherapy and predicting their use of technology. *Journal of Clinical Psychology*, *76*(6), 1151–1172. DOI: 10.1002/jclp.22967 PMID: 32410312

Baker, E., Barlow, C. F., Daniel, L., Morey, C., Bentley, R., & Taylor, M. P. (2023). Psychological health impacts of environmental exposures: A scoping review of evaluative instruments. *The Science of the Total Environment*, *912*(1), 1–10. DOI: 10.1016/j.scitotenv.2023.169063

Balcombe, L., & De Leo, D. (2021). Digital mental health challenges and the horizon ahead for solutions. *JMIR Mental Health*, *8*(3), e26811. DOI: 10.2196/26811 PMID: 33779570

Baldassano, C. F. (2005). Assessment tools for screening and monitoring bipolar disorder. *Bipolar Disorders*, *7*(1), 8–15. DOI: 10.1111/j.1399-5618.2005.00189.x PMID: 15762864

Baluni, P., Bhutani, R., Singh, R., & Singh, A. K. (2024). A systematic literature review for identifying the factors causing prevalences of suicide among youths in India. In Aloka, P. (Ed.), *Student Well-Being in Higher Education Institutions* (pp. 237–266). IGI Global., DOI: 10.4018/979-8-3693-4417-0.ch010

Bandura, A. (1997). *Self-efficacy: The exercise of control.* W. H. Freeman.

Barua, A., Ghosh, M. K., Kar, N., & Basilio, M. A. (2010). Socio-demographic factors of geriatric depression. *Indian Journal of Psychological Medicine*, *32*(2), 87–92. DOI: 10.4103/0253-7176.78503

Baum, N. (2016). Secondary traumatization in mental health professionals: A systematic review of gender findings. *Traumatology*, *22*(2), 144–151. DOI: 10.1177/1524838015584357 PMID: 25964278

Bayat, M. (2007). Evidence of resilience in families of children with autism. *Journal of Intellectual Disability Research*, *51*(9), 702–714. DOI: 10.1111/j.1365-2788.2007.00960.x PMID: 17845239

Beauchamp, T. L., & Childress, J. F. (2019). *Principles of biomedical ethics* (8th ed.). Oxford University Press.

Bechara, A. O., Chen, Z. J., Cowden, R. G.Jr, Worthington, E. L., Toussaint, L., Rodrigquez, N., Murillo, H. G., Ho, M. Y., Mathur, M. B., & VanderWeele, T. J. (2024). Do forgiveness campaign activities improve forgiveness, mental health, and flourishing? *International Journal of Public Health*, *69*(1), 1–15. DOI: 10.3389/ijph.2024.1605341

Beck, A. T., Ward, C. H., Mendelson, M., Mock, J., & Erbaugh, J. (1961). An inventory for measuring depression. *Archives of General Psychiatry*, *4*(1), 561–571. DOI: 10.1001/archpsyc.1961.01710120031004 PMID: 13688369

Bedaso, A., Adams, J., Peng, W., & Sibbritt, D. (2021). The relationship between social support and mental health problems during pregnancy: A systematic review and meta-analysis. *Reproductive Health*, *18*(1), 1–9. DOI: 10.1186/s12978-021-01209-5

Beilharz, J., Maniam, J., & Morris, M. (2015). Diet-induced cognitive deficits: The role of fat and sugar, potential mechanisms and nutritional interventions. *Nutrients*, *7*(8), 6719–6738. DOI: 10.3390/nu7085307 PMID: 26274972

Belsky, J., & Pluess, M. (2009). Beyond diathesis stress: Differential susceptibility to environmental influences. *Psychological Bulletin*, *135*(6), 885–908. DOI: 10.1037/a0017376

Bendall, S., Eastwood, O., Cox, G., Farrelly-Rosch, A., Nicoll, H., Peters, W., Bailey, A. P., McGorry, P. D., & Scanlan, J. N. (2020). A Systematic Review and Synthesis of Trauma-Informed Care Within Outpatient and Counseling Health Settings for Young People. *Child Maltreatment*, *26*(5), 533–545. DOI: 10.1177/1077559520927468 PMID: 32536207

Berger, R. (2015). *Stress, trauma, and posttraumatic growth: Social context, environment, and identities*. Routledge., DOI: 10.4324/9780203118795

Berring, L. L.. (2024). Implementing trauma-informed care—Settings, definitions, models, and outcomes. *International Journal of Mental Health Nursing*, *33*, e130–e149. DOI: 10.1111/inm.13144

Berry, J. W., Worthington, E. L.Jr, Parrott, L.III, O'Connor, L. E., & Wade, N. G. (2001b). Transgression narrative test of forgivingness. *Personality and Social Psychology Bulletin*, *27*(10), 1277–1290. Advance online publication. DOI: 10.1177/01461672012710004

Bhargav, H., Holla, B., Ramakrishna, K. K., Shivakumar, V., Gokulakrishnan, K., Varambally, S., & Gangadhar, B. N. (2022). Yoga and integrative healthcare. *International Journal of Yoga*, *15*(2), 150–157. DOI: 10.4103/ijoy.ijoy_56_22 PMID: 36329771

Bhugra, D., Till, A., & Sartorius, N. (2013). What is mental health? *The International Journal of Social Psychiatry*, *59*(1), 3–4. DOI: 10.1177/0020764012463315 PMID: 23349505

Bloom, S. L. (2019). *Creating sanctuary: Toward the evolution of sane societies*. Routledge.

Bloom, S. L., & Farragher, B. (2018). *Restoring sanctuary: A new operating system for trauma-informed systems of care*. Oxford University Press.

Bonanno, G. A. (2004). Loss, trauma, and human resilience: Have we underestimated the human capacity to thrive after extremely aversive events? *The American Psychologist*, *59*(1), 20–28. DOI: 10.1037/0003-066X.59.1.20 PMID: 14736317

Brady, J. L., Guy, J. D., Poelstra, P. L., & Brokaw, B. F. (1999). Vicarious traumatization, spirituality, and the treatment of sexual abuse survivors: A national survey of women psychotherapists. *Professional Psychology, Research and Practice*, *30*(4), 386–393. https://psycnet.apa.org/doi/10.1037/0735-7028.30.4.386. DOI: 10.1037/0735-7028.30.4.386

Braun, V., & Clarke, V. (2006). Using thematic analysis in psychology. *Qualitative Research in Psychology*, *3*(2), 77–101. DOI: 10.1191/1478088706qp063oa

Bronfenbrenner, U. (1979). *The ecology of human development: Experiments by nature and design*. Harvard University Press. DOI: 10.4159/9780674028845

Brudek, P., Steuden, S., & Kaleta, K. (2023). Wisdom and wellbeing polish older adults: The mediating role of forgiveness. *Frontiers in Psychology*, *14*(1), 1–7. DOI: 10.3389/fpsyg.2023.1163113

Buber, M. (1958). *I and Thou* (2nd ed.). (Smith, R. G., Trans.). Charles Scribner's Sons.

Bunting, L., Montgomery, L., & Mooney, S.. (2021). Implementing trauma-informed approaches in healthcare: A mixed-methods systematic review. *BMJ Open*, *11*, e043817. DOI: 10.1136/bmjopen-2020-043817

Buser, M. C., & Scinicariello, F. (2017). Cadmium, lead, and depressive symptoms: Analysis of national health and nutrition examination survey 2011-2012. *The Journal of Clinical Psychiatry*, *78*(5), 515–521. DOI: 10.4088/JCP.15m10383

Callaghan, A., McCombe, G., Harrold, A., McMeel, C., Mills, G., Moore-Cherry, N., & Cullen, W. (2020). The impact of green spaces on mental health in urban settings: a scoping review. *Journal of Psychological health, 30*(2), 179–193. DOI: 10.1080/09638237.2020.1755027

Carver, C. S., & Connor-Smith, J. (2010). Personality and Coping. *Annual Review of Psychology*, *61*(1), 679–704. DOI: 10.1146/annurev.psych.093008.100352 PMID: 19572784

Carver, C. S., & Vargas, S. (2012). Stress, Coping, and Health. In Friedman, H. S. (Ed.), *The Oxford Handbook of Health Psychology* (1st ed., pp. 163–188). Oxford University Press., DOI: 10.1093/oxfordhb/9780195342819.013.0008

Cedillo, Y. E., Kelly, T., Davis, E., Durham, L., Smith, D. L.Jr, Kennedy, R. E., & Fernandez, J. R. (2023). Evaluation of food security status, psychological well-being, and stress on BMI and diet-related behaviors among a sample college students. *Public Health*, *224*(1), 32–40. DOI: 10.1016/j.puhe.2023.08.015

Çelik, E., & Ertürk, K. (2022). The effect of forgiveness psychoeducation on forgiveness and life satisfaction in high school students. *Counselling & Psychotherapy Research*, *22*(1), 187–196. DOI: 10.1002/capr.12418

Champine, R. B., Johnson, M., & Green, A. (2023). Trauma-informed care: Recent advances, limitations, and future directions. *Journal of Trauma & Dissociation*, *24*(1), 1–17. DOI: 10.1080/15299732.2022.2148474 PMID: 36567526

Chan, J. B., & Sigafoos, J. (2001). Does respite care reduce parental stress in families with developmentally disabled children? *Child and Youth Care Forum*, *30*(5), 253–263. DOI: 10.1023/A:1014467226528

Charan, J. K., Chandra, S., Vaissnave, V., Ragupathi, T., Satyanarayana, P., & Manjunath, T. C. (2025). Impact of Generative AI on Industries and Organizations. In Zhao, J., Kumar, V., Katina, P., & Richards, J. (Eds.), *Humans and Generative AI Tools for Collaborative Intelligence* (pp. 509–528). I Global Scientific Publishing., DOI: 10.4018/979-8-3693-8332-2.ch022

Choudhry, V., Dayal, R., Pillai, D., Kalokhe, A., Beier, K., & Patel, V. (2018). Child sexual abuse in India: A systematic review. *PLoS One*, *13*(10), e0205086. DOI: 10.1371/journal.pone.0205086 PMID: 30300379

Chun, C.-A., Moos, R. H., & Cronkite, R. C. (2006). Culture: A Fundamental Context for the Stress and Coping Paradigm. In Wong, P. T. P., & Wong, L. C. J. (Eds.), *Handbook of Multicultural Perspectives on Stress and Coping* (pp. 29–53). Springer US., DOI: 10.1007/0-387-26238-5_2

Cleary, J. P., Janvier, A., Farlow, B., Weaver, M., Hammel, J., & Lantos, J. (2021). Cardiac interventions for patients with trisomy 13 and trisomy 18: Experience, ethical issues, communication, and the case for individualized family-centered care. *Journal of Patient Experience*, *9*, 1–8. DOI: 10.1177/21501351211044132 PMID: 34919485

Cleverley, K., & Kidd, S. A. (2011). Resilience and suicidality among homeless youth. *Journal of Adolescence*, *34*(5), 1049–1054. DOI: 10.1016/j.adolescence.2010.11.003

Cohen, S., Underwood, L. G., & Gottlieb, B. H. (2000). Social relationships and health. In Cohen, S., Underwood, L. G., & Gottlieb, B. H. (Eds.), *Social Support Measurement and Intervention: A Guide for Health and Social Scientists* (pp. 3–26). Oxford Academic Press., DOI: 10.1093/med:psych/9780195126709.003.0001

Coleman, P. K. (2015). Diagnosis of fetal anomaly and the increased maternal psychological toll associated with pregnancy termination. *Issues in Law & Medicine, 30*(1), 3–23. https://www.researchgate.net/publication/279308414 PMID: 26103706

Comas-Díaz, L., & Jacobsen, F. M. (1991). Ethnocultural transference and countertransference in the therapeutic dyad. *The American Journal of Orthopsychiatry, 61*(3), 392–402. https://psycnet.apa.org/doi/10.1037/h0079267. DOI: 10.1037/h0079267 PMID: 1951646

Compas, B. E., Jaser, S. S., Bettis, A. H., Watson, K. H., Gruhn, M. A., Dunbar, J. P., Williams, E., & Thigpen, J. C. (2017). Coping, emotion regulation, and psychopathology in childhood and adolescence: A meta-analysis and narrative review. *Psychological Bulletin, 143*(9), 939–991. DOI: 10.1037/bul0000110 PMID: 28616996

Courtois, C. A., & Ford, J. D. (2020). *Treating complex traumatic stress disorders (Adults): Scientific foundations and therapeutic models.* Guilford Press.

Coyle, C. T., & Enright, R. D. (1998). Forgiveness education with adult learners. In T. Pourchot, & M. C. Smith (Eds.), *Adult learning and development: Perspectives from Educational Psychology*, 296(1), 1-11. DOI: 10.4324/9781410603418

Cunningham, M. (2003). Impact of trauma work on social work clinicians: Empirical findings. *Social Work, 48*(4), 451–459. DOI: 10.1093/sw/48.4.451 PMID: 14620102

D'Andrea, W., Ford, J. D., & Courtois, C. A. (2020). Integrating trauma-informed care in psychotherapy for complex PTSD. *Journal of Contemporary Psychotherapy, 50*(2), 109–122. DOI: 10.1007/s10879-019-09449-7

Dal, N., & Bilici, S. (2024). An overview of the potential role of nutrition in mental disorders in the light of advances in nutripsychiatry. *Current Nutrition Reports, 13*(2), 69–81. DOI: 10.1007/s13668-024-00520-4 PMID: 38329691

Dan, V. H., Ponnuchamy, L., Anand, N. K., Bhaskarapillai, B., & Sharma, M. K. (2023). Resilience and self-compassion among persons with depressive disorders: Prerequisite for a positive mental health approach. *Journal of Family Medicine and Primary Care, 12*(8), 1621–1628. DOI: 10.4103/jfmpc.jfmpc_2270_22 PMID: 37767454

Das, A., Sharma, M. K., Thamilselvan, P., & Marimuthu, P. (2017). Technology addiction among treatment seekers for psychological problems: Implication for screening in mental health setting. *Indian Journal of Psychological Medicine*, *39*(1), 21–27. DOI: 10.4103/0253-7176.198939 PMID: 28250554

Davidson, R. J., & McEwen, B. S. (2012). Social influences on neuroplasticity: Stress and interventions to promote well-being. *Nature Neuroscience*, *15*(5), 689–695. DOI: 10.1038/nn.3093 PMID: 22534579

Davis, C. G. (2001). The tormented and the transformed: Understanding responses to loss and trauma. In Neimeyer, R. A. (Ed.), *Meaning reconstruction & the experience of loss* (pp. 137–155). American Psychological Association., DOI: 10.1037/10397-007

De Candia, C., Hughes, M., & Hopper, E. K. (2022). Trauma-informed TF-CBT with children exposed to violence: Outcomes and challenges. *Child Abuse & Neglect*, *132*, 105797. DOI: 10.1016/j.chiabu.2022.105797

Degan, T. J., Kelly, P. J., Robinson, L. D., & Deane, F. P. (2018). Health literacy in substance use disorder treatment: A latent profile analysis. *Journal of Substance Abuse Treatment*, *96*(1), 46–52. DOI: 10.1016/j.jsat.2018.10.009

Department of Health and Aged Care. (2021). National digital mental health framework. Retrieved from https://www.health.gov.au/resources/publications/national-digital-mental-health-framework

Dijksman, I., Dinant, G., & Spigt, M. (2017). The perception and needs of psychologists toward blended care. *Telemedicine Journal and e-Health*, *23*(12), 983–995. DOI: 10.1089/tmj.2017.0031 PMID: 28556693

Dimitros, E., Katsarou, D. V., Mantsos, E., Bara, A., Argyriadi, A., Argyriadis, A., & Goupos, T. (2025). Perceptions of primary and secondary school principals on the support, educational forms and methods of gifted students in Greece. *Journal of Research in Special Educational Needs*. Advance online publication. DOI: 10.1111/1471-3802.70045

Donaldson, S. I.. (2021). Future perspectives on positive psychology: A research agenda. *Frontiers in Psychology*, *12*, 760088.

Dunst, C. J., Trivette, C. M., & Deal, A. G. (2007). *Enabling and empowering families: Principles and guidelines for practice*. Brookline Books.

Dzhambov, A. M., Hartig, T., Tilov, B., Atanasova, V., Makakova, D. R., & Dimitrova, D. D. (2019). Residential greenspace is associated with mental health via intertwined capacity-building and capacity-restoring pathways. *Environmental Research*, *178*(1), 1–13. DOI: 10.1016/j.envres.2019.108708

Emerson, E., Hatton, C., Llewellyn, G., Blacher, J., & Graham, H. (2010). Socio-economic position, household composition, health status and indicators of child well-being in families of children with and without intellectual disabilities. *Journal of Intellectual Disability Research, 54*(12), 1086–1098.

Engel, G. L. (1977). The need for a new medical model: A challenge for biomedicine. *Science, 196*(4286), 129–136. DOI: 10.1126/science.847460 PMID: 847460

English, T., John, O. P., Srivastava, S., & Gross, J. J. (2012). Emotion regulation and peer-rated social functioning: A 4-year longitudinal study. *Journal of Research in Personality, 46*(6), 780–784. DOI: 10.1016/j.jrp.2012.09.006 PMID: 23471162

Enright, R. D., Knutson, J. A., Holter, A. C., Baskin, T., & Knutson, C. (2007). Waging peace through forgiveness in Belfast, Northern Ireland II: Educational programs for mental health improvement of children. *Journal of Research in Education, 17*(1), 63–78.

Enright, R. D.The Human Development Study Group (HDSG). (1994). Piaget on the moral development of forgiveness: Reciprocity or identity? *Human Development, 37*(2), 63–80. DOI: 10.1159/000278239

Epel, E. S., Crosswell, A. D., Mayer, S. E., Prather, A. A., Slavich, G. M., Puterman, E., & Mendes, W. B. (2018). More than a feeling: A unified view of stress measurement for population science. *Frontiers in Neuroendocrinology, 49*, 146–169. DOI: 10.1016/j.yfrne.2018.03.001 PMID: 29551356

Epstein, L., Epstein, F., & Kirkilis, R. E. (1998). *Trusting you are loved: Practices for partnerships*. Partnership Foundation.

Erbe, D., Eichert, H., Riper, H., & Ebert, D. (2017). Blending face-to-face and internet-based interventions for the treatment of mental disorders in adults: Systematic review. *Journal of Medical Internet Research, 19*(9), e306. DOI: 10.2196/jmir.6588 PMID: 28916506

Erikson, E. H. (1982). *The life cycle completed.* W. W. Norton & Company.

Farrell, R. M., Nutter, B., & Agatisa, P. K. (2013). Patient-centered prenatal counseling: Aligning obstetric healthcare professionals with needs of pregnant women. *Women & Health, 55*(3), 302–316. DOI: 10.1080/03630242.2014.996724 PMID: 25794055

Feijt, M., de Kort, Y., Bongers, I., & IJsselsteijn, W. (2018). Perceived drivers and barriers to the adoption of eMental health by psychologists: The construction of the levels of adoption of eMental health model. *Journal of Medical Internet Research, 20*(4), e153. DOI: 10.2196/jmir.9485 PMID: 29691215

Felitti, V. J., Anda, R. F., Nordenberg, D., Williamson, D. F., Spitz, A. M., Edwards, V., Koss, M. P., & Marks, J. S. (1998). Relationship of childhood abuse and household dysfunction to many of the leading causes of death in adults. *American Journal of Preventive Medicine, 14*(4), 245–258. DOI: 10.1016/S0749-3797(98)00017-8 PMID: 9635069

Figley, C. R. (1995). *Compassion fatigue: Coping with secondary traumatic stress disorder in those who treat the traumatized.* DOI: 10.4324/9780203777381

Figley, C. R. (2021). Compassion fatigue and secondary trauma: Implications for mental health professionals. *Journal of Clinical Psychology, 77*(11), 2433–2445. DOI: 10.1002/jclp.23121

Fitzgibbons, R. (1998). *Anger and the healing power of forgiveness: A psychiatrist's view. Exploring forgiveness.* University of Wisconsin Press. DOI: 10.2307/jj.36032636.10

Flett, J. A. M., Hayne, H., Riordan, B. C., Thompson, L. M., & Conner, T. S. (2019). Mobile Mindfulness Meditation: A Randomised Controlled Trial of the Effect of Two Popular Apps on Mental Health. *Mindfulness, 10*(5), 863–876. DOI: 10.1007/s12671-018-1050-9

Folkman, S., & Moskowitz, J. T. (2000). Positive affect and the other side of coping. *The American Psychologist, 55*(6), 647–654. DOI: 10.1037/0003-066X.55.6.647 PMID: 10892207

Folkman, S., & Moskowitz, J. T. (2004). Coping: Pitfalls and Promise. *Annual Review of Psychology, 55*(1), 745–774. DOI: 10.1146/annurev.psych.55.090902.141456 PMID: 14744233

Follette, V. M., Polusny, M. M., & Milbeck, K. (1994). Mental health and law enforcement professionals: Trauma history, psychological symptoms, and impact of providing services to child sexual abuse survivors. *Professional Psychology, Research and Practice, 25*(3), 275–282. DOI: 10.1037/0735-7028.25.3.275

Fredrickson, B. L. (2004). The broaden-and-build theory of positive emotions: Resources for successful coping. *Psihologijske Teme, 13*(2), 143–154.

Fredrickson, B. L., Cohn, M. A., Coffey, K. A., Pek, J., & Finkel, S. M. (2008). Open hearts build lives: Positive emotions, induced through loving-kindness meditation, build consequential personal resources. *Journal of Personality and Social Psychology, 95*(5), 1045–1062. DOI: 10.1037/a0013262 PMID: 18954193

Freedman, S. (2007). Forgiveness education with at-risk adolescents: A case study analysis. In Malcom, W., DeCourville, N., & Belicki, K. (Eds.), *Women's reflections on the complexities offorgiveness* (pp. 91–115). Routledge.

Freedman, S. (2018). Forgiveness as an educational goal with at-risk adolescents. *Journal ofMoral Education, 47*(4), 415–431. DOI: 10.1080/03057240.2017.1399869

Freedman, S., & Knupp, A. (2003). The impact of forgiveness on adolescent adjustment to parental divorce. *Journal of Divorce & Remarriage, 39*(1/2), 135–165. DOI: 10.1300/J087v39n01_08

Fusar-Poli, P., De Pablo, G. S., De Micheli, A., Nieman, D. H., Correll, C. U., Kessing, L. V., Pfennig, A., Bechdolf, A., Borgwardt, S., Arango, C., & Van Amelsvoort, T. (2019). What is good mental health? A scoping review. *European Neuropsychopharmacology, 31*(1), 33–46. DOI: 10.1016/j.euroneuro.2019.12.105 PMID: 31901337

Gable, S. L., & Haidt, J. (2005). What (& why) is positive psychology? *Review of General Psychology, 9*(2), 103-110. . 103DOI: <ALIGNMENT.qj></ALIGNMENT>10.1037/1089-2680.9.2

Galderisi, S., Heinz, A., Kastrup, M., Beezhold, J., & Sartorius, N. (2015). Toward a new definition of mental health. *World Psychiatry; Official Journal of the World Psychiatric Association (WPA), 14*(2), 231–233. DOI: 10.1002/wps.20231 PMID: 26043341

Gambaro, M. E. (2002). School-based forgiveness education in the management of trait anger in early adolescents. Unpublished doctoral dissertation, University of Wisconsin-Madison.

Gambaro, M. E., Enright, R. D., Baskin, T. A., & Klatt, J. (2008a). Can school-based forgiveness counselling improve conduct and academic achievement in academically at-risk adolescents? *Journal of Research in Education, 18*(1), 16–27.

García-Vázquez, F. I., Valdés-Cuervo, A. A., Martínez-Ferrer, B., & Parra-Pérez, L. G. (2020). Forgiveness, gratitude, happiness, and prosocial bystander behavior in bullying. *Frontiers in Psychology, 10*(1), 28–37. DOI: 10.3389/fpsyg.2019.02827

Gautam, S., Jain, A., Chaudhary, J., Gautam, M., Gaur, M., & Grover, S. (2024). Concept of mental health and mental well-being, it's determinants and coping strategies. *Indian Journal of Psychiatry, 66*(2, Suppl 2), 231–244. DOI: 10.4103/indianjpsychiatry.indianjpsychiatry_707_23

Godoy, L. D., Rossignoli, M. T., Delfino-Pereira, P., Garcia-Cairasco, N., & De Lima Umeoka, E. H. (2018). A Comprehensive Overview on Stress Neurobiology: Basic Concepts and Clinical Implications. *Frontiers in Behavioral Neuroscience*, *12*, 127. DOI: 10.3389/fnbeh.2018.00127 PMID: 30034327

Gona, J. K., Newton, C. R., Hartley, S., & Bunning, K. (2016). Developing and validating the 'parenting a child with disabilities' scale in a rural context in Kenya. *Disability and Rehabilitation*, *38*(20), 2019–2030.

Grajek, M., Krupa-Kotara, K., Białek-Dratwa, A., Sobczyk, K., Grot, M., Kowalski, O., & Staśkiewicz, W. (2022). Nutrition and mental health: A review of current knowledge about the impact of diet on mental health. *Frontiers in Nutrition*, *9*, 943998. Advance online publication. DOI: 10.3389/fnut.2022.943998 PMID: 36071944

Griffin, B. J., Worthington, E. L., Lavelock, C. R., Wade, N. G., & Hoyt, W. T. (2015). Forgiveness and mental health. In Toussaint, L., Worthington, E., & Williams, D. (Eds.), *Forgiveness and Health*. Springer., DOI: 10.1007/978-94-017-9993-5_6

Gross, J. J. (2015). Emotion Regulation: Current Status and Future Prospects. *Psychological Inquiry*, *26*(1), 1–26. DOI: 10.1080/1047840X.2014.940781

Gruebner, O., Rapp, M. A., Adli, M., Kluge, U., Galea, S., & Heinz, A. (2017). Cities and Psychological health. *Deutsches Ärzteblatt International*, *114*(1), 121–127. DOI: 10.3238/arztebl.2017.0121

Gunjan, G., & Rana, S. S. (2023). Effect of forgiveness on happiness and well-being. *Indian Journal of Positive Psychology*, *14*(3), 360–363.

Gun, S., Titov, N., & Andrews, G. (2011). Acceptability of internet treatment of anxiety and depression. *Australasian Psychiatry*, *19*(3), 259–264. DOI: 10.3109/10398562.2011.562295 PMID: 21682626

Guon, J., Wilfond, B. S., Farlow, B., Brazg, T., & Janvier, A. (2013). Our children are not a diagnosis: The experience of parents who continue their pregnancy after a prenatal diagnosis of trisomy 13 or 18. *American Journal of Medical Genetics. Part A*, *164A*(2), 308–318. DOI: 10.1002/ajmg.a.36298 PMID: 24311520

Gupta, A., & Singhal, N. (2005). Psychosocial support for families of children with intellectual disabilities. *British Journal of Special Education*, *31*(4), 214–221.

Guru Basava Aradhya, S., Chithambar Gupta, V., Raman, M. S., Singh, J., Manjunath, T. C., & Sharma, M. (2025). Health Crises and Digitalization: Digital Health. In Yıldırım, D., Yıldırım, S., & Kandpal, V. (Eds.), *Sustainable Digitalization Strategies in Business and Healthcare* (pp. 171–198). IGI Global Scientific Publishing., DOI: 10.4018/979-8-3373-5087-5.ch007

Haber, N.. (2023). Dangers of large language models in mental health care. *ACM Conference on Fairness, Accountability, and Transparency*.

Hailes, H. P., Yu, R., Danese, A., & Fazel, S. (2019). Long-term outcomes of childhood sexual abuse: An umbrella review. *The Lancet. Psychiatry*, *6*(10), 830–839. DOI: 10.1016/S2215-0366(19)30286-X PMID: 31519507

Hamilton, M. (1960). Hamilton depression rating scale (HDRS). *Journal of Neurology, Neurosurgery, and Psychiatry*, *23*(1), 56–62. DOI: 10.1136/jnnp.23.1.56 PMID: 14399272

Harmanpreet, C. S., Kalshetti, P., Satyanarayana, P., Sharma, M., & Manjunath, T. C. (2025). Digital Transformation in the Public Sector Entities. In A. Santos Ferreira & C. Lourenço dos Santos (Eds.), Enhancing Public Sector Accountability and Services Through Digital Innovation (pp. 353-380). IGI Global Scientific Publishing. DOI: 10.4018/979-8-3693-9251-5.ch011

Hartley, S. L., Barker, E. T., Seltzer, M. M., Floyd, F. J., Greenberg, J. S., Orsmond, G. I., & Bolt, D. (2012). The relative risk and timing of divorce in families of children with an autism spectrum disorder. *Journal of Family Psychology*, *24*(4), 449–457. DOI: 10.1037/a0019847 PMID: 20731491

Hastings, R. P., & Beck, A. (2004). Practitioner review: Stress intervention for parents of children with intellectual disabilities. *Journal of Child Psychology and Psychiatry, and Allied Disciplines*, *45*(8), 1338–1349. DOI: 10.1111/j.1469-7610.2004.00357.x PMID: 15482495

Hastings, R. P., & Brown, T. (2002). Behavior problems of children with autism, parental self-efficacy, and mental health. *American Journal of Mental Retardation*, *107*(3), 222–232. DOI: 10.1352/0895-8017(2002)107<0222:BPOCWA>2.0.CO;2 PMID: 11966335

Hastings, R. P., Kovshoff, H., Brown, T., Ward, N. J., Espinosa, F. D., & Remington, B. (2005). Coping strategies in mothers and fathers of preschool and school-age children with autism. *Autism*, *9*(4), 377–391. DOI: 10.1177/1362361305056078 PMID: 16155055

Hastings, R. P., & Taunt, H. M. (2002). Positive perceptions in families of children with developmental disabilities. *American Journal of Mental Retardation*, *107*(2), 116–127. DOI: 10.1352/0895-8017(2002)107<0116:PPIFOC>2.0.CO;2 PMID: 11853529

Haugen, P. T., McCrillis, A. M., Smid, G. E., & Nijdam, M. J. (2017). Mental health stigma and barriers to mental health care for first responders: A systematic review and meta-analysis. *Journal of Psychiatric Research*, *94*(1), 218–229. DOI: 10.1016/j.jpsychires.2017.08.001 PMID: 28800529

Haug, S., Goldstein, M., Cummins, D., Fayard, E., & Merritt, A. (2017). Using patient-centered care after a prenatal diagnosis of trisomy 18 or trisomy 13: A review. *JAMA Pediatrics*, *171*(4), 382–387. https://jamanetwork.com/journals/jamapediatrics/article-abstract/2601244. DOI: 10.1001/jamapediatrics.2016.4798 PMID: 28192554

Held, B. S. (2002). The tyranny of the positive attitude in America: Observation and speculation. *Journal of Clinical Psychology*, *58*(9), 965–991. DOI: 10.1002/jclp.10093 PMID: 12209859

Helgeson, V. S., & Zajdel, M. (2022). Psychosocial interventions for people newly diagnosed with a chronic disease. *Health Psychology Review*, *16*(3), 333–353.

Hemanth Kumar, T., Naga Kumari, Y. V., & Narasimha Rao, A. (2024). Child sexual abuse in India: Understanding the problem, responding to the challenges, and charting a way forward. In Shaik, A., Thota, S. L., & Atmakuri, L. R. (Eds.), *Child sexual abuse* (pp. xx–xx). Springer., DOI: 10.1007/978-981-99-8745-0_5

Henriksen, I. O., Ranøyen, I., Indredavik, M. S., & Stenseng, F. (2017). The role of self-esteem in the development of psychiatric problems: A three-year prospective study in a clinical sample of adolescents. *Child and Adolescent Psychiatry and Mental Health*, *11*(1), 1–13. DOI: 10.1186/s13034-017-0207-y PMID: 29299058

Herman, J. P., Nawreen, N., Smail, M. A., & Cotella, E. M. (2020). Brain mechanisms of HPA axis regulation: Neurocircuitry and feedback in context Richard Kvetnansky lecture. *Stress (Amsterdam, Netherlands)*, *23*(6), 617–632. DOI: 10.1080/10253890.2020.1859475 PMID: 33345670

Hilvert-Bruce, Z., Rossouw, P., Wong, N., Sunderland, M., & Andrews, G. (2012). Adherence as a determinant of effectiveness of internet cognitive behavioural therapy for anxiety and depressive disorders. *Behaviour Research and Therapy*, *50*(7–8), 463–468. DOI: 10.1016/j.brat.2012.04.001 PMID: 22659155

Hodgson, J., Pitt, P., Metcalfe, S., Halliday, J., Menezes, M., Fisher, J., Hickerton, C., Petersen, K., & McClaren, B. (2016). Experiences of prenatal diagnosis and decision-making about termination of pregnancy: A qualitative study. *Australian and New Zealand Journal of Obstetrics and Gynaecology*, *56*(6), 605–613. DOI: 10.1111/ajo.12501 PMID: 27402530

Hofmann, S. G., Asnaani, A., Vonk, I. J. J., Sawyer, A. T., & Fang, A. (2012). The Efficacy of Cognitive Behavioral Therapy: A Review of Meta-analyses. *Cognitive Therapy and Research, 36*(5), 427–440. DOI: 10.1007/s10608-012-9476-1 PMID: 23459093

Hollander-Goldfein, B., Isserman, N., & Goldenberg, J. E. (2012). *Transcending trauma: Survival, resilience and clinical implications in survivor families.* Routledge.

Horesh, D., & Brown, A. D. (2020). Traumatic stress in the age of COVID-19: A call to close critical gaps and adapt to new realities. *Psychological Trauma: Theory, Research, Practice, and Policy, 12*(4), 331–335. DOI: 10.1037/tra0000592 PMID: 32271070

Huber, M., Knottnerus, J. A., Green, L., Horst, H. V. D., Jadad, A. R., Kromhout, D., Leonard, B., Lorig, K., Loureiro, M. I., Meer, J. W. M. V. D., Schnabel, P., Smith, R., Weel, C. V., & Smid, H. (2011). How should we define health? *BMJ (Clinical Research Ed.), 343*(2), 41–63. DOI: 10.1136/bmj.d4163 PMID: 21791490

Hughes, K., Ford, K., & Bellis, M. A.. (2021). Health impacts of adverse childhood experiences: A systematic review and meta-analysis. *The Lancet. Public Health, 6*(11), e848–e858. DOI: 10.1016/S2468-2667(21)00232-2 PMID: 34756168

Hunter, A. (2007). Forgiveness: Hindu and western perspectives. *Journal of Hindu-Christian Studies, 20*(1), 11. DOI: 10.7825/2164-6279.1386

Hwang, W., Myers, H., Abekim, J., & Ting, J. (2007). A conceptual paradigm for understanding culture's impact on mental health: The cultural influences on mental health (CIMH) model. *Clinical Psychology Review, 28*(2), 211–227. DOI: 10.1016/j.cpr.2007.05.001

Hyman, S. E. (2000). The genetics of mental illness: Implications for practice. *Bulletin of the World Health Organization, 78*(4), 455–463.

Institute for Health Metrics and Evaluation (IHME). Global Burden of Disease (GBD). (2021). [Online]. https://vizhub.healthdata.org/gbd-results/

Iodice, J. A., Malouff, J. M., & Schutte, N. S. (2021). The effects of gratitude interventions on anxiety and depression: A systematic review and meta-analysis. *Einstein (Sao Paulo, Brazil), 19*, eRW5887.

Isobel, S., & Edwards, C. (2017). Using trauma informed care as a framework to promote the positive mental health of people with intellectual disability. *Journal of Intellectual Disabilities, 21*(3), 228–248. DOI: 10.1177/1744629517716738

Isobel, S., Goodyear, M., Furness, T., & Foster, K. (2021). Individual and organizational change: Trauma-informed care implementation in mental health services. *Issues in Mental Health Nursing*, *42*(9), 821–832. DOI: 10.1080/01612840.2021.1962485

Jacobs, M., Cooper, S. A., McGowan, R., Nelson, S. M., & Pell, J. (2016). Pregnancy outcome following prenatal diagnosis of chromosomal anomaly: A record linkage study of 26,261 pregnancies. *PLoS One*, *11*(1), e0166909. DOI: 10.1371/journal.pone.0166909 PMID: 27907018

Jayasankar, P., Manjunatha, N., Rao, G. N., Gururaj, G., Varghese, M., & Benegal, V.NMHS India National Collaborator Group. (2022). Epidemiology of common mental disorders: Results from "National Mental Health Survey" of India, 2016. *Indian Journal of Psychiatry*, *64*(1), 13–19. DOI: 10.4103/indianjpsychiatry.indianjpsychiatry_865_21 PMID: 35400745

Jha, A. P., Stanley, E. A., Kiyonaga, A., Wong, L., & Gelfand, L. (2010). Examining the protective effects of mindfulness training on working memory capacity and affective experience. *Emotion (Washington, D.C.)*, *10*(1), 54–64. DOI: 10.1037/a0018438 PMID: 20141302

Johansson, R., Björklund, M., Hornborg, C., Karlsson, S., Hesser, H., Ljótsson, B., Rousseau, A., Frederick, R. J., & Andersson, G. (2013). Affect-focused psychodynamic psychotherapy for depression and anxiety through the Internet: A randomized controlled trial. *PeerJ*, *1*, e102. DOI: 10.7717/peerj.102 PMID: 23862104

Johnson, L. M., West, C., & Lange, B. (2021). Trauma-informed cognitive-behavioral therapy: Clinical outcomes in adult survivors of abuse. *Psychotherapy Research*, *31*(8), 1094–1108. DOI: 10.1080/10503307.2020.1865078

Jones, J., & Passey, J. (2004). Family adaptation, coping and resources: Parents of children with developmental disabilities and behavior problems. *Journal on Developmental Disabilities*, *11*(1), 31–46.

Joormann, J., & Stanton, C. H. (2016). Examining emotion regulation in depression: A review and future directions. *Behaviour Research and Therapy*, *86*, 35–49. DOI: 10.1016/j.brat.2016.07.007 PMID: 27492851

Juster, R.-P., & Misiak, B. (2023). Advancing the allostatic load model: From theory to therapy. *Psychoneuroendocrinology*, *154*, 106289. DOI: 10.1016/j.psyneuen.2023.106289 PMID: 37202225

Kagan, J. (1991). Etiologies of adolescents at risk. *The Journal of Adolescent Health*, *12*(1), 591–596. DOI: 10.1016/1054-139X(91)90006-J

Kapoor, A. R., Patel, A., & Nair, V. P. (2024). Exploring the neurobiological mechanisms mediating the impact of air pollution on cognitive and emotional health in urban residents of New Delhi. *Studies in Psychological Science*, *2*(2), 21–31. DOI: 10.56397/SPS.2024.06.03

Kashdan, T. B., & Rottenberg, J. (2010). Psychological flexibility as a fundamental aspect of health. *Clinical Psychology Review*, *30*(7), 865–878. DOI: 10.1016/j.cpr.2010.03.001 PMID: 21151705

Katsarou, D., Kougioumtzis, G., Efthymiou, E., Sofologi, M., & Mantsos, E. (2025). School-based mental health interventions for adolescents: supporting typically developing students and students with neurodevelopmental disorders. *Review of Clinical Pharmacology and Pharmacokinetics, International Edition*, 39(1), 11-22.

Katsarou, D., Efthymiou, E., Kougioumtzis, G., Sofologi, M., & Theodoratou, M. (2024). Identifying Language Development in Children with ADHD: Differential Challenges, Interventions, and Collaborative Strategies. *Children (Basel, Switzerland)*, *11*(7), 841–850. DOI: 10.3390/children11070841 PMID: 39062289

Katsarou, D., Mantsos, E., Papadopoulou, S., Sofologi, M., Efthymiou, E., Vasileiou, I., Megari, K., Theodoratou, M., & Kougioumtzis, G. (2025). Exploring AI technology in grammar performance testing for children with learning disabilities. *Education Sciences*, *15*(3), 351–365. DOI: 10.3390/educsci15030351

Kawachi, I., & Berkman, L. F. (2001). Social Ties and Psychological health. *Journal of Urban Health*, *78*(3), 458–467. DOI: 10.1093/jurban/78.3.458

Kay, S. R., Fiszbein, A., & Opler, L. A. (1987). The positive and negative syndrome scale (PANSS) for schizophrenia. *Schizophrenia Bulletin*, *13*(2), 261–276. DOI: 10.1093/schbul/13.2.261 PMID: 3616518

Kemmeren, L. L., van Schaik, A., Smit, J. H., Ruwaard, J., Rocha, A., Henriques, M., Ebert, D. D., Titzler, I., Hazo, J.-B., Dorsey, M., Zukowska, K., & Riper, H. (2019). Unraveling the black box: Exploring usage patterns of a blended treatment for depression in a multicenter study. *JMIR Mental Health*, *6*(7), e12707. DOI: 10.2196/12707 PMID: 31344670

Kendler, K. S., Myers, J. M., Maes, H. H., & Keyes, C. L. M. (2011). The relationship between the genetic and environmental influences on common internalizing psychiatric disorders and mental well-being. *Behavior Genetics*, *41*(5), 641–650. DOI: 10.1007/s10519-011-9466-1

Kern, M. L.. (2014). A holistic approach to measuring well-being: The PERMA-Profiler. *The Journal of Positive Psychology*, *10*(3), 226–236. PMID: 25745508

Khalifeh, H., Dean, K., & Osborn, D. (2022). Reducing coercion through trauma-informed psychiatric care: A multicenter study. *European Psychiatry : the Journal of the Association of European Psychiatrists, 65*(1), e21. DOI: 10.1192/j.eurpsy.2022.21 PMID: 35189997

Kim, J. J., Payne, E. S., & Tracy, E. L. (2022). Indirect effects of forgiveness on psychological health through anger and hope: A parallel mediation analysis. *Journal of Religion and Health, 61*(5), 3729–3746. DOI: 10.1007/s10943-022-01518-4

Kim, J., & Kim, H. (2017). Demographic and environmental factors associated with mental health: A cross-sectional study. *International Journal of Environmental Research and Public Health, 14*(4), 1–12. DOI: 10.3390/ijerph14040431

Kim, J., Lee, H., & Park, S. (2023). Trauma-informed approaches in school-based mental health programs: A meta-analysis. *School Psychology International, 44*(3), 235–256. DOI: 10.1177/01430343221149983

Knight, C. (2021). Trauma-informed practice and care: Implications for social work. *Clinical Social Work Journal, 49*(4), 433–445. DOI: 10.1007/s10615-021-00792-z

Knott, V., Habota, T., & Mallan, K. (2020). Attitudes of Australian psychologists towards the delivery of therapy via video conferencing technology. *Australian Psychologist, 55*(6), 606–617. Advance online publication. DOI: 10.1111/ap.12464

Kok, B. E., & Fredrickson, B. L. (2010). Upward spirals of the heart: Vagal tone, positive emotions, and upward spirals of health. *Biological Psychology, 84*(3), 432–436. DOI: 10.1016/j.biopsycho.2010.09.005 PMID: 20851735

Kozlowska, K., Walker, P., McLean, L., & Carrive, P. (2015). Fear and the Defense Cascade: Clinical Implications and Management. *Harvard Review of Psychiatry, 23*(4), 263–287. DOI: 10.1097/HRP.0000000000000065 PMID: 26062169

Kravchuk, S. (2021). The relationship between psychological resilience and tendency to forgiveness. *Academic Journal of Interdisciplinary Studies, 10*(1), 11–21. DOI: 10.36941/ajis-2021-0002

Kumari, S., Malik, M., Florival, C., Manalai, P., & Sonje, S. (2018). An Assessment of Five (PANSS, SAPS, SANS, NSA-16, CGI-SCH) commonly used Symptoms Rating Scales in Schizophrenia and Comparison to Newer Scales (CAINS, BNSS). *Journal of Addiction Research & Therapy, 8*(3), 1–14. DOI: 10.4172/2155-6105.1000324 PMID: 29430333

Kuo, B. C. H. (2013). Collectivism and coping: Current theories, evidence, and measurements of collective coping. *International Journal of Psychology, 48*(3), 374–388. DOI: 10.1080/00207594.2011.640681 PMID: 22335198

Lafarge, C., Mitchell, K., & Fox, P. (2013). Women's experiences of coping with pregnancy termination for fetal abnormality. *Qualitative Health Research, 23*(7), 924–936. DOI: 10.1177/1049732313484198 PMID: 23558712

Laishram, J., Fernandez, S., Devi, P. A., Bhowmick, M. R., Heigrujam, R., & Devi, H. S. (2025). Sleep quality and mental health among medical students in Imphal, Manipur: A cross-sectional study. *Journal of Family Medicine and Primary Care, 14*(1), 276–282. DOI: 10.4103/jfmpc.jfmpc_1160_24 PMID: 39989537

Lakhan, S. E., & Vieira, K. F. (2008). Nutritional therapies for mental disorders. *Nutrition Journal, 7*(2), 1–11. DOI: 10.1186/1475-2891-7-2

Lakovschek, I. C., Streubel, B., & Ulm, B. (2011). Natural outcome of trisomy 13, trisomy 18, and triploidy after prenatal diagnosis. *American Journal of Medical Genetics. Part A, 155*(11), 2616–2626. DOI: 10.1002/ajmg.a.34284 PMID: 21990236

Lal, S., & Adair, C. (2014). E-Mental health: A rapid review of the literature. *Psychiatric Services (Washington, D.C.), 65*(1), 24–32. DOI: 10.1176/appi.ps.201300009 PMID: 24081188

LaMonica, H., Davenport, T., Braunstein, K., Ottavio, A., Piper, S., Martin, C., Hickie, I. B., & Cross, S. (2019). Technology-enabled person-centered mental health services reform: Strategy for implementation science. *JMIR Mental Health, 6*(9), e14719. DOI: 10.2196/14719 PMID: 31538938

Lazarus, R. S., & Folkman, S. (1984). *Stress, appraisal, and coping*. Springer. https://link.springer.com/rwe/10.1007/978-1-4419-1005-9_215

Lazarus, R. S., & Folkman, S. (1984). *Stress, appraisal, and coping*. Springer.

Lazarus, R. S., & Folkman, S. (1984). *Stress, Appraisal, and Coping*. Springer.

Lee, M. S., Shin, J. S., Lee, J., Lee, Y. J., Kim, M. R., Park, K. B., Shin, D., Cho, J. H., & Ha, I. H. (2015). The association between mental health, chronic disease and sleep duration in Koreans: A cross-sectional study. *BMC Public Health, 15*(1), 1–13. DOI: 10.1186/s12889-015-2542-3

Lee, Y. R., & Enright, R. D. (2009). Fathers' forgiveness as a moderator between perceived unfair treatment by a family of origin member and anger with own children. *The Family Journal (Alexandria, Va.), 17*(1), 22–31. DOI: 10.1177/1066480708328474

Leitch, L. (2022). The evolution of trauma-informed care: Moving toward relational safety. *Frontiers in Psychology, 13*, 853730. DOI: 10.3389/fpsyg.2022.853730

Lenin, B. P. (in progress). *Therapist experiences in counselling sexually abused children* (Unpublished doctoral thesis). Martin Luther Christian University.

Lickenbrock, D. M., Ekas, N. V., & Whitman, T. L. (2011). Feeling good, feeling bad: Influences of maternal perceptions of the child and child behavior problems on maternal affect in families of children with autism spectrum disorders. *Journal of Autism and Developmental Disorders, 41*(7), 848–858. DOI: 10.1007/s10803-010-1105-9 PMID: 20839039

Lijo, K. J. (2018). Forgiveness: Definitions, perspectives, contexts and correlates. *Journal of Psychology & Psychotherapy, 8*(3), 342–350. DOI: 10.4172/2161-0487.1000342

Lim, S. Y., Kim, E. J., Kim, A., Lee, H. J., Choi, H. J., & Yang, S. J. (2016). Nutritional factors affecting mental health. *Clinical Nutrition Research, 5*(3), 1–15. DOI: 10.7762/cnr.2016.5.3.143

Linley, P. A., Joseph, S., & Loumidis, K. (2005). Positive and negative changes following vicarious trauma: Associations with sense of coherence. *Journal of Traumatic Stress, 18*(6), 751–758. DOI: 10.1002/jts.20083 PMID: 16382431

Lloyd, T., & Hastings, R. P. (2008). Psychological variables as correlates of adjustment in mothers of children with intellectual disabilities: Cross-sectional and longitudinal relationships. *Journal of Intellectual Disability Research, 52*(1), 37–48. DOI: 10.1111/j.1365-2788.2007.00974.x PMID: 18173571

Lotzin, A., Buth, S., & Sehner, S.. (2022). A systematic review and meta-analysis on the effects of trauma-informed care. *European Journal of Psychotraumatology, 13*(2), 2067891. DOI: 10.1080/20008198.2022.2067891 PMID: 38872598

Loveland, J. M., Lounsbury, J. W., Welsh, D., & Buboltz, W. C. (2007). The validity of physical aggression in predicting adolescent academic performance. *The British Journal of Educational Psychology, 77*(1), 167–176. DOI: 10.1348/000709905X79563

Lugli, L., Rossi, C., Berardi, A., Pugliese, M., Ceccarelli, P., Sileo, G., Chiossi, G., Contu, G., Calabrese, O., Marca, A., & Bertucci, E. (2024). Prenatal multidisciplinary counseling for fetal congenital anomalies: A narrative review. *International Journal of Gynaecology and Obstetrics: the Official Organ of the International Federation of Gynaecology and Obstetrics, 160*(1), 45–55. DOI: 10.1002/ijgo.16068 PMID: 39660910

Maguire, M., Light, A., Kuppermann, M., Dalton, V. K., Steinauer, J. E., & Kerns, J. L. (2015). Grief after second-trimester termination for fetal anomaly: A qualitative study. *Contraception, 91*(3), 234–239. DOI: 10.1016/j.contraception.2014.11.015 PMID: 25499590

Makwana, N. (2019). Disaster and its impact on mental health: A narrative review. *Journal of Family Medicine and Primary Care*, *8*(10), 1–9. DOI: 10.4103/jfmpc.jfmpc_893_19

Manwell, L. A., Barbic, S. P., Roberts, K., Durisko, Z., Lee, C., Ware, E., & McKenzie, K. (2015). What is mental health? Evidence towards a new definition from a mixed methods multidisciplinary international survey. *BMJ Open*, *5*(6), 1–12. DOI: 10.1136/bmjopen-2014-007079 PMID: 26038353

Martin, L., Gitsels-van der Wal, J. T., Pereboom, M. T., Spelten, E. R., Hutton, E. K., & van Dulmen, S. (2016). Clients' psychosocial communication and midwives' verbal and nonverbal communication during prenatal counseling for anomaly screening. *Patient Education and Counseling*, *99*(1), 85–91. DOI: 10.1016/j.pec.2015.07.020 PMID: 26298217

Maslow, A. H. (1958). A dynamic theory of human motivation. In Stacey, C. L., & DeMartino, M. (Eds.), *Understanding human motivation* (pp. 26–47). Howard Allen Publishers., DOI: 10.1037/11305-004

Masten, A. S. (2014). *Ordinary magic: Resilience in development*. Guilford Press.

Masten, A. S. (2018). Resilience theory and research on children and families: Past, present, and promise. *Journal of Family Theory & Review*, *10*(1), 12–31. DOI: 10.1111/jftr.12255

McCabe, H. (2007). Parent advocacy in the face of adversity: Autism and families in the People's Republic of China. *Focus on Autism and Other Developmental Disabilities*, *22*(1), 39–50. DOI: 10.1177/10883576070220010501

McConnell, D., & Savage, A. (2015). Stress and resilience among families caring for children with intellectual disability: Expanding the research agenda. *Current Developmental Disorders Reports*, *2*(2), 100–109. DOI: 10.1007/s40474-015-0040-z

McCoyd, J. L. M. (2007). Pregnancy interrupted: Loss of a desired pregnancy after diagnosis of fetal anomaly. *Health Care for Women International*, *28*(1), 3–18. DOI: 10.1080/01674820601096153 PMID: 17148106

McCullough, M. (2001). Forgiveness: Who does it and how do they do it? *Current Directions in Psychological Science*, *10*(6), 194–197. 194-197.doi.org/10.1111/1467-8721.00147. DOI: 10.1111/1467-8721.00147

McCullough, M. (2008). *Beyond revenge: The evolution of the forgiveness instinct*. John Wiley & Sons.

McCullough, M. E. (2000). Forgiveness as human strength: Theory, measurement, and links to well-being. *Journal of Social and Clinical Psychology*, *19*(1), 43–55. DOI: 10.1521/jscp.2000.19.1.43

McEwen, B. S. (2012). Brain on stress: How the social environment gets under the skin. *Proceedings of the National Academy of Sciences of the United States of America*, *109*(supplement_2), 17180–17185. DOI: 10.1073/pnas.1121254109 PMID: 23045648

McEwen, B. S. (2021). Neurobiology of stress and resilience: Implications for trauma recovery. *Nature Reviews. Neuroscience*, *22*(7), 420–433. DOI: 10.1038/s41583-021-00495-9

McKenzie, K., Murray, G., Murray, A., Delahunty, L., Hutton, L., Murray, K., & O'Hare, A. (2018). Child and adolescent intellectual disability screening questionnaire to identify children with intellectual disability. *Developmental Medicine and Child Neurology*, *61*(4), 444–450. DOI: 10.1111/dmcn.13998 PMID: 30146754

Mcloughlin, C. S., Kubick, R. J., & Lewis, M. (2002). Best practices in promoting safe schools. In Thomas, A., & Grimes, J. (Eds.), *Best Practices in School Psychology IV* (pp. 1181–1194). NASP Publications.

McRae, K., & Gross, J. J. (2020). Emotion regulation. *Emotion (Washington, D.C.)*, *20*(1), 1–9. DOI: 10.1037/emo0000703 PMID: 31961170

Menschner, C., & Maul, A. (2023). Building a trauma-informed workforce: Evaluation of professional training outcomes. *The Journal of Behavioral Health Services & Research*, *50*(2), 210–225. DOI: 10.1007/s11414-022-09821-0

Mental Health Foundation (MHF). (2008). What works for you? London. [online]. https://www.mentalhealth.org.uk/sites/default/files/2022-09/MHF-What-Works-For-You-study.pdf

Merritt, T. A., Catlin, A., Wool, C., Peverini, R., Goldstein, M., & Oshiro, B. (2012). Trisomy 18 and trisomy 13: Treatment and management decisions. *NeoReviews*, *13*(1), e40–e48. DOI: 10.1542/neo.13-1-e40

Miron, A.. (2023). Theoretical and methodological critiques of positive psychology: Issues with measurement and self-report bias. *The Journal of Positive Psychology*, *18*(4), 501–518.

Mohd, T. A. M. T., Yunus, R. M., Hairi, F., Hairi, N. N., & Choo, W. Y. (2019). Social support and depression among community dwelling older adults in Asia: A systematic review. *BMJ Open*, *9*(7), 1–10. DOI: 10.1136/bmjopen-2018-026667 PMID: 31320348

Morgan, N., & Mall, S. (2019). Pathways between urbanization and harmful substance use. *Current Opinion in Psychiatry*, *32*(3), 218–223. DOI: 10.1097/YCO.0000000000000488 PMID: 30695003

Myers, C. A. (2020). Food insecurity and psychological distress: A review of the recent literature. *Current Nutrition Reports*, *9*(2), 107–118. DOI: 10.1007/s13668-020-00309-1

National Mental Health (NMH). (2010). *National survey confirms that youth are disproportionately affected by mental disorders*. [online]. https://www.nimh.nih.gov/health/statistics/mental-illness

Negi, S., Singh, R., & Singh, A. K. (2025). Natural disaster: prevalence of post - traumatic stress and psychological outcome of Survivors in Joshimath, Uttarakhand, India. In Kurebwa, J., & Makwerere, D. (Eds.), *Managing the Health Risks of Climate Change* (pp. 107–134). IGI Global Scientific Publishing., DOI: 10.4018/979-8-3693-4183-4.ch005

Ngan, O. M. Y., Yi, H., Bryant, L., Sahota, D. S., Chan, O. Y. M., & Ahmed, S. (2020). Parental expectations of raising a child with disability in decision-making for prenatal testing and termination of pregnancy: A mixed methods study. *Patient Education and Counseling*, *103*(11), 2373–2383. DOI: 10.1016/j.pec.2020.05.010 PMID: 32507714

Niedhammer, I., Bertrais, S., & Witt, K. (2021). Psychosocial work exposures and health outcomes: A meta-review of 72 literature reviews with meta-analysis. *Scandinavian Journal of Work, Environment & Health*, *47*(7), 489–508. DOI: 10.5271/sjweh.3968 PMID: 34042163

Ojha, R., & Syed, S. (2020). Challenges faced by mental health providers and patients during the coronavirus 2019 pandemic due to technological barriers. *Internet Interventions : the Application of Information Technology in Mental and Behavioural Health*, *21*, 100330. DOI: 10.1016/j.invent.2020.100330 PMID: 32542180

Olshansky, S. (1962). Chronic sorrow: A response to having a mentally defective child. *Social Casework*, *43*(4), 190–193. DOI: 10.1177/104438946204300404

Orman, J., & O'Dea, B. (2018). e-Therapy in primary care mental health. *Australian Journal of General Practice*, *47*(4), 168–172. DOI: 10.31128/AJGP-11-17-4410 PMID: 29621855

Padhy, S., Sarkar, S., Panigrahi, M., & Paul, S. (2015). Psychological health effects of climate change. *Indian Journal of Occupational and Environmental Medicine*, *19*(1), 3–13. DOI: 10.4103/0019-5278.156997

Palmer, C. A., & Alfano, C. A. (2017). Sleep and emotion regulation: An organizing, integrative review. *Sleep Medicine Reviews, 31*, 6–16. DOI: 10.1016/j.smrv.2015.12.006 PMID: 26899742

Pandey, R., Tiwari, G. K., Pandey, R., Mandal, S. P., Mudgal, S., Parihar, P., & Shukla, M. (2020). The relationship between self-esteem and self-forgiveness: *Understanding the mediating role of positive and negative self-compassion.* DOI: 10.22541/au.158981530.01103201

Parihar, P., Tiwari, G. K., & Rai, P. K. (2020). Understanding the relationship between self-compassion and interdependent happiness of the married Hindu couples. *Polish Psychological Bulletin, 51*(4), 260–272. DOI: 10.24425/ppb.2020.135458

Park, C. L. (2010). Making sense of the meaning literature: An integrative review of meaning making and its effects on adjustment to stressful life events. *Psychological Bulletin, 136*(2), 257–301. DOI: 10.1037/a0018301 PMID: 20192563

Park, M., Kim, D., Lee, U., Na, E., & Jeon, H. (2019). A literature overview of virtual reality (VR) in treatment of psychiatric disorders: Recent advances and limitations. *Frontiers in Psychiatry, 10*, 505. Advance online publication. DOI: 10.3389/fpsyt.2019.00505 PMID: 31379623

Pearlman, L. A., & Saakvitne, K. W. (1995). *Trauma and the therapist: Countertransference and vicarious traumatization in psychotherapy with incest survivors.* W. W. Norton. https://wwnorton.com/books/Trauma-and-the-Therapist/

Peen, J., Schoevers, R. A., Beekman, A. T., & Dekker, J. (2009). The current status of urban-rural differences in psychiatric disorders. *Acta Psychiatrica Scandinavica, 121*(2), 84–93. DOI: 10.1111/j.1600-0447.2009.01438.x PMID: 19624573

Peiro, P., et al. (2023). Defining positive health as a "reserve in capacities." *European Journal of Public Health, 33*(4), ckae144.834.

Penberthy, J. K., Cox, D., Breton, M., Robeva, R., Kalbfleisch, M. L., Loboschefski, T., & Kovatchev, B. (2005). Calibration of ADHD Assessments across studies: A meta-analysis tool. *Applied Psychophysiology and Biofeedback, 30*(1), 31–51. DOI: 10.1007/s10484-005-2172-0 PMID: 15889584

Pinto, R. Q., Soares, I., Carvalho-Correia, E., & Mesquita, A. R. (2015). Gene–environment interactions in psychopathology throughout early childhood. *Psychiatric Genetics, 25*(6), 223–233. DOI: 10.1097/YPG.0000000000000106 PMID: 26313931

Porges, S. W. (2022). Polyvagal theory and the biology of safety. *Frontiers in Integrative Neuroscience, 16*, 871227. DOI: 10.3389/fnint.2022.871227 PMID: 35645742

Prasko, J., Ociskova, M., Vanek, J., Burkauskas, J., Slepecky, M., Bite, I., Krone, I., Sollar, T., & Juskiene, A. (2022). Managing transference and countertransference in cognitive behavioral supervision: Theoretical framework and clinical application. *Psychology Research and Behavior Management, 15*, 2129–2155. DOI: 10.2147/PRBM.S369294 PMID: 35990755

Raine, A., Ling, S., Streicher, W., & Liu, J. (2022). The conduct and oppositional defiant disorder scales (CODDS) for disruptive behaviour disorders. *Psychiatry Research, 316*(1), 1–15. DOI: 10.1016/j.psychres.2022.114744 PMID: 35961152

Raman, M. S., Koppa, K. B., Chithambar Gupta, V., Bhat, V. A., & Guru Basava Aradhya, S. (2025). Digital Transformation and Sustainability Artificial Intelligence and Sustainable Development. In Yıldırım, D., Yıldırım, S., & Kandpal, V. (Eds.), *Effects of Digitalization and Circular Economy on Sustainable Policy and Climate Change Prevention* (pp. 69–96). IGI Global Scientific Publishing., DOI: 10.4018/979-8-3693-9909-5.ch003

Rao, T. S. (2008). Understanding nutrition, depression and mental illnesses. *Indian Journal of Psychiatry, 50*(2), 77–88. DOI: 10.4103/0019-5545.42391

Rashid, T., & Ostermann, R. F. (2010). Strength-based assessment in clinical practice. *Journal of Clinical Psychology, 66*(6), 488–498. PMID: 19294732

Rauf, T., & Freese, J. (2024). Genetic influences on depression and selection into adverse life experiences. *Social Science & Medicine, 344*(1), 1–11. DOI: 10.1016/j.socscimed.2024.116633 PMID: 38324978

Reddy, V. (2019). Mental health issues and challenges in India: A review. [IJSSME]. *International Journal of Social Sciences Management and Entrepreneurship, 3*(2), 1–11.

Reddy, V. (2019). Psychological health issues and challenges in India: A review. [IJSSME]. *International Journal of Social Sciences Management and Entrepreneurship, 3*(2), 1–11.

Reed, G., & Enright, R. D. (2006). The effects of forgiveness therapy on depression anxiety, and post-traumatic stress for women after spousal emotional abuse. *Journal of Consulting and Clinical Psychology, 74*(5), 920–929. DOI: 10.1037/0022-006X.74.5.920

Reynolds, J., Griffiths, K., Cunningham, J., Bennett, K., & Bennett, A. (2015). Clinical practice models for the use of E-Mental health resources in primary health care by health professionals and peer workers: A conceptual framework. *JMIR Mental Health, 2*(1), e6. DOI: 10.2196/mental.4200 PMID: 26543912

Richardson, G. E. (2002). The metatheory of resilience and resiliency. *Journal of Clinical Psychology*, *58*(3), 307–321. DOI: 10.1002/jclp.10020 PMID: 11836712

Ritchie, Z., Teachman, G., Shaul, R. Z., & Smith, M. J. (2024). "She was finally mine": The moral experience of families in the context of trisomy 13 and 18–a scoping review with thematic analysis. *BMC Medical Ethics*, *25*(1), 94. DOI: 10.1186/s12910-023-00994-x PMID: 38431625

Rose, M., & Devine, J. (2014). Assessment of patient-reported symptoms of anxiety. *Dialogues in Clinical Neuroscience*, *16*(2), 197–211. DOI: 10.31887/DCNS.2014.16.2/mrose PMID: 25152658

Rose, S., McCusker, P., Mitchell, M., Roesch-Marsh, A., Jian, M., & Petrova, L. (2025). Self-care in social work: An imperative or beyond reach? *British Journal of Social Work*, *55*(3), 1455–1473. DOI: 10.1093/bjsw/bcae204

Rutter, M. (2012). Resilience as a dynamic concept. *Development and Psychopathology*, *24*(2), 335–344. DOI: 10.1017/S0954579412000028 PMID: 22559117

Ryff, C. D. (1989). Happiness is everything, or is it? Explorations on the meaning of psychological well-being. *Journal of Personality and Social Psychology*, *57*(6), 1069–1081. DOI: 10.1037/0022-3514.57.6.1069

SAMHSA. (2014). *SAMHSA's concept of trauma and guidance for a trauma-informed approach*. U.S. Department of Health and Human Services.

Sanjari, M., Bahramnezhad, F., Fomani, F. K., Shoghi, M., & Cheraghi, M. A. (2014). Ethical challenges of researchers in qualitative studies: The necessity to develop a specific guideline. *Journal of Medical Ethics and History of Medicine*, *7*, 14. PMID: 25512833

Sappok, T., Heinrich, M., & Underwood, L. (2015). Screening tools for autism spectrum disorders. *Advances in Autism*, *1*(1), 12–29. DOI: 10.1108/AIA-03-2015-0001

Schotanus-Dijkstra, M.. (2024). Efficacy of strengths-based positive psychology interventions in enhancing well-being. *Applied Psychology. Health and Well-Being*.

Schwarz, L. E., Corrigan, F. M., & Hull, A. M. (2021). Trauma-focused psychotherapies: Mechanisms of change and outcome evidence. *Journal of Contemporary Psychotherapy*, *51*(2), 119–130. DOI: 10.1007/s10879-020-09481-6

Scott, M., Watermeyer, J., & Wessels, T.-M. (2024). A balancing act: Non-directive communication, risk perceptions, and meeting patient needs in genetic counseling: A South African case study. *Journal of Genetic Counseling*, *33*(2), 1741–1752. DOI: 10.1002/jgc4.1741 PMID: 37323090

Segerstrom, S. C., & Miller, G. E. (2004). Psychological Stress and the Human Immune System: A Meta-Analytic Study of 30 Years of Inquiry. *Psychological Bulletin, 130*(4), 601–630. DOI: 10.1037/0033-2909.130.4.601 PMID: 15250815

Seligman, M. E. P. (2011). *Flourish: A visionary new understanding of happiness and well-being*. Free Press.

Shapiro, S. L., Brown, K. W., & Biegel, G. M. (2007). Teaching self-care to caregivers: Effects of mindfulness-based stress reduction on mental health of therapists in training. *Training and Education in Professional Psychology, 1*(2), 105–115. https://psycnet.apa.org/doi/10.1037/1931-3918.1.2.105. DOI: 10.1037/1931-3918.1.2.105

Sheppes, G., Scheibe, S., Suri, G., Radu, P., Blechert, J., & Gross, J. J. (2014). Emotion regulation choice: A conceptual framework and supporting evidence. *Journal of Experimental Psychology. General, 143*(1), 163–181. DOI: 10.1037/a0030831 PMID: 23163767

Sheppes, G., Suri, G., & Gross, J. J. (2015). Emotion Regulation and Psychopathology. *Annual Review of Clinical Psychology, 11*(1), 379–405. DOI: 10.1146/annurev-clinpsy-032814-112739 PMID: 25581242

Shin, J. Y., Nhan, N. V., Crittenden, K. S., Hong, H. T., Flory, M., & Ladinsky, J. (2006). Parenting stress of mothers and fathers of young children with cognitive delays in Vietnam. *Journal of Intellectual Disability Research, 50*(10), 748–760. DOI: 10.1111/j.1365-2788.2006.00840.x PMID: 16961704

Singha, R. (2024b). Fostering mindfulness and compassion: Strategies, benefits, and challenges. In S. Watson (Ed.), *Applications of service learning in higher education* (pp. 45–64). IGI Global Scientific Publishing. https://doi.org/DOI: 10.4018/979-8-3693-2133-1.ch00

Singh, A., Singh, R., & Singh, A. K. (2025). A review-based theoretical analysis on somatization of psychological symptoms and physical manifestation of trauma in youths. In Sofologi, M., Katsarou, D., & Efthymiou, E. (Eds.), *Exploring Cognitive and Psychosocial Dynamics Across Childhood and Adolescence* (pp. 273–294). IGI Global., DOI: 10.4018/979-8-3693-4022-6.ch014

Singha, R. (2024). Mindfulness and social cognitive processing. In Reddy, K. (Ed.), *Principles and clinical interventions in social cognition* (pp. 104–124). IGI Global Scientific Publishing., DOI: 10.4018/979-8-3693-1265-0.ch007

Singha, R. (2025). Empowering students through mindfulness and meditation practices. In Gonçalves, S. (Ed.), *Nurturing student well-being in the modern world* (pp. 141–170). IGI Global Scientific Publishing., DOI: 10.4018/979-8-3693-1455-5.ch006

Singha, R. (2026). Resilience in education: Addressing addiction and cultivating mindfulness for well-being. In Collister, R. (Ed.), *Facing precarity in adult, community, and vocational education: Role of meaningful work* (pp. 253–278). IGI Global Scientific Publishing., DOI: 10.4018/979-8-3693-1099-1.ch011

Singha, R., & Kanna, Y. S. (2022). Women's empowerment, mindfulness, and role of women in eradicating alcohol and drug addiction from Indian society. *Journal of International Women's Studies*, *24*(7), 7. https://vc.bridgew.edu/jiws/vol24/iss7/7

Singha, R., & Singha, S. (2024). Mindfulness-Based Interventions: Applications in Western and Indian Psychology. In Sathiyaseelan, A., & Balasundaram, S. (Eds.), *Global Applications of Indian Psychology: Therapeutic and Strategic Models* (pp. 192–212). IGI Global Scientific Publishing., DOI: 10.4018/978-1-6684-9778-4.ch011

Singha, R., & Singha, S. (2024b). Mindfulness in the Age of Populism. In Chennattuserry, J. C., Deshpande, M., & Hong, P. (Eds.), *Encyclopedia of New Populism and Responses in the 21st Century*. Springer., DOI: 10.1007/978-981-99-7802-1_437

Singha, R., & Singha, S. (2024c). Understanding neurodiversity and mindfulness: A holistic approach to addiction in professional preparation programs. In Jamanis, S., & Vogler-Elias, D. (Eds.), *Autism, neurodiversity, and equity in professional preparation programs* (pp. 255–275). IGI Global Scientific Publishing., DOI: 10.4018/979-8-3693-0163-0.ch012

Singh, K., Junnarkar, M., & Jain, A. (2017). Factors affecting mental health of north Indian adolescents. *Psychological Studies*, *62*(2), 168–177. DOI: 10.1007/s12646-017-0398-6

Singh, R., Thapliyal, C., & Chowdhury, K. (2021). Emotion regulation, parenting style, and satisfaction with life in adult. *Webology*, *1*(1), 1441–1448. DOI: 10.29121/WEB/V18I1/25

Siste, K., Hanafi, E., Sen, L. T., Murtani, B. J., Christian, H., Limawan, A. P., Siswidiani, L. P., & Adrian, N. (2021). Implications of COVID-19 and lockdown on internet addiction among adolescents: Data from a developing country. *Frontiers in Psychiatry*, *12*(1), 1–13. DOI: 10.3389/fpsyt.2021.665675

Sivanand, R., Selvakumar, P., & Sharma, N. (2025). Nanotechnology Applications in Cancer Drug Delivery Systems: A Review. *Journal of Environmental Nanotechnology*, *14*(2), 458–470. DOI: 10.13074/jent.2025.06.2511221

Skinner, D., Correa, V., Skinner, M., & Bailey, D. (2001). Role of religion in the lives of Latino families of young children with developmental delays. *American Journal of Mental Retardation*, *106*(4), 297–313. DOI: 10.1352/0895-8017(2001)106<0297:RORITL>2.0.CO;2 PMID: 11414871

Skirton, H., & Barr, O. (2007). Influences on uptake of antenatal screening for down syndrome: A review of the literature. *Evidence-Based Midwifery*, *5*(1), 4–10.

Smith, L. E., Seltzer, M. M., Tager-Flusberg, H., Greenberg, J. S., & Carter, A. S. (2013). A comparative analysis of well-being and coping among mothers of children with autism spectrum disorder, Down syndrome, and fragile X syndrome. *American Journal on Intellectual and Developmental Disabilities*, *118*(4), 273–292.

Snyder, C. R. (2002). Hope theory: Rainbows in the mind. *Psychological Inquiry*, *13*(4), 249–275. DOI: 10.1207/S15327965PLI1304_01

Solomon, M., Pistrang, N., & Barker, C. (2001). The benefits of mutual support groups for parents of children with disabilities. *American Journal of Community Psychology*, *29*(1), 113–132. DOI: 10.1023/A:1005253514140 PMID: 11439824

Song, H. T., Sun, X. Y., Yang, T. S., Zhang, L. Y., Yang, J. L., & Bai, J. (2015). Effects of sleep deprivation on serum cortisol level and mental health in servicemen. *International Journal of Psychophysiology*, *96*(3), 169–175. DOI: 10.1016/j.ijpsycho.2015.04.008 PMID: 25913092

Soto-Icaza, P., Aboitiz, F., & Billeke, P. (2015). Development of social skills in children: Neural and behavioral evidence for the elaboration of cognitive models. *Frontiers in Neuroscience*, *9*(1), 1–12. DOI: 10.3389/fnins.2015.00333 PMID: 26483621

Souka, A. P., Michalitsi, V. D., Skentou, H., Euripioti, H., Papadopoulos, G. K., Kassanos, D., Messinis, I. E., & Salamalekis, E. E. (2010). Attitudes of pregnant women regarding termination of pregnancy for fetal abnormality. *Prenatal Diagnosis*, *30*(10), 977–980. DOI: 10.1002/pd.2600 PMID: 20730784

Southwick, S. M., & Charney, D. S. (2012). The Science of Resilience: Implications for the Prevention and Treatment of Depression. *Science*, *338*(6103), 79–82. DOI: 10.1126/science.1222942 PMID: 23042887

Spahn, K. C.. (2022). Guidelines for the cultural adaptation of positive psychology interventions (PPIs) when working with non-Western populations. *Frontiers in Psychology*, *13*, 809362.

Statham, H. (2002). Prenatal diagnosis of fetal abnormality: The decision to terminate the pregnancy and the psychological consequences. *Fetal and Maternal Medicine Review*, *13*(4), 213–247. DOI: 10.1017/S0965539502000414

Steger, M. F. (2012). Making meaning in life. *Psychological Inquiry*, *23*(4), 381–385. DOI: 10.1080/1047840X.2012.720832

Stoewen, D. L. (2022). Nature, nurture, and mental health Part 1: The influence of genetics, psychology, and biology. *The Canadian Veterinary Journal = La Revue Vétérinaire Canadienne*, *63*(4), 427–430. PMID: 35368400

Sundquist, K., Johansson, L., DeMarinis, V., Johansson, S., & Sundquist, J. (2005). Posttraumatic stress disorder and psychiatric co-morbidity: Symptoms in a random sample of female Bosnian refugees. *European Psychiatry : the Journal of the Association of European Psychiatrists*, *20*(2), 158–164. DOI: 10.1016/j.eurpsy.2004.12.001 PMID: 15797701

Sutton, P. M. (2013). The Enright process model of psychological forgiveness.

Sweeney, A., Clement, S., Filson, B., & Kennedy, A. (2018). Trauma-informed mental healthcare in the UK: What is it and how can we further its development? *Mental Health Review (Brighton)*, *23*(3), 131–144. DOI: 10.1108/MHRJ-01-2018-0008

Taddi, V. V., Kohli, R. K., & Puri, P. (2024). Perception, use of social media, and its impact on the mental health of Indian adolescents: A qualitative study. *World Journal of Clinical Pediatrics*, *13*(3), 1–9. DOI: 10.5409/wjcp.v13.i3.97501

Tang, Y. Y., Tang, R., & Gross, J. J. (2019). Promoting psychological well-being through an evidence-based mindfulness training program. *Frontiers in Human Neuroscience*, *13*(1), 1–5. DOI: 10.3389/fnhum.2019.00237

Tare, S., Verma, H., & Jahagirdar, D. (2025). A Correlation Between Resilience and Positive Mental Health. *International Journal of Indian Psychology*, *3*(1), 1–13. DOI: 10.25215/1301.017

Tater, B., & John, K. (2024). Effects of smartphone addiction on the physical and mental well-being of Indian students. *Indian Journal of Science and Technology*, *17*(25), 2622–2634. DOI: 10.17485/IJST/v17i25.1355

Taubman-Ben-Ari, O. (2014). Well-being and personal growth in emerging motherhood: and what about meaning? In Batthyany, A., & Russo-Netzer, P. (Eds.), *Meaning in positive and existential psychology* (pp. 417–438). Springer. DOI: 10.1007/978-1-4939-0308-5_21

Tedeschi, R. G., & Calhoun, L. G. (2004). Posttraumatic growth: Conceptual foundations and empirical evidence. *Psychological Inquiry*, *15*(1), 1–18. DOI: 10.1207/s15327965pli1501_01

Temoshok, L. R. (2005). *Forgiveness and health in persons living with HIV/AIDS. Handbook of Forgiveness*. Routledge.

Thapliyal, C., Singh, R., & Singh, A. K. (2025). Association of forgiveness with learning: for social and psychological wellbeing. In Benoit, S. (Ed.), *Cultivating Flourishing Practices and Environments by Embracing Positive Education* (pp. 335–360). IGI Global Scientific Publishing., DOI: 10.4018/979-8-3693-9466-3.ch011

Thoits, P. A. (2011). Mechanisms linking social ties and support to physical and mental health. *Journal of Health and Social Behavior*, *52*(2), 145–161. DOI: 10.1177/0022146510395592 PMID: 21673143

Thompson, T., Tisher, J., Davis, S., Miller, C., Kirk, J., Tartaglia, N., & Howell, S. (2024). The emotional journey of adapting to prenatally identified trisomy X. *Journal of Genetic Counseling*, *33*(1), 177–190. DOI: 10.1002/jgc4.1778 PMID: 37691399

Thomson, G., & Schmied, V. (2017). *Psychosocial resilience and risk in the perinatal period*. Routledge., DOI: 10.4324/9781315656854

Tielman, M. L.. (2024). Efficacy of chatbot-delivered interventions for mental health and well-being: A meta-analysis. *JMIR Mental Health*, *1*(1), e59560.

Tikka, S. K., Garg, S., & Siddiqui, M. A. (2020). Prescribing physical activity in psychological health: A focused review on the latest evidence, recommendations, challenges, and relevance to India. *Indian Journal of Psychological Medicine*, *43*(6), 535–541. DOI: 10.1177/0253717620972330

Titzler, I., Saruhanjan, K., Berking, M., Riper, H., & Ebert, D. D. (2018). Barriers and facilitators for the implementation of blended psychotherapy for depression: A qualitative pilot study of therapists' perspective. *Internet Interventions : the Application of Information Technology in Mental and Behavioural Health*, *12*, 150–164. DOI: 10.1016/j.invent.2018.01.002 PMID: 30135779

Tiwari, G. K., Kashyap, A. K., Rai, P. K., Tiwari, R. P., & Pandey, R. (2022). Collective affirmation in action: Understanding the success of lockdown in India during the first wave of the COVID-19 pandemic. *Journal of Research and Health*, *12*(3), 137–150. DOI: 10.32598/JRH.12.3.1992.1

Topooco, N., Riper, H., Araya, R., Berking, M., Brunn, M., Chevreul, K., Cieslak, R., Ebert, D. D., Etchmendy, E., Herrero, R., Kleiboer, A., Krieger, T., García-Palacios, A., Cerga-Pashoja, A., Smoktunowicz, E., Urech, A., Vis, C., & Andersson, G. (2017). Attitudes towards digital treatment for depression: A European stakeholder survey. *Internet Interventions : the Application of Information Technology in Mental and Behavioural Health*, *8*, 1–9. DOI: 10.1016/j.invent.2017.01.001 PMID: 30135823

Torous, J., Jän Myrick, K., Rauseo-Ricupero, N., & Firth, J. (2020). Digital Mental Health and COVID-19: Using Technology Today to Accelerate the Curve on Access and Quality Tomorrow. *JMIR Mental Health*, *7*(3), e18848. DOI: 10.2196/18848 PMID: 32213476

Tøssebro, J. (2016). Scandinavian disability policy: From deinstitutionalisation to non-discrimination and beyond. *Alter (Paris)*, *10*(2), 111–123. DOI: 10.1016/j.alter.2016.03.003

Totsika, V., Hastings, R. P., Emerson, E., Lancaster, G. A., & Berridge, D. M. (2011). A population-based investigation of behavioral and emotional problems and maternal mental health: Associations with autism spectrum disorder and intellectual disability. *Journal of Child Psychology and Psychiatry, and Allied Disciplines*, *52*(1), 91–99. DOI: 10.1111/j.1469-7610.2010.02295.x PMID: 20649912

Toussaint, L. L., Worthington, E. L., Williams, D. R., & Webb, J. R. (2020). Forgiveness and physical health. In Worthington, E. L.Jr, & Wade, N. G. (Eds.), *Handbook of Forgiveness* (2nd ed., pp. 178–187).

Tripathi, A., & Mullet, E. (2010). Conceptualizations of forgiveness and forgivingness among Hindus. *The International Journal for the Psychology of Religion*, *20*(4), 255–266. DOI: 10.1080/10508619.2010.507694

Troy, A. S., Wilhelm, F. H., Shallcross, A. J., & Mauss, I. B. (2010). Seeing the silver lining: Cognitive reappraisal ability moderates the relationship between stress and depressive symptoms. *Emotion (Washington, D.C.)*, *10*(6), 783–795. DOI: 10.1037/a0020262 PMID: 21058843

Túry, F., Güleç, H., & Kohls, E. (2009). Assessment methods for eating disorders and body image disorders. *Journal of Psychosomatic Research*, *69*(6), 601–611. DOI: 10.1016/j.jpsychores.2009.05.012 PMID: 21109049

Uchino, B. N.. (2003). Social support and health outcomes: A meta-analysis. *Psychological Bulletin*, *129*(2), 273–295.

Ungar, M. (2011). The social ecology of resilience: Addressing contextual and cultural ambiguity of a nascent construct. *The American Journal of Orthopsychiatry*, *81*(1), 1–17. https://psycnet.apa.org/doi/10.1111/j.1939-0025.2010.01067.x. DOI: 10.1111/j.1939-0025.2010.01067.x PMID: 21219271

UNICEF. (2017). *A familiar face: Violence in the lives of children and adolescents.* United Nations Children's Fund. https://www.unicef.org/media/48671/file/Violence_in_the_lives_of_children_and_adolescents.pdf

van der Kolk, B. A. (2014). *The body keeps the score: Brain, mind, and body in the healing of trauma.* Penguin Books. https://www.penguinrandomhouse.com/books/313183/the-body-keeps-the-score-by-bessel-van-der-kolk-md/

van der Kolk, B. A. (2014). *The body keeps the score: Brain, mind, and body in the healing of trauma.* Viking Press.

van der Steen, S. L., Houtman, D., Bakkeren, I. M., Galjaard, R.-J., Polak, M., Busschbach, J., Tibben, A., & Riedjik, S. (2019). Offering a choice between NIPT and invasive PND in prenatal genetic counseling: The impact of clinician characteristics on patients' test uptake. *European Journal of Human Genetics : EJHG*, *27*(1), 103–111. DOI: 10.1038/s41431-018-0287-z PMID: 30297905

Van Lange, P. A., Rusbult, C. E., Drigotas, S. M., Arriaga, X. B., Witcher, B. S., & Cox, C. L. (1997). Willingness to sacrifice in close relationships. *Journal of Personality and Social Psychology*, *72*(6), 1373–1395. DOI: 10.1037/0022-3514.72.6.1373

Van Oosten, K. (2008). Kamma and forgiveness with some thoughts on Cambodia. *Exchange*, *37*(3), 237–262. DOI: 10.1163/157254308X311974

Wadsworth, M. E. (2015). Development of Maladaptive Coping: A Functional Adaptation to Chronic, Uncontrollable Stress. *Child Development Perspectives*, *9*(2), 96–100. DOI: 10.1111/cdep.12112 PMID: 26019717

Walker, L. V., Miller, V. J., & Dalton, V. K. (2008). The health-care experiences of families given the prenatal diagnosis of trisomy 18. *Journal of Perinatology*, *28*(1), 12–19. DOI: 10.1038/sj.jp.7211860 PMID: 18165828

Walsh, F. (2016). *Strengthening family resilience* (3rd ed.). Guilford Press.

Warale, P. N., Limbore, N. V., Anute, N., Ahluwalia, G. K., & Raut, A. (2025). AI-Enhanced Customer Engagement and Experience: Chatbots, Virtual Assistants, and AI-Powered Customer Interactions. In Hussain, Z., Khan, A., Uzir, M., Sharipudin, M., & Shaheen, A. (Eds.), *Impacts of AI-Generated Content on Brand Reputation* (pp. 335–362). IGI Global Scientific Publishing., DOI: 10.4018/979-8-3373-4327-3.ch014

Webb, T. L., Miles, E., & Sheeran, P. (2012). Dealing with feeling: A meta-analysis of the effectiveness of strategies derived from the process model of emotion regulation. *Psychological Bulletin*, *138*(4), 775–808. DOI: 10.1037/a0027600 PMID: 22582737

Werner-Seidler, A., Wong, Q., Johnston, L., O'Dea, B., Torok, M., & Christensen, H. (2019). Pilot evaluation of the Sleep Ninja: A smartphone application for adolescent insomnia symptoms. *BMJ Open*, *9*(5), e026502. DOI: 10.1136/bmjopen-2018-026502 PMID: 31133584

White, M., & Epston, D. (1990). *Narrative means to therapeutic ends*. Norton.

Wind, T. R., Joshi, P. C., Kleber, R. J., & Komproe, I. H. (2013). The impact of recurrent disasters on mental health: A study on seasonal floods in northern India. *Prehospital and Disaster Medicine*, *28*(3), 279–285. DOI: 10.1017/S1049023X13000290

Winn, P., Acharya, K., Peterson, E., & Leuthner, S. (2018). Prenatal counseling and parental decision-making following a fetal diagnosis of trisomy 13 or 18. *Journal of Perinatology*, *38*(5), 588–595. DOI: 10.1038/s41372-018-0107-x PMID: 29740195

World Health Organisation (WHO). Global Health Estimation (GHE). (2019). [Online]. https://www.who.int/data/gho/data/themes/mortality-and-global-health-estimates

World Health Organization (WHO). (1992). *The ICD-10 classification of mental and behavioural disorders: Diagnostic criteria for research*. [Online]. https://www.who.int/publications/i/item/9241544554

World Health Organization (WHO). (2024a). Health and Well-being. [Online]. https://www.who.int/data/gho/data/major-themes/health-and-well-being

World Health Organization (WHO). (2024b). Mental health [Online]. https://www.who.int/india/health-topics/mental-health

World Health Organization (WHO). (2024c). Mental health Impact [Online]. https://www.who.int/health-topics/mental-health#tab=tab_2

World Health Organization (WHO). (2024d). Mental health of adolescents [Online]. https://www.who.int/news-room/fact-sheets/detail/adolescent-mental-health

World Health Organization (WHO). (2024e). Mental health of adolescents [Online]. https://www.who.int/news-room/fact-sheets/detail/mental-health-of-older-adults

World Health Organization. (2013). *Mental health action plan 2013–2020*. WHO Press. https://www.who.int/publications/i/item/9789241506021

Worthington, E. L., Mazzeo, S. E., & Canter, D. E. (2006). Forgiveness-promoting approach: Helping clients REACH forgiveness through using a longer model that teaches reconciliation. In *American Psychological Association eBooks* (pp. 235–257). DOI: 10.1037/10886-010

Worthington, E. L. (2001). *Five steps to forgiveness: The art and science of forgiving*. Crown.

Worthington, E. L.Jr., (Ed.). (2007). *Handbook of forgiveness*. Routledge. DOI: 10.4324/9780203955673

Worthington, E. L.Jr, & Scherer, M. (2004). Forgiveness is an emotion-focused coping strategy that can reduce health risks and promote health resilience: Theory, review, and hypotheses. *Psychology & Health, 19*(1), 385–405. DOI: 10.1080/0887044042000196674

Yehuda, R., Lehrner, A., & Bierer, L. M. (2023). Cultural and epigenetic influences in trauma response. *Current Opinion in Psychology, 48*, 101481. DOI: 10.1016/j.copsyc.2022.101481

Yuen, E. Y., Liu, W., Karatsoreos, I. N., Feng, J., McEwen, B. S., & Yan, Z. (2009). Acute stress enhances glutamatergic transmission in prefrontal cortex and facilitates working memory. *Proceedings of the National Academy of Sciences of the United States of America, 106*(33), 14075–14079. DOI: 10.1073/pnas.0906791106 PMID: 19666502

Zakrzewski, V. (2015). Social-emotional learning: why now? Greater Good Magazine. https://greatergood.berkeley.edu/article/item/social_emotional_learning_why_now

About the Contributors

Agathi Argyriadi is a Psychologist with specialization on Cognitive – Behavioral Psychotherapy and Developmental Psychology. Her PhD thesis is entitled "The effects of "Aesthetic flow experiences" in school's environment of first graders. A psycho-educational approach". She also holds a M.Ed. on Special Education and a second Master on Counseling. She is an Assistant Professor at the Department of Psychology, American University in Dubai and a Lecturer in the Department of Education at Frederick University, teaching developmental and cognitive psychology. In the past she has also taught at Cyprus University of Technology (Therapeutic communication), at the East London University (Research Methods and Statistics) and at the Technological Educational Institute of Peloponnese at the department of Speech Pathology (teaching Developmental Psychology and Clinical Neuropsychology), for 3 years. She has acted as a self- employed Psychologist and for a 3-year project against violence at the Ministry of Internal Affairs of the Hellenic Republic. She has also acted for two years, as an external associate at a private school in Greece, with the aim of monitoring and supporting students with learning difficulties, psychological problems and counseling of parents. Agathi Argyriadi was also a professor at the Foundation for Youth and Lifelong Learning and specifically at the Institute for Vocational Training of the Ministry of Education. She has published articles in international journals and she has participated in numerous of training seminars. She is the writer of 10 scientific books in the field of psychology. Her research interests focus on optimizing learning environments using positive psychology and aesthetic theories, developmental psychological issues, special education field, social inclusion issues. She teaches in the Distance Learning Program of Special Education.

Alexandros Argyriadis is an Assistant Professor in mental health at the Hellenic Mediterranean University in Crete, Greece.

***

Rajshri Chalakh is currently working as an Assistant Professor of Law in MSS Law College Hyderabad which is affiliated to Osmania University. She is also pursuing PhD from National Law University Nagpur. Having completed her LLM from National Law University Nagpur in Corporate and Commercial Laws, she has an expertise in Corporate Laws. She has academic experience of around 2 years. She has worked as an Associate Editor for the ISBN book published by Asia Law House titled "75 Years of Working of Supreme Court of India" in June 2025.

Anindita Das is an esteemed Associate Professor of the Department of Physical Education Pedagogy at Lakshmibai National Institute of Physical Education (LNIPE), Gwalior. With a prolific career, Dr. Das has authored numerous research papers, patents, and books, contributing significantly to the field of physical education. Her work emphasizes innovative teaching methodologies and educational strategies, aimed at fostering excellence in physical education pedagogy. Renowned for her dedication to advancing knowledge and practice in sports education, Dr. Das continues to inspire students and professionals through her leadership, research, and unwavering commitment to academic excellence.

Efthymia Efthymiou, Associate Professor at Zayed University (UAE), studies inclusive teaching, classroom discourse, and learning environments that enable every student with disabilities to belong and participate. She brings this lens to medical education, promoting disability-competent, technology-enhanced training. She also works with UAE federal schools to turn research on inclusion and digital access into classroom practice.

Shreya Ghosh is an Assistant Professor at PES University, Bangalore, and a research scholar with a strong passion for inquiry and innovation. Her interests lie in neuroscience, psychology, human relations, and sustainable development.

Dimitra V. Katsarou is a permanent Assistant Professor in the Department of Sciences of Preschool Education and Educational Design at the University of the Aegean, Greece. Her academic and research interests focus on developmental psychopathology, language disorders, neurodevelopmental conditions, special and inclusive education, developmental psychology, and early childhood development. Her work emphasizes interdisciplinary approaches to the assessment, diagnosis, and intervention of children with developmental and communication disorders, with particular attention to evidence-based practices that promote learning, mental health, and social inclusion. Dr. Katsarou has authored and edited numerous scientific books, book chapters, and peer-reviewed publications in international journals. She has also edited several international volumes on developmental disorders, psycholinguistics, bilingualism, and educational inclusion. She actively participates in international research collab.

Awesh Khati is a committed Ph.D. scholar in Physical Education Pedagogy at the prestigious Lakshmibai National Institute of Physical Education (LNIPE), Gwalior. With a strong academic background and a deep passion for advancing the field of physical education, he has authored several research papers and book chapters, including publications in Scopus-indexed journals. He is also the author of a published book on football, reflecting his blend of academic rigor and practical insight. Alongside his scholarly work, Mr. Khati is an accomplished football player, bringing valuable on-field experience to his research. His contributions demonstrate a dedication to promoting holistic physical development and enriching sports education, positioning him as a promising voice in the realm of physical education and sports science.

Prince Kouassi is an Assistant Professor of Psychology and Chair of the Psychology Department at the American University in Dubai. His work focuses on applied behavioural science, mental health, and higher education practice. He has led the development of the university's first behavioural research lab, advanced departmental teaching and learning frameworks, and fostered collaborations supporting student research and professional development. Dr Kouassi's scholarship spans research methods, stigma in mental health, and consumer behaviour, and he regularly supervises undergraduate research projects. He is committed to advancing evidence informed practice in psychology education across the Middle East.

Georgios Kougioumtzis is an Associate Professor of Counseling, ICT, and Teaching Methodology, in the Department of Turkish and Modern Asian Studies, at National and Kapodistrian University of Athens, Greece; a Visiting Professor in the School of Psychology, at Neapolis University Pafos, Cyprus, in the field of Counseling / Educational Psychology, and Specific Learning Difficulties, and a Visiting Academic in the School of Social Sciences, at Hellenic Open University, Patras, Greece, in the field of Psychology / Counseling. He holds a Ph.D. in Pedagogics, Teaching Methodology, and Counseling / Teacher Mentoring, from the Department of Philosophy, Pedagogy, and Psychology - National and Kapodistrian University of Athens. He has published 12 books by IGI Global Scientific Publishing (USA) and Grigori Publications (Greece) in the fields of Educational Psychology, Counseling Psychology, Specific Learning Difficulties, and Teaching Methodology and ICT, and over than two hundred (200) papers. He is married and the father of three daughters.

Blessy Lenin is a PhD Scholar of Martin Luther Christian University.

Seema Mulmule is currently working as an Assistant Professor in Marwadi Shiksha Samithi, Osmania University. She pursued bachelors in Arts and then she completed L lb and practised in High court and district court of Maharashtra and Nagapur. She dealt matrimonial and cheque bounce cases and civil matters . She also dealt with Consumer matters. She has 10 years experience in dealing with different areas in court of law. As she was always want to depart knowledge so joined in teaching field. She has two years experience in teaching.she also has worked as legal officer in sriram city finance.. she also worked as arbitrator in few matters.

Radhika P is an Assistant Professor in the Department of Electronics and Communication Engineering at SRM Institute of Science and Technology. She is actively involved in teaching, research, and academic development, with a strong commitment to imparting quality technical education. Her areas of expertise and interest contribute to both undergraduate and postgraduate programs, and she continually strives to enhance student learning through innovative teaching methodologies and research-oriented practices.

Selvakumar P is currently an Associate Professor in the Department of Science and Humanities at Nehru Institute of Technology, Coimbatore, Tamil Nadu, India. Prior to joining Nehru Institute of Technology, he held positions as an Assistant Professor in the Department of Science and Humanities various engineering colleges in Coimbatore, Tamil Nadu, India, spanning from 2011 to 2023. Dr.P. Selvakumar's academic and research interests lie primarily in the field of phytochemistry. He has made significant contributions to his field, with an impressive record that includes 30 journal publications, 12 patents, and 20 conference papers. Additionally, he has organized 5 seminars and conferences, further demonstrating his commitment to academic and scientific exchange. Throughout his career, Dr. P.Selvakumar has been recognized for his dedication and excellence in teaching, having been honored with several awards, including the Best Teacher Awards. He holds a prominent position in the academic community, contributing actively to research.

Sohom Saha is a dedicated academic and sports psychology scholar currently pursuing his Ph.D. in Physical Education at LNIPE, Gwalior. He holds an M.P.Ed. from LNIPE and a B.P.Ed. and B.A. in Physical Education from Visva-Bharati University, Shantiniketan. Specializing in Sports Psychology, Volleyball, and Yoga, he blends scientific insight with hands-on experience. Mr. Saha has competed in national-level sports, including All-India Inter-University events and NCC championships. He has published extensively in Scopus, Web of Science, and peer-reviewed journals, with research interests in emotional resilience, psychological well-being, and performance enhancement. He has also authored books on sports psychology and technology and serves as a reviewer for international journals. A member of the Sports Psychology Association of India, his work advocates mental toughness, inclusivity, and athlete development, aiming to inspire future educators and researchers in the sporting field.

Lalitha Saipogu is currently working as an Assistant Professor in the Department of Computer Science and Engineering (Data Science) at CVR College of Engineering, Hyderabad, Telangana (Postal Code: 501510). She is passionate about emerging technologies and has a keen interest in the areas of Deep Learning, Machine Learning, and Blockchain. With her strong academic background and commitment to teaching, Lalitha plays a vital role in guiding students and contributing to the academic excellence of the department.

Vijeta Sharma is an accomplished academic professional with over 9 years of experience in higher education, currently serving as Assistant Professor and Program Coordinator at CU Online, Chandigarh University. A PhD holder and UGC-NET qualified, she specializes in People Management, Organizational Behavior, Banking & Finance, and Business Environment, with a strong focus on case-based teaching using Harvard Manage Mentor. She is actively involved in curriculum design, digital content development, student mentoring, and academic quality assurance, and is a recognized podcast protagonist and keynote speaker. Her work spans research publications, AI-based granted patents, and continuous engagement in NEP 2020–aligned faculty development, reflecting her commitment to academic excellence, innovation, and learner-centric education.

Ajay Kumar Singh is working as an Associate Professor (Research) in the Department of Humanities and Social Science, Graphic Era (Deemed to be University) Dehradun. He has worked as Assistant Professor (Economics) in the School of Liberal Arts & Management, DIT University Dehradun for 6 years. He did Post-Doctorate Research with EDI of India, Ahmedabad, Gujarat (India). He received MPhil (Economics) from DAVV Indore (India), and PhD (Economics) from IIT Indore (India. He has published several research papers in the diversified area such as climate change, agricultural productivity, assessment of food security; estimation of GFSI, development of environmental sustainability index (ESI) and its association with socio-economic indicators; measurement and determinants of entrepreneurship ecosystem, and dimension of sustainable development and its interlinkages with economic development.

Ravindra Singh has completed his Ph.D. from Banaras Hindu University (Institute of Eminence). Currently, he is working as an Assistant Professor of

Psychology at Magadh University, Bodh Gaya, Bihar. Earlier he was Indian Youth Ambassador at BRICS. Beijing China 2017 during Indian delegation. Dr. Singh has also worked as a Junior Project Fellow, a funded project, in New Delhi in 2018. He worked as a Former Teaching Assistant at IIT, BHU. Recently he was the Youth Member at G20 Youth for India's G-20 Presidency. He served as an Independent Reviewer in Frontiers in Psychology Journal and a Member of APA, International Affiliate, Washington DC, and a member of the prestigious National Academy of Psychology, (NAOP) India. He has 7 Years of teaching experience and supervising 3 PhD candidates along with many posts' graduate thesis supervision.

Maria Sofologi is an Adjunct Ass. Professor at the Department of Early Childhood and Education at the University of Ioannina in Greece. She delivers the courses "Cognitive Psychology", and "Developmental Psychology". She is also a postdoctoral researcher at the University of Ioannina in Greece. She holds a Ph.D. in Cognitive Psychology from the Aristotle University of Thessaloniki. She also holds a Master of Science degree in Cognitive Psychology from the Aristotle University of Thessaloniki. During her master's degree years she trained and practiced different assessment cognitive tools to evaluate all cognitive functions like memory, attention, language, executive functions both in adults and children. She is the key speaker in many European and Hellenic conferences concerning cognitive psychology, educational psychology, special education in children and adults, as well. Her academic work includes a series of many scientific publications, books, and book chapters concerning Cognitive Psychology, Special Education, Educational Psychology, and Cognitive impairments in children and adults as well.

Chitralekha Thapliyal is currently pursuing a Doctor of Philosophy in Psychology at Graphic Era (Deemed to be University). She completed her masters in psychology. The has keen to address the various phenomena related to affected process especially emotions and motivation. As a doctoral student, she started to do research in pursuit of knowledge and more understanding of the psychological field. Her research started with exploring various psychological challenges faced by children during elementary education.

Index

Q

R

S

T

V

www.ingramcontent.com/pod-product-compliance
Lightning Source LLC
LaVergne TN
LVHW080858300926
849162LV00003B/460